P

MW00908188

Pathways to Fitness

FOUNDATIONS, MOTIVATION, APPLICATIONS

Nolan A. Thaxton

Medgar Evers College of the
City University of New York

1817

HARPER & ROW, PUBLISHERS, New York
Cambridge, Philadelphia, San Francisco, Washington,
London, Mexico City, São Paulo, Singapore, Sydney

Sponsoring Editor: Claudia M. Wilson
Project Editor: Lauren G. Shafer
Text Design: Suzanne Dyer Company/Lurelle Cheverie
Cover Design: Brenda Booth
Text Art: RDL Artset, Ltd.
Production: Kewal K. Sharma
Compositor: ComCom Division of Haddon Craftsmen, Inc.
Printer and Binder: The Murray Printing Company

Pathways to Fitness: Foundations, Motivation, Applications

Copyright © 1988 by Harper & Row, Publishers, Inc.

All rights reserved. Printed in the United States of America. No part of this book may be used or reproduced in any manner whatsoever without written permission, except in the case of brief quotations embodied in critical articles and reviews. For information address Harper & Row, Publishers, Inc., 10 East 53d Street, New York, NY 10022.

Library in Congress Cataloging-in-Publication Data

Thaxton, Nolan A.
    Pathways to fitness.

    Includes Index.
    1. Exercise.   2. Physical Fitness.   3. Health.
I. Title.
RA781.T395   1988   613.7   87-8665
ISBN 0-06-046618-9

87 88 89 90 9 8 7 6 5 4 3 2 1

CONTENTS

The increased interest and participation in physical fitness activities that began in the 1960s continues unabated. Besides the multimillion-dollar industry for equipment, clothing, health food, and other products associated with the health and fitness boom are the hundreds of books written on health and fitness. Some are written by persons who lack the technical knowledge to write on the topic. However, because many are well-known personalities, their books are read by thousands of individuals. Jane Fonda and Richard Simmons are two examples of persons who are not physical educators or physical fitness experts but who have written books on health and fitness that have sold in the millions.

In some cases some of these books present an unsuspecting public with misleading and sometimes inaccurate information regarding health and fitness. Fitness programs based on information in some of these books are often unsuccessful, and they also result in unnecessary injuries to persons who use the books as their only "factual" information.

The author, who has a doctorate degree in health and physical education and has been teaching health and fitness courses for more than 20 years, wrote this book to present a scientifically based resource for persons interested in health and fitness. A further reason for writing this book was to dispel some of the myths associated with health and fitness and to replace them with factual information.

Audience

The text is designed for use by a wide and diverse audience: college students in a general fitness class, students majoring in physical education, older adults returning to college after many years out of school, and individuals who wish to develop their own fitness programs outside of a formal classroom setting.

Objectives

The overall objective is to present current, authoritative information on health and fitness. Specific objectives are to present a rationale for developing organized fitness programs and the scientific basis for developing such programs, to present motivational strategies and procedures for developing fitness programs, and to provide recommended activities for the development of optimal fitness.

Organization

The book contains fourteen chapters, organized into three distinct yet interrelated sections: foundations for fitness, motivation for fitness, and applications for fitness. Section One, "Foundations for Fitness," contains an introductory chapter on physical fitness in modern society, one that clarifies selected fitness concepts, and one that discusses the body as an exercise machine. Chapters on exercise, nutrition, and weight control and on evaluating physical fitness also are included in Section One.

In the chapter on the human body, highly technical terms are defined and examples and nontechnical information are presented to clarify the material. In addition, be aware that this chapter can stand alone. Persons using this book do not have to read the entire chapter before reading other parts of the book.

Section Two, "Motivation for Fitness," which contains three chapters, focuses on the motivational aspects of developing and adhering to a fitness program. The keystone of this section is Chapter 8, "Behavior Change through Behavior Modification," and the centerpiece of the chapter is a plan for self-modification of behavior. Although the author feels that each person is responsible for his or her own actions, he recognizes that some people need help in developing positive exercise and health behaviors; the self-modification of behavior plan is presented to provide assistance for these individuals. The other two chapters in Section Two are "Risk Factors in Cardiovascular Disease" and "Values of Physical Activity."

Section Three, "Applications for Fitness," contains six chapters. Chapter 9 discusses the principles and procedures for developing a scientifically based program of physical fitness. Chapters 10 through 13 recommend specific pathways to cardiorespiratory endurance; pathways to flexibility, strength, and muscular endurance; pathways to weight control; and pathways to fitness for individuals with selected handicapping conditions. A final chapter deals with special considerations and concerns, such as gynecological problems that might result from participation in fitness programs, fitness for children and older adults, and exercising under extreme environmental conditions (in extreme heat or cold, at high altitude, and so on).

Special Features

The following special features are included to enhance the usefulness of the book:

1. *Chapter highlights and key words.* At the beginning of each chapter are chapter highlights to provide a focus for important information in the chapter and key words that should be understood.
2. *Section overviews.* Before each section is a brief descriptive overview and titles of the chapters in the section.

3. *Illustrations.* Numerous illustrations in the form of charts, line drawings, photographs, and so on are presented to help clarify the narrative information in the text. Line art describes the heart, blood vessels, and other organs of the body. Photographs demonstrating various fitness activities amplify the verbal explanation of these activities.

4. *Appendixes.* Eleven appendixes complement and supplement information presented in the chapters of the text. In addition to similar information contained in some other fitness books, such as the nutritive values of foods and recommended daily dietary allowances, these appendixes provide information on the nutrients in vegetarian foods, a step-by-step procedure for constructing a t scale, a series of exercises designed primarily to help prevent postural deviations and lower back problems, and fitness forms. The pages containing the fitness forms can be photocopied and used as separate worksheets.

5. *Glossary.* A glossary of technical terms serves as a ready reference guide.

Acknowledgments

The publication of a textbook is a complex undertaking, requiring the cooperative workings of many individuals with varying areas of expertise. I was fortunate enough to have had many persons, each of whom made significant contributions to the project, help with the production of this textbook. A few deserve formal thanks.

I would like to sincerely thank Professor Paul Bobb, formerly my colleague at Medgar Evers College, and now Athletic Director at the City College of New York, for his assistance in preparing the prospectus for the book, and for developing the outline and bibliography for Chapter 4, "Nutrition, Exercise, and Weight Control."

The many fine photographs in the book were taken by photographers Tony Akeem, Suzanne Sheehy, Steven Marks, and Charles McClary. A special thanks is also extended to Tina Torres, Greg Cochrane, Curtis Cooper, Charlene Brown, Vina Mizell, and Walter Mosley, students at Medgar Evers College who posed for many of the photo illustrations in the book.

Joanne Alexander and Troy Frank drafted many of the art illustrations for the book; Doug Jeffers entered the first draft of the manuscript on his computer; Joyce Cannady, secretary of the Health Sciences Division at Medgar Evers College, helped to tie up many loose ends during the preparation of the first draft of the manuscript; and Iola Thompson, Instructor of Health and Physical Education at Medgar Evers College, wrote the aerobic dance routine and provided invaluable assistance with other areas of the book. The help of all of these individuals is deeply appreciated.

I would also like to express my appreciation to Claudia Wilson and Lauren Shafer, editors at Harper and Row, for their help and direction during the production of the textbook. Also, thanks to the reviewers: Ruth H. Alexander, University of Florida, Gainesville; W. Larry Kenney, The Pennsylvania State University; Clayre K. Petray, California State University, Long Beach; Lisa Plummer, University of Illinois at Urbana-

Champaign; Karl G. Stoedefalke, The Pennsylvania State University; Walter R. Welsch, University of Florida, Gainesville; and Robb Williams, University of Cincinnati.

Finally, a special word of thanks and appreciation is extended to my wife and best friend, Ann Thaxton, for the countless hours she spent proofreading every draft of the manuscript, and for offering many insightful suggestions for improving the textbook.

Nolan A. Thaxton

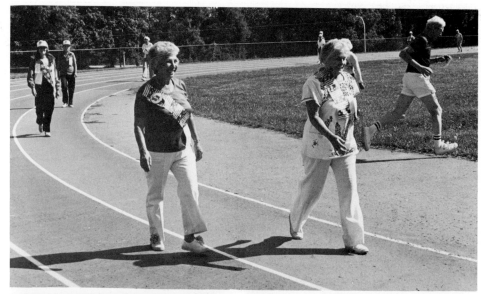

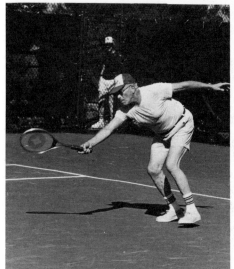

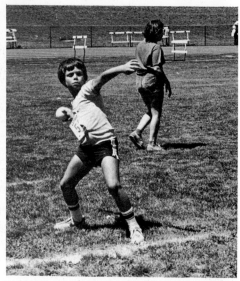

It is important for people of all ages and both sexes to engage in some form of physical activity on a regular basis.

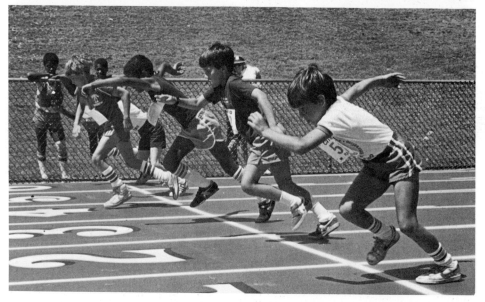

FOUNDATIONS FOR FITNESS

Section One contains the rationale for developing fitness programs and the basic theoretical information to support such programs. The need for organized fitness programs is discussed in relationship to the automated and mechanized society of modern America. Physical fitness is defined, and the relationship among physical fitness, health, and wellness is discussed. Information is presented on the human body as well as material on procedures for fitness evaluation.

CHAPTER 1

Physical Fitness in Modern Society

atrophy   hypokinetic disease
hypertrophy

Key Words

After reading this chapter, you should be able to:
1. Define and/or explain the key words listed above.
2. List and discuss eight reasons for the low level of participation in physical activity by a majority of adult Americans.
3. Identify and discuss two legitimate barriers to physical fitness participation.
4. List and discuss nine myths regarding physical activity.
5. Summarize the benefits of regular physical activity.
6. List and discuss the problems caused by physical inactivity and the alternative lifestyle suggested by the author.

Chapter Highlights

Increasing numbers of Americans have become preoccupied during the past 20 years with achieving a higher level of *physical fitness,* defined in this text as the ability of the body's systems (particularly the cardiorespiratory, muscular, and skeletal systems) to function at their optimal level. To achieve optimal physical fitness, more adults today (compared with a decade or two ago) are participating in various physical activities. (The meaning of physical fitness is clarified further in Chapter 2.)

What is the level of participation in physical activity by Americans today? It is difficult to indicate the exact percentage of the population that participates in physical activities on a regular basis, due to the variable definitions of *active participation,* among other things, but it is estimated that approximately 20 percent of the population exercises at a level generally recommended for cardiovascular benefit.[1] The authors of that study also concluded that another 40 percent of the population is active at a lower intensity or frequency, and 40 percent is completely sedentary.[2] These conclusions were based on the results of eight national surveys on leisure-time physical activity conducted in the United States and Canada between 1972 and 1983.

Although the percentage of the population engaging in physical activities was only an approximation, several factors regarding participation in leisure-time activities by the population were revealed as facts. These include the following:

Males and females are equally likely to participate in conditioning activities (such as walking, bicycling, and calisthenics), but males are more likely to be involved in sports, intense activities, or activities performed frequently.

Decreasing proportions of the population are classified as physically active with increasing age, but this is not necessarily an inevitable outcome of aging.

The proportion of the population classified as physically active in its leisure time is positively related to socioeconomic status as indicated by income, education, and occupation. That is, the activity level of the highest socioeconomic groups exceeds that of the lowest groups.

Six activities consistently account for the largest numbers of participants: walking, swimming, calisthenics, bicycling, jogging or running, and bowling.

The proportion of the population that is physically active during its leisure time has increased substantially in recent years.[3]

Money spent on exercise-related products is at an all-time high. One estimate is that more than $30 billion is spent each year on products related to recreational and sports activity.[4] The market for sports shoes alone has reached $1 billion. Additional expenditures include $5 billion for health foods and vitamins, $50 million for diet and exercise books, $1 billion for cosmetic surgery, $6 billion for diet drinks, and $240 million for barbells and aerobic dance programs. Health clubs and corporate fitness centers add another $5 billion to the fitness market.[5]

Although there has been a substantial increase in the proportion of the population in recent years who engage in some physical activity and more is being spent on fitness-related products, the majority of the American adult population is not engaged in regular programs of physical activity of an aerobic nature. The increase in participation in exercise programs results mainly from an increase in physical activity by persons in the higher socioeconomic groups.

Why is only approximately 20 percent of the adult American population* engaged in regular programs of aerobic physical activity? This is

---

* The focus in this chapter is the level of physical activity for adult Americans. Equally important, however, is the need for increased participation in physical activity by more children and youth, particularly since the results of recent studies indicate that about half of American children and

a difficult question; however, part of the answer was provided by the reasons people give for not participating in physical activity. Some of the reasons are based on myth and misconception, and some are simply excuses not to exercise.

Reasons for the Low Level of Participation in Physical Activity

The reasons for not participating in physical activities by adult Americans, including those offered by college students, college graduates, and the general public, are as follows:

1. Not enough time
2. Health reasons
3. Family obligations
4. Lack of motivation (too lazy)
5. The weather
6. Lack of facilities or partners
7. Negative attitude toward physical activity
8. Lack of knowledge regarding physical activity

The first six reasons were given by respondents to a Harris survey on fitness in America in 1978.[6] The last two reasons, along with many of the others, were given by people who responded to my questions on this topic. In my view, the only legitimate barriers to participation in physical activity programs are a lack of knowledge or information regarding physical activity and specific health problems that prompt a physician to proscribe activity for individuals with such problems. Although I don't consider them legitimate, the majority of the reasons given are perceived as real problems by the respondents. Therefore, they must be considered by all of us who plan programs of physical fitness or write books on the subject.

The negative attitude toward physical activity, which results in some individuals not participating in various forms of physical activity, deserves special comment. A negative attitude toward physical activity may be the result of several factors (such as the myths that are discussed in this chapter). Chief among these factors is the negative view of physical activity that is fostered during the early school years by some physical education teachers.

Many people have been exposed to a physical educator who made them run three extra laps or perform five additional push-ups because

Negative Attitude Toward Physical Activity

adolescents are not receiving adequate exercise to develop healthy hearts and lungs. Physical activity for children and youth is presented as a topic of special concern in Chapter 14.

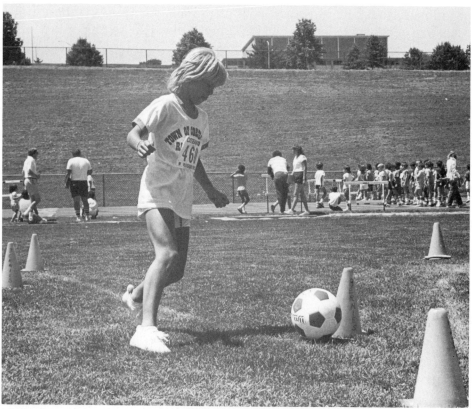

(a)

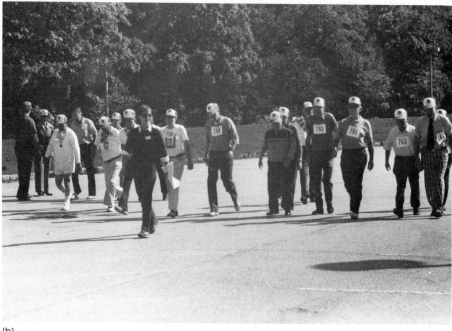

(a) Regular participation in physical activity should be started during childhood. (b) More Americans should be engaged in aerobic activities. Walking is an excellent aerobic activity.

(b)

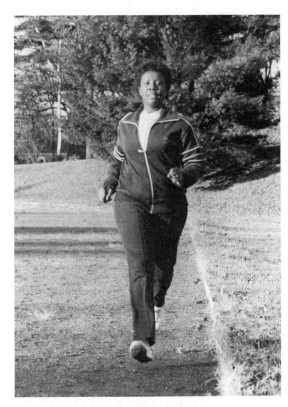

Jogging is an
excellent activity for
cardiorespiratory
endurance
development, and it
can be performed
alone.

they "acted up" in gym or did not perform with the skill in a physical
activity that the teacher required. This is typical of behavior that instills
a negative attitude toward physical activity during youngsters' formative
years. Regardless of the situation, exercise should never be used as a
punishment; instead, fitness leaders should encourage participation in
physical activity as a positive pathway to physical fitness.

Myths Regarding Physical Activity

Let us now focus on some myths that generally foster negative attitudes
toward physical activity.

The following nine negative statements against participation in physical activity programs are presented in descending order, according to
the percentage of 1590 respondents who agreed with each statement in
the 1978 Harris survey.[7] (See Table 1.1 for the percentage of the total
sample as well as the "high actives"—people who exercise at least five
days a week—and "low actives"—people who do not exercise—who
agreed with each statement. Note that a higher percentage of the low
actives agreed with each statement than did the high actives.) Each
statement is followed by a summary of the facts that prove the statement
wrong.

*The trouble with participating in a sport is that I can only do it now
and then, and too much physical exertion at one time is bad for people.*
It is true that participation in a strenuous sport or physical activity on

a sporadic basis is not beneficial and in fact may be harmful to the body. However, one need not participate in a sport to become physically fit. Participation in an aerobic activity (such as walking, jogging, aerobic dance, swimming, or bicycling) at an acceptable intensity level for 15 to 60 minutes a day, three to five days a week, will provide enough physical activity for physiological benefits to be realized by the systems of the body.[8]

Too many people, such as joggers and weight lifters, become fanatical about physical fitness, which is not healthy. For the vast majority of participants, exercise is a positive factor in the development of physical fitness and the reduction of stress. In rare instances, however, some people who participate in physical activity programs become overly

TABLE 1.1   **Perceptions Toward Nine Myths About Fitness Activities**

	Public (1590) (%)	High Actives (220) (%)	Low Actives (620) (%)
The trouble with participating in a sport is that I can only get to do it every now and then, and too much physical exertion at one time like this is bad for people.	54	44	58
Too many people, such as joggers and weight lifters, become fanatical about physical fitness, which is not healthy.	47	30	54
I'm so busy that I don't have enough energy left when I get around to thinking about exercising.	33	15	47
In the things I have to do every day, I get enough exercise without doing any sports or athletics.	31	12	49
These fads about physical fitness come and go, and I'm not impressed by this current emphasis on it.	30	17	41
Too much exercising can enlarge the heart, and this is bad when you stop exercising.	29	26	32
People who exercise work up big appetites and then eat too much, making the exercise useless.	28	10	38
The key to staying fit is not exercise but to control how much you eat.	27	15	36
Middle-aged and older people don't really need exercise other than walking.	18	6	28

Source: Louis Harris and Associates, The Perrier Study: Fitness in America *(New York: Perrier–Great Waters of France, Inc., 1979), p. 25. Reprinted by permission.*

obsessed with such participation. Although small in number, these individuals become unduly preoccupied with the development of physical fitness. Cases have been reported, for example, where runners have experienced the need to run more miles and to increase the number of days per week they run to receive physical and psychological benefits from the exercise. They place running ahead of family responsibilities, jobs, even their own health. Such people are said to be "negatively addicted" to running.[9] People who suffer from negative addiction manifest withdrawal symptoms if deprived of exercise. The withdrawal symptoms may lead to anxiety and depression accompanied by restlessness, insomnia, and overall fatigue.

Although a few people do become negatively addicted to exercise, the majority receive beneficial effects. A sensible program of physical activity designed according to the principles and procedures discussed in Chapter 9 will produce optimal results for the individual participant.[10]

I'm so busy that I don't have enough energy left when I get around to thinking about exercising. Just the opposite is true of many people who are engaged in a regular program of physical activity. They report that they feel better and have more energy. For example, over 90 percent of the 237 participants in a federally sponsored exercise program reported that they felt better and about 89 percent said they had greater stamina.[11]

It is recommended that people who feel that they will be too tired to participate in a physical activity at the end of the day should work out at other times. Scheduling physical activity sessions in the morning or during the lunch break can alleviate this perceived listlessness. Starting with moderate levels of physical activity and progressing to more strenuous levels will elicit feelings of having more energy rather than less.

I get enough exercise without doing any sports or athletics. With the mechanized and automated society in which we live, and the resultant reduction in physical labor, the vast majority of Americans do not get enough physical activity during their daily activities. Even people engaged in heavy labor, such as loggers in Oregon, do not get enough aerobic activity to stimulate adequately the heart, blood vessels, and lungs enough to improve cardiorespiratory endurance significantly. A planned program of physical activity of the aerobic type is necessary to supplement the development of strength and muscular endurance achieved through heavy work activity. The need for a planned program of physical activity is greater for those segments of the population whose daily activities are less strenuous than those who perform physically demanding tasks.

These fads about physical fitness come and go, and I'm not impressed by this current emphasis. This is a perception held by some people who are not active (in the 1978 Harris survey, for instance, only 17 percent of the high actives believed this claim, compared with 41 percent of the nonactives[12]). There is no factual information to either support or reject the claim. However, the steady increase in the number of Americans who exercise regularly does not seem to indicate that it is a fad. According to the 1984 Gallup Poll, for example, 47 percent of the American population reported that they exercised regularly in 1983, compared with 24 percent in 1961 when the question regarding participation in physical activity was first asked.[13] It is hoped that this increased participation in physical activity is the result of an increased knowledge of the benefits of exercise and the ability to design an activity program, and that many more Americans will begin to exercise on a regular basis.

Too much exercising can enlarge the heart, and this is bad when you stop exercising. First, I do not recommend overexercising (strenuous exercise every day of the week). Endurance training programs in which increased demands are placed on the heart will enlarge it (muscle *hypertrophy*). But rather than being bad for a person, the increase in the size of the heart muscle as it adapts to the increased work demands of endurance training results in a stronger heart. This type of heart is capable of producing a larger stroke volume (the amount of blood pumped from the heart with each beat).[14] There is no scientific evidence that a normal heart is adversely affected by physical activity, if the demands on the heart are progressively increased.

When one discontinues endurance exercise programs, the heart will reduce in size (*atrophy*) according to the law of use and disuse. However, I am not aware of any scientific evidence that damage to the heart results because of its atrophied condition. Furthermore, the knowledge that a muscle will reduce in size and functional capacity due to disuse should motivate individuals to engage in regular programs of physical activity throughout their life.

People who exercise work up big appetites and then eat too much, making exercise useless. There is no scientific evidence to support this assertion. The opposite is actually true. Research on both animal and human subjects by Jean Mayer[15] has demonstrated that moderately active people eat less than those who are inactive. Individuals who are engaged in strenuous endurance activities eat more to supply the extra calories needed for the increased activity.

The key to staying fit is not exercise but to control how much you eat. One should not equate slimness or obesity with fitness or unfitness. A person could be slim and not fit in terms of aerobic functioning—the optimal working of the heart, blood vessels, and lungs. This type of fitness is developed by engaging in endurance-type activities of the proper intensity, frequency, and duration. Furthermore, research has demonstrated that a significant percentage of individuals who engage in aerobic or endurance exercise programs have less fat weight per total body weight than their sedentary counterparts.[16]

Middle-aged and older people don't really need exercise other than walking. Walking is an excellent form of exercise and is recommended for some individuals (those who are obese or who have certain types of cardiovascular problems, for example), but it should not be recommended for all middle-aged and older persons as a matter of course. The exercise prescription, including the type of activity, should be based on the results of a medical examination, which should include an exercise stress test. Jogging, swimming, cross-country skiing, and tennis have proved successful supplements to walking as physical activities for middle-aged and older adults desirous of developing and maintaining optimal health.

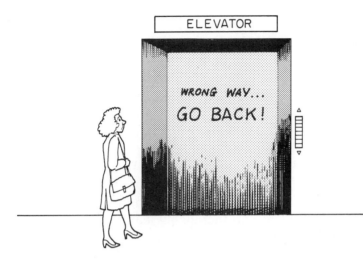

Try using the stairs
instead of the elevator.

The Need for Physical Activity

Our increasingly mechanized and automated society, with its corresponding decrease in physical labor, requires that individuals engage in more planned programs of physical activity. By and large, jobs today require much less physical effort than those of our forebears before World War II. In the late 1800s and early 1900s, when most jobs involved farming or industrial work, hard physical labor was the norm. One estimate is that as a result of mechanization during the past hundred years, human and animal effort has declined drastically—from 90 percent of the total muscle power to produce goods to 10 percent.[17] Today human beings are controllers of mechanical power rather than mere sources of power as in years past.

As the majority of the population shifted from an agrarian to an urban and suburban society, the workweek as well as the nature of the work force changed. In comparison to the type of work and the 60 to 70 hours a week that people worked in an earlier generation, our workweek of 40 hours of sedentary labor is indeed a radical change. Furthermore, the advent of mechanization and automation has produced automobiles, buses, subways, elevators, and escalators and the many labor-saving devices, such as washing machines and dryers, vacuum cleaners, floor waxers, and electric can openers. All these machines have helped to foster decreased physical activity in humans.

Automation has even helped to make recreational activities less active. For example, many people will use a motor-powered boat instead of a rowboat when they go fishing. Golfers ride motorized carts rather than get the exercise of walking during a golf match.

Benefits of Physical Activity

A summary of the benefits of regular physical activity (discussed in some detail in Chapter 7) is presented here. A program of physical activity of the aerobic type will improve the functioning of the heart, blood vessels, and lungs, thereby improving cardiorespiratory endurance. Strength, muscular endurance, and flexibility will be improved as a result of a properly designed physical activity program. A regular program of physical activity will improve body composition as it aids in weight control by reducing fat weight and increasing lean body weight. Research has demonstrated that regular exercise plays a vital role in protecting against coronary heart disease by improving cardiovascular functioning through improved blood flow, enlarged size, and decreased tendency of blood clotting in the coronary arteries.[18]

Although the psychological benefits of physical activity are less well documented than the physiological benefits, there have been reports of reduced anxiety and depression, improved self-image, and a general feeling of wellness as a result of participation in regular, vigorous physical activity. It has been reported that vigorous physical activity has been a means of helping some people to cope with the many stressors of modern society.

Problems Associated with Inactivity

In contrast to regular physical activity, inactivity causes a deterioration of many physiological systems of the body. Research evidence linking inactivity to obesity (having a greater percentage of fat weight than normal for one's height and body weight) is becoming more definitive. Obesity and inactivity are identified as risk factors in cardiovascular disease. The vast number of obese people in the United States—estimated to be between 25 and 50 million—and the positive relationship of inactivity to obesity are compelling reasons for advocating more physical activity for greater numbers of Americans.

Another problem in America is the increased incidence of a variety of pathological conditions, collectively termed "hypokinetic disease" by Kraus and Rabb, which are said to be due to some degree to the generally prevailing lack of exercise.[19] These authors further state: "These diseases, disorders, aches and pains concern chiefly the muscular and cardiovascular systems, metabolism and emotional patterns."[20] In a more specific reference to the degenerative afflictions caused by insufficient exercise, Kraus states that "underexercise is a major factor causing back pain and tension syndrome (stiff neck and headache) and even emotional instability, duodenal ulcers, and heart disease."[21]

Choose the Active Life

The alternative to inactivity and all the problems associated with it is increased physical activity and the documented benefits that can be gained from such activity. It cannot be emphasized too strongly that regular activity programs must be instituted with the establishment of sensible behavior patterns in other risk factor areas. In other words, to achieve optimal wellness, individuals should (besides regular exercise) eat a nutritiously balanced diet, exercise moderation in the consumption of alcohol, avoid other drugs (unless prescribed), and eliminate smoking anything. The increased physical fitness that will accrue from these combined efforts will lead to a fuller and more enjoyable life for a greater number of Americans.

Notes

1. Thomas Stephens, David R. Jacobs, Jr., and Craig C. White, "A Descriptive Epidemiology of Leisure-Time Physical Activity," *Public Health Reports,* 100 (March 1985):147–158.
2. Ibid., p. 149.
3. Ibid., pp. 154–155.
4. J. D. Reed, "America Shapes Up," *Time,* November 2, 1981, p. 103.
5. Ibid.
6. Louis Harris and Associates, *The Perrier Study: Fitness in America* (New York: Perrier–Great Waters of France, Inc., 1979).
7. Ibid., p. 4.
8. American College of Sports Medicine, "The Recommended Quantity and Quality of Exercise for Developing and Maintaining Fitness in Healthy Adults," *Medicine and Science in Sports* 10 (1978):vii–x.
9. William P. Morgan, "Negative Addiction in Runners," *Physician and Sports-medicine* 7 (February 1979):57–70.
10. James O. Mason and Kenneth E. Powell, "Physical Activity, Behavioral Epidemiology, and Public Health," *Public Health Reports* 100 (1985):113.
11. Donald C. Durbeck et al., "The National Aeronautics and Space Adminis-tration–U.S. Public Health Service Evaluation and Enhancement Program," *American Journal of Cardiology,* 30 (1972):789.
12. Harris and Associates.
13. George H. Gallup, "Jogging/Exercise," in *The Gallup Poll* (Wilmington, Del.: Scholarly Resources, Inc., 1984), pp. 6–17.
14. William D. McArdle, Frank I. Katch, and Victor L. Katch, *Exercise Physiol-ogy: Energy, Nutrition, and Human Performance* (Philadelphia: Lea & Febiger, 1981), pp. 229–230.
15. Jean Mayer and F. J. Stare, "Exercise and Weight Control: Frequent Mis-conceptions," *Journal of the American Dietetic Association* 29 (1953):-340–343; Jean Mayer et al., "Exercise, Food Intake and Body Weight in Normal Rats and Genetically Obese Adult Mice," *American Journal of Physiology* 177 (1954):544; Jean Mayer, "Exercise and Weight Control," in Warren R. Johnson, ed., *Science and Medicine of Exercise and Sports* (New York: Harper & Row, 1960), pp. 301–310.
16. Steven N. Blair, David R. Jacobs, Jr., and Kenneth E. Powell, "Relationships

Between Exercise or Physical Activity and Other Health Behaviors," *Public Health Reports* 100 (1985):172–180.

17. John Diebold, "Automation," in *Collier's Encyclopledia,* vol. 3 (New York: Crowell-Collier Educational Corp., 1969), p. 325.

18. "Public Health Aspects of Physical Activity and Exercise," *Public Health Reports,* 100 (1985):113–225.

19. Hans Kraus and Wilhelm Raab, *Hypokinetic Disease* (Springfield, Ill.: Thomas, 1961), p. 173.

20. Ibid.

21. Hans Kraus, "Backache," in *Stress and Tension* (New York: Simon & Schuster, 1965), p. 8.

CHAPTER 2

Clarifying Selected Fitness Concepts

body composition
cardiorespiratory endurance
health
health-related fitness components
isometric contraction
isotonic contraction
joint flexibility

muscular endurance
optimal fitness
physical fitness
skill-related fitness
  components
strength
wellness

Chapter Highlights

After reading this chapter, you should be able to:
1. Define and/or explain the key words listed above.
2. Distinguish between optimal fitness development and maximum fitness development.
3. Identify and discuss the essential differences between strength and muscular endurance and between muscular endurance and cardiorespiratory endurance.
4. Describe the relationship between physical fitness and health and between physical fitness and wellness.

It was pointed out in Chapter 1 that although more Americans are exercising today, the percentage who are engaged in aerobic-type exercise is still smaller than those who do not. One reason some people do not become engaged in an exercise program is that they lack the knowledge of how to design an exercise program and are unknowledgeable about exercise and fitness itself.

This chapter will clarify important concepts related to physical fitness. Information regarding the design and implementation of a fitness

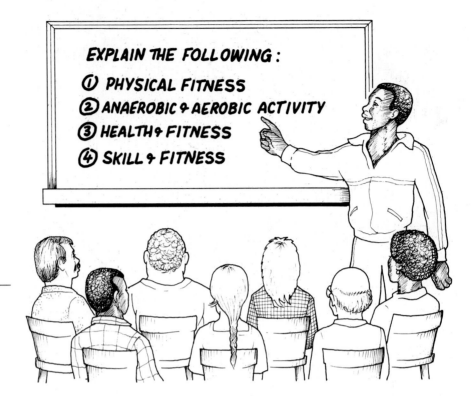

An understanding of certain concepts related to fitness is important in the development of a fitness program.

program is presented in other chapters. This information will provide the knowledge and the motivation to enable more Americans to adopt an active lifestyle that includes participation in a fitness program.

What Is Physical Fitness?

There is no universally accepted definition of fitness. In fact, the concept of physical fitness changes as views of society and its people change. Persons have been thought of as being fit at various periods of time if they had a muscular physique, could lift heavy weights, and were able to pass a physical fitness test consisting of items such as push-ups, sit-ups, vertical jumps, and chin-ups. The ability to pursue daily activities without undue fatigue and have enough energy left for emergencies has also been a popular definition of physical fitness.

Varying conceptions of physical fitness persist. In the cover story in *Time* magazine of August 30, 1982, the new ideal of beauty for women is described as "taut, toned, and coming on strong."[1] The fit female is depicted as one with a body that is thin but strong. The lithe bodies of Jane Fonda and Debbie Allen and the muscular physique of Martina Navratilova, among others, were the examples given to depict fitness. Granted, these women certainly do not portray the Arnold Schwarzeneg-

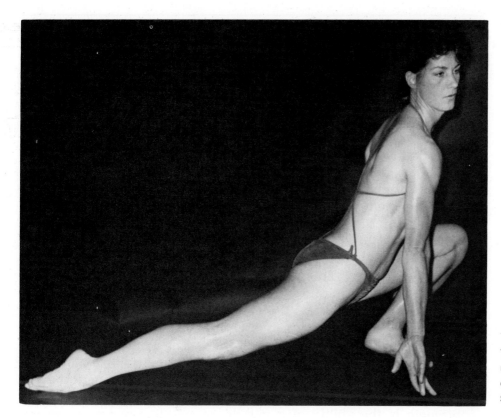

This young woman used body building to develop a lithe yet strong body.

ger type of strength with bulging muscles; but the idea of equating strength with fitness is a limiting concept. Strength is only one component of physical fitness.

Physical fitness is a condition whereby the systems of the body are able to function at their optimal efficiency. Although all body systems must function properly for total fitness, the cardiorespiratory, muscular, and skeletal systems are the focus in the discussion of fitness in this textbook. This means that the heart, blood vessels, lungs, muscles, and joints must function at an optimal level in our concept of physical fitness.

The term *optimal* in this definition of fitness is important. It indicates that each person should strive to develop his or her body's systems to the highest degree possible. There is no single maximum level that all people must attain. In this sense fitness is an individual matter. One should strive to attain the highest fitness level possible, recognizing individual capacity, interests, and fitness goals.

I focus on the cardiorespiratory, muscular, and skeletal systems because research findings associate inactivity and obesity with coronary heart disease and other cardiovascular diseases. Both inactivity and obesity are recognized as risk factors in coronary heart disease. By engaging in activities that will improve the functioning of the three systems of the body mentioned, a person will develop cardiorespiratory endurance, strength, and muscular endurance, flexibility, and lean body mass (desired instead of the fat weight associated with obesity).

Components of Physical Fitness

Components of physical fitness may be thought of as health-related or skill-related.

Health-related Components of Fitness

These components relate to the development of an efficient heart, blood vessels, lungs, muscles, and joints and to a body with a relatively high percentage of lean weight compared to fat weight. Specific health-related components are cardiorespiratory endurance, strength, muscular endurance, joint flexibility, and body composition.

Cardiorespiratory endurance is the ability of the heart, lungs, and blood vessels to deliver essential nutrients, especially oxygen, to the working muscles and to remove waste materials from the body. A characteristic of cardiorespiratory endurance is the body's ability continuously to take in and process the amount of oxygen that is needed for demanding physical tasks for long periods. Examples of activities to improve cardiorespiratory endurance are jogging a mile or more, swimming several laps in a pool one after the other, and riding a bicycle for ten minutes or longer. (Each of these activities should be performed at an intensity level high enough to produce physiological benefits.)

Strength is the ability of a muscle or muscle group to exert one maximal force against a resistance. There are two general types of muscle contractions for strength, isotonic and isometric. In isotonic contraction, a muscular contraction results in body movement. In isometric contraction, the muscle or muscle group does not change in length, and

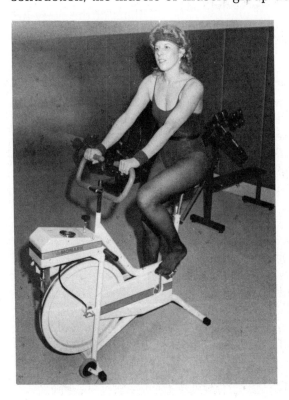

Riding a stationary bicycle is one way to develop cardiorespiratory endurance.

no joint movement occurs. Curling a 50-pound dumbbell with the right hand one time demonstrates the isotonic strength of the biceps muscle in that arm. Pushing against a wall or pushing the palms of the hands against each other for one maximum effort are examples of isometric strength. Strength development, though important, should not be considered the only component of physical fitness.

Rather than being thought of as the embodiment of physical fitness, strength should be considered an important adjunct of other components in performing daily tasks, both work and recreational. Abdominal strength is necessary to hold the body erect; adequate leg strength is required to climb stairs; upper body strength is required to lift objects while doing housework. Jogging requires the development of minimal strength in the muscles of the legs. The development of adequate strength should be an important consideration in the overall physical fitness development process.

Muscular endurance is the ability of a muscle or muscle group to exert repeated contractions against a resistance for an extended period of time or to maintain an isometric contraction for an extended period of time. Examples of activities requiring muscular endurance include performing sit-ups, push-ups, and half squats. Muscular endurance is distinguished from cardiorespiratory endurance by the emphasis on the body system or systems being stressed—the heart, lungs, and blood vessels are stressed in cardiovascular endurance activities, and specific muscle groups (for example, the arms and shoulder muscles in push-ups) are stressed in muscular endurance activities. Muscular endurance is distinguished from strength by the ratio of intensity to duration of the activity—long duration and low intensity characterize muscular endurance, whereas strength involves activities of short duration and high intensity.

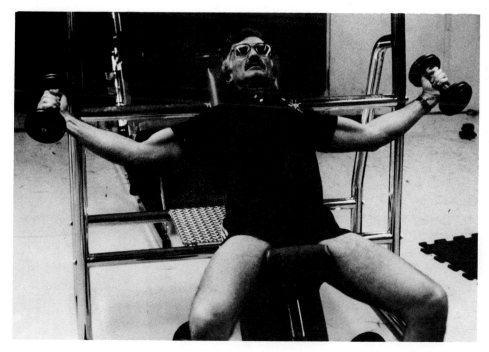

Weight training develops strength and muscular endurance, two components of fitness.

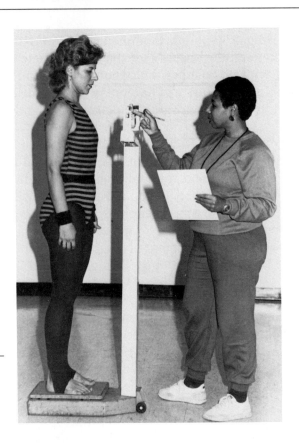

What is a desirable percentage of lean body mass to total body weight?

Joint flexibility is the ability of the joints to move throughout the full range of motion. Flexibility is specific to each joint and is limited primarily by the structure of the joint. For example, persons with good flexibility in the lower back and hamstring muscles of the legs will be able to touch their toes without bending their knees. On the other hand, flexibility of the arm and shoulder is required for individuals to scratch their backs. Practicing progressive stretching routines and participating in activities requiring joints to move through their full range of motion will improve flexibility.

Body composition refers to the relative percentages of lean body weight (or mass) and body fat (or adipose tissue). The inclusion of body composition as a component of physical fitness is a recent occurrence. The American Alliance for Health, Physical Education, Recreation and Dance, a professional organization for persons in physical education and allied areas, developed a Health Related Fitness Test in 1980 that included body composition as a fitness component.

Desirable body composition is a relatively high percentage of lean body tissue in relationship to fat tissue. A general rule of thumb is to keep the percentage of body fat for males below 25 and for females below 30; these are the thresholds of obesity.[2] Individuals should strive to keep the percentage of body fat to about 15 percent of total body weight for males and 20 percent for females. Methods of appraising body composition are discussed in Chapter 5.

These components are associated with a high degree of athletic ability. They include speed, power, agility, balance (or coordination), and reaction time. The development of skill-related components of fitness will increase the range of possible activities that can be used to develop fitness. However, their development is not mandatory for fitness gains. If one wanted to use swimming to develop cardiorespiratory endurance, for example, one would obviously need to possess the necessary swimming skills. The same could be said for other sport skills. The fact remains, however, that activities such as walking, jogging, and hiking, which require no high level of skill development, can be used to develop cardiorespiratory endurance. A high level of athletic skill is *not* necessary for physical fitness development.

Skill-related Components of Fitness

The Relationship of Physical Fitness to Health

How does physical fitness fit into the scheme of overall health? First, an explanation of health is necessary. Health is used in the broad, dynamic sense espoused by the World Health Organization. Health is defined by this recognized body as "a state of complete physical, mental, and social well-being and not merely the absence of disease or infirmity." This is a holistic view of health.

In this context, physical fitness is one important facet of health. Research evidence suggests that when one is physically fit, one is able to lead a more enjoyable life because of improved mental, emotional,

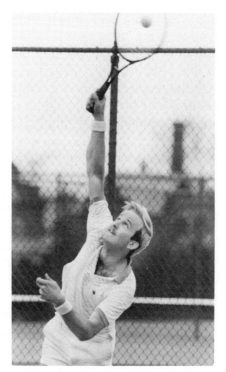

The ability to play tennis is necessary if this activity is to be used to develop physical fitness.

and social development as well as physical development. Participation in activities that promote physical fitness also has been shown to reduce depression and anxiety and to increase a person's self-image and ability to deal with stress in a positive manner.[3]

A final important point regarding both physical fitness and health is that they should be viewed from a preventive and maintenance perspective rather than a rehabilitative perspective. Developing sensible habits that include an active lifestyle, consumption of a nutritiously balanced diet, elimination or moderation of alcohol and smoking, and removal of psychological stressors will result in a healthier, happier existence. Physical fitness and dynamic health are inextricably interrelated. A dynamic state of physical fitness is a necessary part of holistic health as an evolving, ongoing process of development.

Physical Fitness and the Concept of Wellness

The increased attention to active lifestyles, fitness, and preventive health has resulted in a recent concept of *wellness,* a term that is associated with "optimal health" or the "highest level of health." Ryan and Travis depict health as a continuum, with high-level wellness at one extreme and premature death at the other.[4] Wellness education stresses the preventive aspects of making choices that will provide the most enjoyable living conditions and mitigate one's chances of illness. Developing an optimal level of physical fitness can be an important aspect of achieving high-level wellness.

The Wellness Clinic in Salina, Kansas, is one example of the positive relationship between physical fitness and wellness. This midwestern town of 40,000 people has been quietly transformed by the Wellness Clinic. According to an article in *Time* magazine, the program has "many of the people in Salina exercising every day and feeling healthier than ever."[5] The goal of the Wellness Clinic in Salina is to get people in good enough physical condition so that they will not have to go to their doctors so often.

A desirable concept of wellness is one that involves taking control of your life and making the most of each day, despite personal handicaps and the vicissitudes of life over which no control is possible. This means, for instance, that the wheelchair-bound individual can accept his or her condition and still engage in activities that will foster high-level wellness. Developing an optimal level of fitness as well as adopting other sensible habits of living to achieve a satisfying and meaningful existence are goals of dynamic fitness and high-level wellness.

Notes

1. "The New Ideal of Beauty," *Time,* August 30, 1982, p. 72.
2. A. W. Sloan, "Estimation of Body Fat in Young Men," *Journal of Applied Physiology* 23 (1967):311–315; A. W. Sloan, J. J. Burt, and C. S. Blyth, "Estima-

tion of Body Fat in Young Women," *Journal of Applied Physiology* 17 (1962):967–970.

3. James O. Mason and Kenneth E. Powell, "Physical Activity, Behavioral Epidemiology, and Public Health," *Public Health Reports* 100 (1985):113–116.

4. Regina S. Ryan and John W. Travis, *The Wellness Workbook: A Guide to Obtaining High-Level Wellness* (Berkeley, Calif.: Ten Speed Press, n.d.), p. 122.

5. J. D. Reed, "America Shapes Up," *Time,* November 2, 1981, p. 95.

CHAPTER 3

Understanding the Human Body as an Exercise Machine

aerobic metabolism
afferent neurons
agonist
anaerobic metabolism
antagonist
cardiac output
efferent neurons
external respiration
homeostasis

internal respiration
metabolism
neuron
pulmonary ventilation
stroke volume
tidal volume
total lung capacity
vital capacity

Chapter Highlights

After reading this chapter,* you should be able to:
1. Define and/or explain the key words listed above.
2. Identify the basic structural and functional unit of life for humans.
3. List the five functions of the skeletal system.
4. Identify the agonist and antagonist muscles in a specific movement.
5. Identify the two structural and two functional divisions of the nervous system and indicate the role each plays in regulating movement.
6. Discuss the role of the sympathetic and parasympathetic nervous systems in regulating body actions.

* Despite attempts at simplification, this chapter may be technical for a person who does not have a good background in the biological sciences or anatomy and physiology. The intent is to present a comprehensive coverage of the human body as a foundation for a complete understanding of how the body reacts and adapts to varying frequencies, intensities, and durations of physical activity. It is designed to be useful for persons with different backgrounds and interests in fitness.

7. Explain the nervous system mechanisms involved in involuntary and voluntary movement.
8. List the three types of neurons and explain the function of each.
9. Trace the general circulation of blood throughout the body during a complete cardiac cycle.
10. Compare and contrast the cardiac output in a sedentary and a trained individual performing the same physical task.
11. Differentiate between a person with an "athlete's heart" and a pathologically malfunctioning heart.
12. Identify the components of the vascular bed.
13. Explain how partial pressure gradients affect blood flow.
14. List and discuss two factors besides partial pressure that affect external respiration.
15. Explain the concepts of "stitch" in the side, second wind, steady state, and oxygen debt.
16. Explain how the heart muscle gets its oxygen and nutrients.

The human body is an incredible machine that adapts to varying intensities and types of physical activity with efficiency and effectiveness. It has specialized systems for body support, protection, and movement; the regulation of body activities; the supply and distribution of nutrients and removal of waste material; and many more systems that are involved indirectly during exercise.

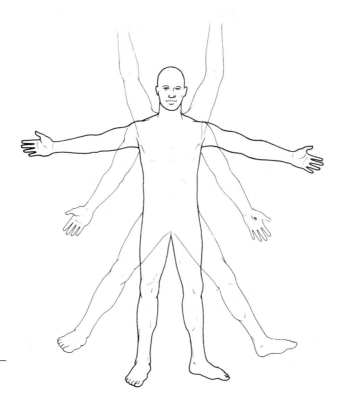

The body in motion.

These systems are comprised of organs, which are composed of tissues, which are themselves made up of cells. Cells are the basic structure and functional units of life in the human organism. There are some one trillion (1,000,000,000,000) cells in the human organism. Each cell type has a specific function and purpose. For example, nerve cells carry messages to muscle cells, which cause movement, and blood cells carry nutrients to working muscles and remove wastes from the tissues.

Homeostasis

There must be an integrated working of all body systems for the human organism to function effectively and efficiently. Regardless of the type or nature of the activity the body is required to perform, it seeks to maintain an equilibrium or constancy of its internal environment, a condition known as *homeostasis*. For this homeostatic condition to exist, the internal environment must have precise concentrations of gases, nutrients, ions, and water; an optimum temperature; and an optimum pressure for the health of the cells.[1]

While working in an integrated manner to help maintain a constant internal environment, each system of the body has specialized functions. An important homeostatic function of the respiratory system, for example, is to provide the cells with enough oxygen to keep the extracellular fluid from falling below normal limits and to remove carbon dioxide from the cells. When the body goes from a resting to an active state, the respiratory system must work faster to keep the fluid level adequate for homeostasis to exist. The cardiovascular system also has a vital role to play in maintaining homeostatic conditions of the body. It must keep an adequate amount of blood moving throughout the body. During increased activity the heart may be required to increase its pumping action significantly, sometimes from 80 beats a minute to 200 beats a minute. On receiving carbon dioxide and other wastes through internal respiration, the cardiovascular system also removes these materials from the cells.

The remainder of the chapter focuses on body systems directly responsible for human movement: the skeletal and muscular systems as the basic movement team, the nervous system as the controller of movement, and the respiratory and cardiovascular systems as the transformers and users of energy for movement.

The Basic Movement Team:
The Skeletal and Muscular Systems

The skeletal and muscular systems work together to produce movement. More than 600 voluntary muscles and precisely 206 bones in the human body provide various kinds of movement.

The Skeletal System: Structure

The skeletal system forms the framework of the body. The 206 bones of the adult human skeleton are grouped in two principle divisions, the *axial* and the *appendicular* (see Figure 3.1). The axial skeleton includes the head, neck, and trunk; the appendicular skeleton contains the bones of the free appendages, which are the upper and lower extremities and the girdles that connect the free appendages to the axial skeletal.

Bones contain hard, osseous tissue that makes them sturdy and durable. However, they are pliable and light enough to permit many types of movement requiring tremendous pressure without breaking. Calcium phosphate, the basic chemical of bones, is necessary in the diet to keep bones strong and resilient.

Movement occurs at the *joint,* the point or position where two or more bones articulate or join. The amount of movement in a joint depends on the structure and function of the joint. The two basic types of joints for movement are ball-and-socket joints and hinge joints. Joints of the hip and shoulder are examples of ball-and-socket joints. Many types of movements (flexion, extension, abduction, adduction, rotation) are possible in ball-and-socket joints. The hinge joint is usually limited to flexion and extension. An example of a hinge joint is the elbow. Try moving this joint and you will notice the limited movement that can be made.

Some joints permit little or no movement (such as the bones of the skull), but we are primarily concerned with the joints that permit free movement. Such joints have three physical characteristics: (1) Between the articulating bones is a space, called the *synovial cavity* (synovial fluid helps to lubricate the action of the moving bones), (2) an articular cartilage covers the ends of the bones to keep them from rubbing directly on each other, and (3) dense, tough connective tissues, called *ligaments,* connect the bones to each other and provide stability to the joint. Bones are attached to muscles by *tendons,* which are white fibrous cords of dense connective tissue.

The Skeletal System: Functions

The skeletal system performs the following five basic functions:

1. It provides support for the soft tissues of the body to keep the body in an erect posture.
2. It protects internal organs of the body such as the brain, heart, and lungs.
3. It provides the surfaces for the attachment of muscles and serves as levers for body movement during muscular contraction.
4. The bones serve as store houses for calcium and phosphorus.

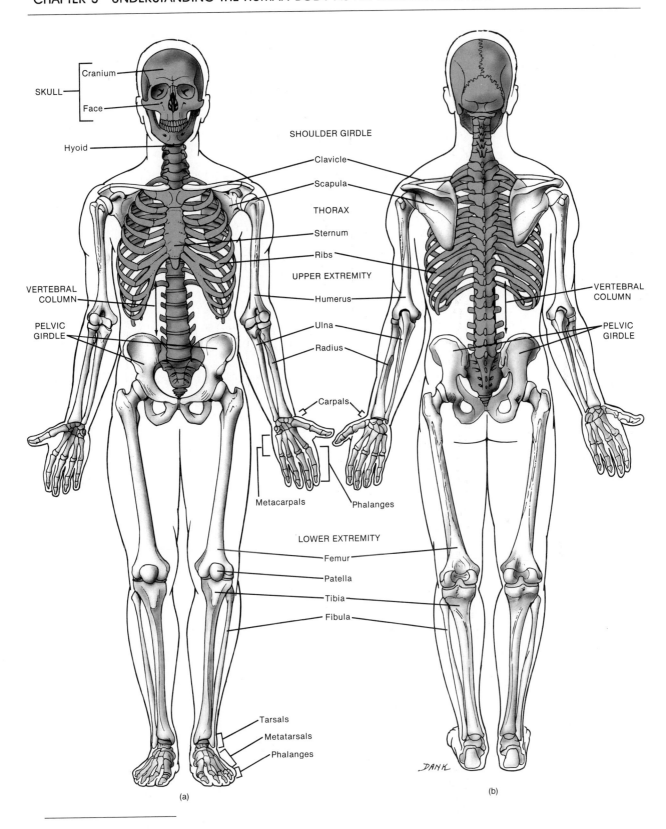

Figure 3.1
Divisions of the skeletal system. The axial skeletal is shaded; the remainder is the appendicular skeleton. (a) Anterior view. (b) Posterior view.

Source: Principles of Anatomy and Physiology, *5th edition by Gerard J. Tortora and Nicholas P. Anagnostakos. Reprinted by permission of Harper & Row, Publishers, Inc.*

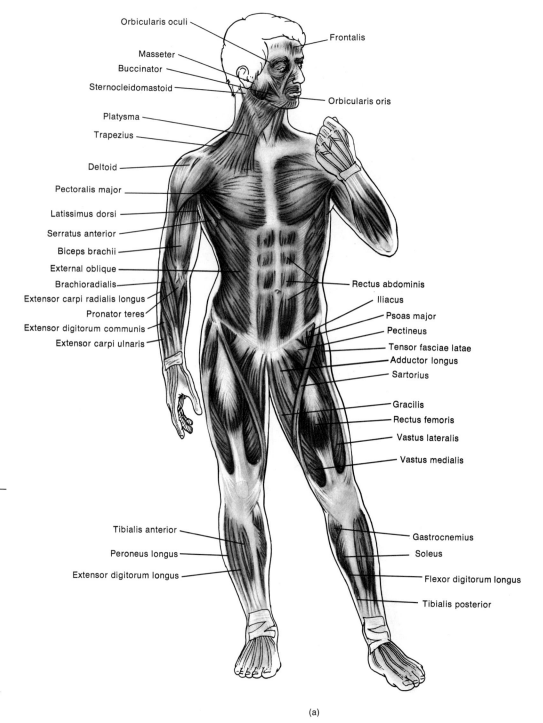

Orbicularis oculi
Frontalis
Masseter
Buccinator
Sternocleidomastoid
Orbicularis oris
Platysma
Trapezius
Deltoid
Pectoralis major
Latissimus dorsi
Serratus anterior
Biceps brachii
External oblique
Brachioradialis
Extensor carpi radialis longus
Pronator teres
Extensor digitorum communis
Extensor carpi ulnaris
Rectus abdominis
Iliacus
Psoas major
Pectineus
Tensor fasciae latae
Adductor longus
Sartorius
Gracilis
Rectus femoris
Vastus lateralis
Vastus medialis
Tibialis anterior
Peroneus longus
Extensor digitorum longus
Gastrocnemius
Soleus
Flexor digitorum longus
Tibialis posterior

(a)

Figure 3.2
Principal superficial muscles of the body. (a) Anterior view. (b) Posterior view.

Source: Principles of Anatomy and Physiology, *5th edition* by Gerard J. Tortora and Nicholas P. Anagnostakos. Reprinted by permission of Harper & Row, Publishers, Inc.

5. It contains chemical laboratories in the red marrow of the bones where red cells are produced.

The Muscular System: Structure

There are three types of muscle tissue in the human body—smooth, cardiac, and skeletal—and they are characterized by location, microscopic structure, and nervous control. Smooth muscle, which is nonstriated and involuntary, lines the blood vessels, the stomach, and the intestines. Cardiac muscle tissue forms the walls of the heart. It is stria-

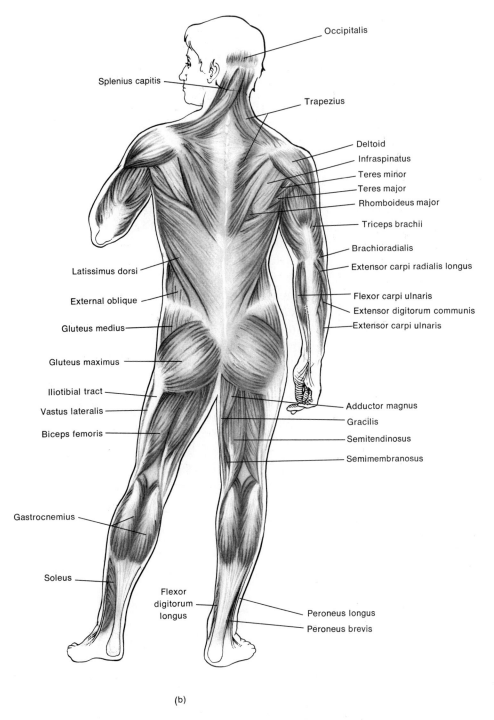

Occipitalis

Splenius capitis

Trapezius

Deltoid
Infraspinatus
Teres minor
Teres major
Rhomboideus major

Triceps brachii

Brachioradialis
Extensor carpi radialis longus

Flexor carpi ulnaris
Extensor digitorum communis
Extensor carpi ulnaris

Latissimus dorsi

External oblique

Gluteus medius

Gluteus maximus

Iliotibial tract
Vastus lateralis
Biceps femoris

Adductor magnus
Gracilis
Semitendinosus
Semimembranosus

Gastrocnemius

Soleus

Flexor
digitorum
longus

Peroneus longus
Peroneus brevis

(b)

ted and involuntary. Skeletal muscle tissue is striated and voluntary. It
is attached to bones and contains the contractile elements necessary to
produce movement. We will focus on the skeletal muscles.

A muscle is a collection of cylindrical cells called *muscle fibers* that
lie parallel to one another and may vary in size from a fraction of an inch
to a foot or more in length. Each muscle fiber is enclosed in a sheath of
connective tissue. Groups of muscle fibers are bound together to form a
primary bundle of muscle tissue (called a *fasciculus*), and these in turn
are wrapped in additional bundles (secondary, tertiary) of connective

tissue to form the muscle itself. The connective tissue that surrounds the various bundles of muscle fibers attaches at the end to form a muscle *tendon.* The tendons attach to the bones.

Figure 3.2 shows the superficial muscles of the body (both anterior and posterior views). It has been estimated that there are 250 million muscle fibers in the human body. The biceps muscle alone has some 600,000 fibers. Skeletal muscles constitute about 45 percent of the body weight of males and about 36 percent in females.

The Muscular System: Functions

The basic function of the muscular system is to work with the skeletal system to produce movement; however, it also enables the body to maintain posture and aids in heat production. An obvious example of movement of the body is walking, which involves the coordinated action of many muscles. The movement of a body part, such as flexion of the forearm at the elbow joint, results from contraction of the biceps muscle and relaxation of the triceps muscle.

Contraction of skeletal muscles holds the body in a stationary position. Without such contractions, the body would fall in a heap. Muscular contractions also produce heat by their movements and thereby play an important role in maintaining normal body temperature.

Types of Muscular Contraction.   As you recall from Chapter 2, there are two types of muscular contractions, isotonic and isometric. In an isotonic contraction, the muscles shorten or lengthen, and movement of body parts or the entire body takes place. The performance of a sit-up can be used to describe both types of contractions. An example of an isotonic contraction in which the muscle shortens is the beginning of a sit-up. The abdominal muscles lengthen as the body is returned from the sit-up position to a supine position. When the body is held in the middle of a sit-up position, the abdominal muscles will remain at a fixed length, and no additional movement will occur. This is an example of a isometric contraction.

Group Actions of Muscles.   Human movements are the results of skeletal muscles acting mainly in groups rather than individually. Muscles attach to bones as members of a team to perform movement, to help steady or support the lever, or to neutralize the undesired action of some muscles. Muscles are thus classified according to their action as *movers* and *synergists* or *fixators.*

A muscle that is primarily responsible for a movement is called an *agonist* or *prime mover.* For example, the biceps brachii is the prime mover in forearm flexion (see Figure 3.2a). During contraction of the biceps brachii in forearm flexion, the triceps brachii muscle, called the *antagonist,* relaxes (see Figure 3.2b). Movement occurs when one muscle group contracts and the opposite muscle group relaxes.

Synergists or fixators assist the prime mover or agonist by reducing undesired action or unnecessary movements in the less mobile articulating joint. In the example of forearm flexion, the deltoid and pectoralis muscles assist in the movement by reducing undesired action or unnecessary movement in the arm and shoulder girdle (see Figure 3.2a).

The Controller of Movement: The Nervous System

The nervous system is responsible for receiving, interpreting, and responding to various stimuli from both the internal and external environment. To perform these functions the nervous system is equipped with a brain and 12 pairs of cranial nerves, a spinal cord and 31 pairs of spinal nerves, and the billions of nerve fibers that spread in a vast network to all parts of the body.

Organization of the Nervous System

The nervous system is divided into two major divisions, the central nervous system and the peripheral nervous system. The central nervous system consists of the brain and spinal cord, and the peripheral component consists of nerve processes that connect the brain and spinal cord with receptors, muscles, and glands. The peripheral nervous system may be divided into two components, the afferent component and the efferent component. The efferent system may be further subdivided into the somatic and autonomic nervous systems. The autonomic nervous system is further subdivided into the sympathetic and parasympathetic nervous system. The two principal divisions, the central nervous system and the peripheral nervous system, and their subdivisions are summarized in Figure 3.3.

The *central nervous system* (CNS) is the control center for thought,

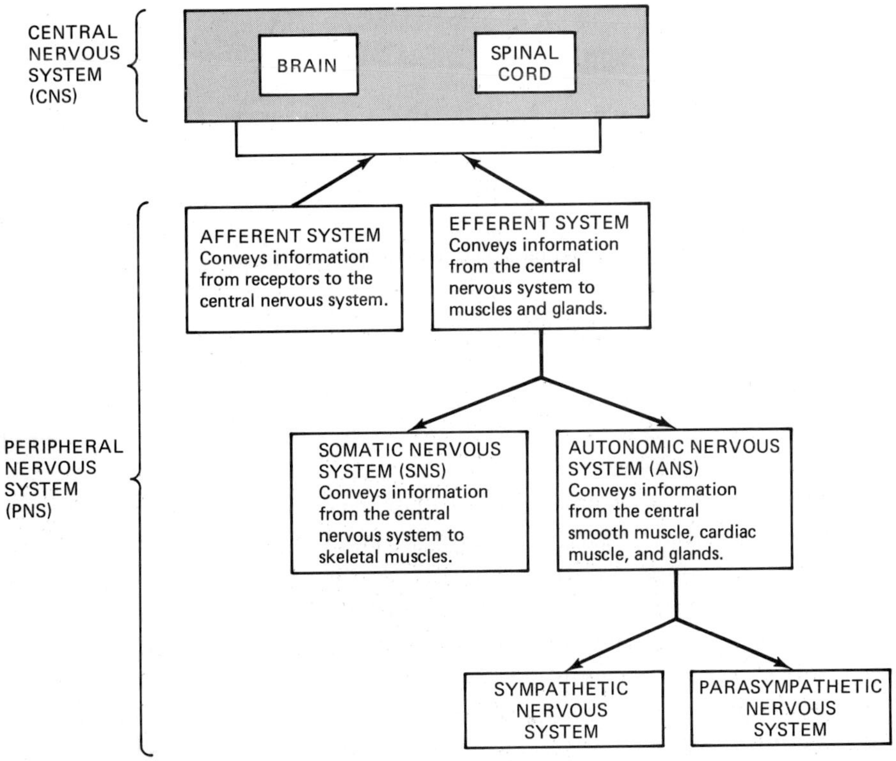

CENTRAL NERVOUS SYSTEM (CNS)

BRAIN   SPINAL CORD

AFFERENT SYSTEM
Conveys information from receptors to the central nervous system.

EFFERENT SYSTEM
Conveys information from the central nervous system to muscles and glands.

PERIPHERAL NERVOUS SYSTEM (PNS)

SOMATIC NERVOUS SYSTEM (SNS)
Conveys information from the central nervous system to skeletal muscles.

AUTONOMIC NERVOUS SYSTEM (ANS)
Conveys information from the central smooth muscle, cardiac muscle, and glands.

SYMPATHETIC NERVOUS SYSTEM

PARASYMPATHETIC NERVOUS SYSTEM

Figure 3.3
Organization of the nervous system.

speech, and muscle action. All body sensations must be relayed from sense receptors in various parts of the body to the central nervous system if they are to be interpreted and acted on.

The *peripheral nervous system* (PNS) consists of all the nerve processes (nerve cells and fibers) outside the CNS that connect the brain and spinal cord with sense receptors, muscles, and glands. The vast network of neurons that comprises the afferent and efferent components of the peripheral nervous system is discussed under a separate heading as the concluding section of the nervous system.

The *somatic nervous system,* a subdivision of the efferent nervous system, is responsible for activity of the skeletal muscles, speech, and thought processes. These are voluntary actions under the conscious will of the body. Conversely, the *autonomic nervous system,* also a subdivision of the efferent system, is considered involuntary since it conveys information to the heart muscle, smooth muscle tissue, and glands, actions over which the body has no voluntary control.

Sometimes the body needs to speed up actions in some organs and at other times it needs to restrict or slow down organ activity. These tasks are accomplished by two divisions of the autonomic nervous system, the *sympathetic division* and the *parasympathetic division.* For example, when preparing to run a marathon, the sympathetic component acts to speed up heart action; when preparing to go to sleep, the parasympathetic component acts to slow down the action of the heart. The actions of these two divisions are integrated to help maintain the internal equilibrium of the body (homeostasis).

Neurons: The Vital Communication Link. A neuron, a specialized nerve cell, is the basic unit of the nervous system. It contains the necessary structural and chemical properties to receive and transmit messages between the central nervous system and the rest of the body. A neuron may vary in length from a fraction of an inch to 6 feet long.

Neurons, grouped according to function, are of three kinds: *sensory* or *afferent* neurons, *motor* or *efferent* neurons, and *connecting* or *internuncial* neurons. Sensory neurons carry messages from sense receptors in the periphery of the body to the central nervous system. Motor neurons relay information from the central nervous system to the muscles and glands. The connecting neurons link sensory to motor neurons and are housed entirely in the central nervous system.

Involuntary and Voluntary Movement. A marvelous thing about the nervous system is that it is capable of monitoring both simple and complex movements. Many of the simple movements performed by humans are involuntary. Reflex movements are in this category; a *reflex* is an involuntary motor response to a sensory stimulus. A most widely recognized human reflex is the jerking response of the knee to being tapped on the tendon of that joint. Other examples of reflex movements include blinking of the eyes when a foreign body strikes the eyeball and the removal of the hand from a hot surface on contact.

In the simplest reflex, the stretch reflex, the impulse travels from the stretched muscle over the sensory nerve fiber to the synapse in the spinal cord and then to the motor nerve fiber of the stretched muscle where that muscle contracts.

Besides such simple movement patterns, the nervous system is completely capable of controlling complex movements and thought processes involving the highest levels of brain activity. Physical activities such as hitting a tennis ball, performing a somersault in gymnastics, and playing the violin and mental acts such as solving a complex problem in calculus or a chemical equation are examples of actions requiring input from the brain.

Transformation and Use of Energy for Movement: The Cardiorespiratory System

The cardiorespiratory system is a combination of the cardiovascular system (consisting of the heart and vascular bed) and the respiratory system (consisting of the lungs and other respiratory apparatus). Before we discuss the structural and functional aspects of these two systems, we should understand the breakdown and use of nutrients to provide energy for movement.

Metabolism

The energy needed for body movement is provided by the breakdown and utilization of three primary food groups—proteins, carbohydrates, and fats. From carbohydrates and fats the body gets the necessary energy for body functions, and from proteins the body gets the nutrients to build and repair tissue. The process through which energy is produced from these food sources is one aspect of *metabolism*—the sum of all the biochemical reactions that occur within the human organism.

Aerobic and Anaerobic Metabolism.   The energy for muscular work is not produced directly through the breakdown of food but is used to manufacture another chemical compound called *adenosine triphosphate* (ATP). Two types of metabolism for muscular contraction and thus movement are *aerobic* metabolism and *anaerobic* metabolism.

Aerobic metabolism involves the breakdown of glucose into pyruvic acid and the release of ATP molecules (a process called *glycolysis*) in the presence of oxygen. In aerobic metabolism, additional chemical reactions produce more ATP (for energy), carbon dioxide, water, and heat. In anaerobic metabolism, which involves the breakdown of glucose without adequate oxygen, a small number of ATP molecules are also produced. However, in contrast to aerobic metabolism, anaerobic metabolism results in the production of lactic acid, and there is no further energy production. High accumulation of lactic acid causes muscle fatigue and a consequent discontinuance of muscle contractions.

The intensity and duration of the activity will determine the degree

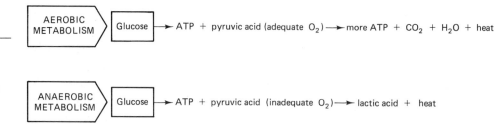

Figure 3.4
Aerobic and
anaerobic metabolic
pathways for energy
production.

to which each metabolic pathway is used to provide the necessary energy for muscular contraction. Since both ATP and glycogen can be metabolized without oxygen, *anaerobic* metabolism is the primary process used to provide quick energy supplies for high-intensity (maximal-effort) activities of relatively short duration. Running sprints (100- and 200-meter dashes, for instance), and performing push-ups and squat thrusts are examples of high-intensity, short-duration activities.

On the other hand, an adequate supply of oxygen is needed for endurance activities of relatively long duration that require only submaximal effort, such as walking, lap swimming, and bicycle riding at a leisurely pace. The ATP for these activities is supplied mainly through *aerobic* metabolism. The body metabolizes both carbohydrates and fats to generate ATP for these endurance activities.

This discussion has centered on the breakdown of carbohydrates for energy production because glucose is the preferred source of energy for the body. However, remember that fats and proteins can also be metabolized. See Figure 3.4 for a summary of energy production through aerobic and anaerobic metabolism.

The relative energy values for one gram of each of the three main food groups are as follows:

$$1 \text{ g of carbohydrate } = 4 \text{ kilocalories}$$
$$1 \text{ g of fat } \qquad\quad = 9 \text{ kilocalories}$$
$$1 \text{ g of protein } \qquad = 4 \text{ kilocalories}$$

The Heart and Blood Circulation

The heart is the main organ of the cardiovascular system, whose job it is to transport nutrients to the working muscles and to remove waste products via blood circulation. The heart is a muscular pump that weighs about one pound and works continuously, pumping 4 to 6 liters of blood throughout the body 1500 times a day. This means that the heart pumps about 7500 liters of blood through the body each day.

Structure and Functioning of the Heart

The heart, situated mostly to the left of the body's midline in the upper chest cavity, is a muscle (called *myocardium*). The heart is enclosed in a loose-fitting membrane called the *pericardium* or *pericardial sac*. It has four chambers to receive and expel blood. The right and left *atria* are the thin-walled top chambers of the heart. They act mainly as receiving cavities for blood. The right and left *ventricles* are the thick-walled bottom chambers, which are responsible for pumping blood from the heart (see Figure 3.5 for a description of the structural aspects of the heart and the path of blood flow through the heart.)

The atria and ventricles are separated by valves, known as *atrioventricular* (AV) *valves.* These valves provide a one-way passage of blood between the right atrium and right ventricle (tricuspid valve) and between the left atrium and right ventricle (bicuspid or mitral valve). Another set of valves, called *semilunar valves,* are situated at the opening where the pulmonary trunk leaves the right ventricle and at the opening between the left ventricle and the aorta. These valves prevent blood from flowing back into the heart's chambers.

For functional purposes the heart may be thought of as two linked pumps, or a right and left heart. The left heart receives oxygenated blood from the lungs and pumps it into the aorta for distribution throughout the body. Simultaneously, the right heart receives deoxygenated blood from all parts of the body via the venae cavae and pumps it to the lungs by way of the pulmonary artery.

Coronary Arteries.   The heart muscle itself must receive nutrients to survive and function properly. A network of blood vessels in the wall of the heart is designed to provide the heart muscle with oxygen and nutrients and remove carbon dioxide and wastes. This array of arteries throughout the heart muscle is a network of *coronary arteries,* and the circulation of blood through these vessels is known as *coronary circulation.*

Cardiac Cycle.   The cardiac cycle is the sequence of events that occur during a complete heartbeat. There are two general phases of the cardiac cycle: the *diastole* or resting phase and the *systole* or contraction phase. A cardiac cycle, or complete heartbeat, consists of a contraction and relaxation phase of both atria and ventricles.

In the atrial diastole phase, blood is flowing into the right and left atria through the venae cavae and pulmonary veins, respectively. (The ventricles are contracted during this period.) The atria then contract (systolic period), forcing the remainder of the blood into the ventricles, which are now relaxed, through the AV valves. As the blood fills the ventricles, they contract, sending deoxygenated blood from the right ventricle to the lungs via the pulmonary artery and oxygenated blood from the left ventricle to the body via the aorta. The AV valves between the atria and ventricles are closed during the first part of atrial diastole, and they open only when the pressure in the atria exceeds that in the ventricles. At the end of ventricular contraction, the valves guarding the pulmonary artery and aorta (semilunar valves) close, and both atria and ventricles relax. The cardiac cycle is ready to be repeated.

Cardiac Output.   A critical factor in the development of cardiorespiratory endurance is the ability of the heart to pump increasing amounts of blood and thus get nutrients to the working muscles. This is accomplished through the cardiac output (CO), which is the amount of blood ejected from the heart (usually measured from the left ventricle) per minute.

The cardiac output is the product of stroke volume (SV) times heart

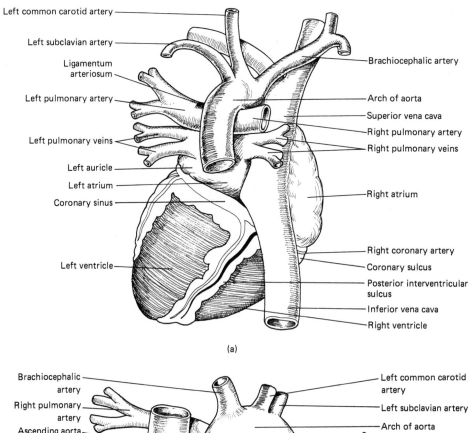

(a)

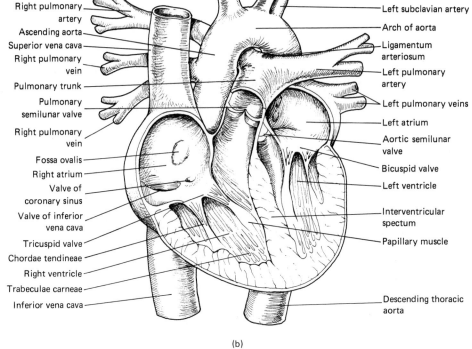

(b)

Figure 3.5
Structure of the heart.
(a) Diagrammatic
posterior external view.
(b) Diagrammatic
anterior internal view.
(c) Path of blood flow
through the heart.

Source: Principles of
Anatomy and
Physiology, *5th Edition
by Gerard J. Tortora
and Nicholas P.
Anagnostakos.
Reprinted by
permission of Harper &
Row, Publishers, Inc.*

rate. Stroke volume is the amount of blood pumped from the heart with
each beat or stroke, and heart rate refers to the number of times the heart
beats per minute.

The cardiac output in an adult at rest, which is similar for both
trained and untrained persons, averages about 5 or 6 liters of oxygen per

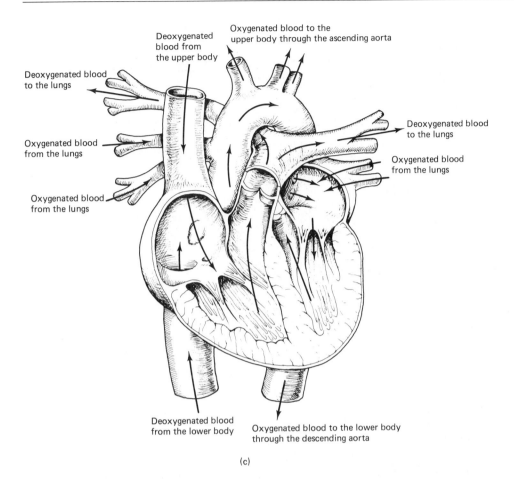

(c)

minute. A resting heart rate may vary between 50 and 100 beats per minute, with an average of about 78 in an adult. Stroke volume averages about 70 milliliters in an untrained adult at rest. Based on these figures, the cardiac output for a relatively sedentary adult would be:

$$\begin{aligned} \text{Cardiac output} &= \text{stroke volume} \times \text{heart rate} \\ &= 70 \text{ ml} \times 78 \text{ beats/min} \\ &= 5460 \text{ ml/min, or } 5.46 \text{ liters/min} \end{aligned}$$

The average resting heart rate for a trained athlete is lower than that of a sedentary person, but the stroke volume is higher. Therefore, the trained person will be able to produce about the same cardiac output as the untrained person. For example, resting pulse rates of 64 to 76 have been recorded for one former world-class miler.[2] Using the lower resting pulse rate value in the cardiac output equation, this world-class endurance athlete would need to have a stroke volume of 85 milliliters per beat to produce a cardiac output equal to that of the average untrained person. Values for resting cardiac output, heart rate, and stroke volume for untrained persons and one world-class miler are summarized here:

	Cardiac Output	= Stroke Volume	× Heart Rate
Untrained:	5460 ml/min	= 70 ml/beat	× 78 beats/min
Athlete:	5460 ml/min	= 85 ml/beat	× 64 beats/min

Cardiac output increases as one goes from a resting state to exercise states requiring increasingly higher work demands or exercise intensity. Unlike the similar cardiac output for trained and untrained persons at rest, cardiac output varies widely between the two during strenuous, endurance-type activities requiring maximum workloads. For example, increases in cardiac output for untrained persons during strenuous work have been reported to be four times the average resting rate, with an average maximum of 20 to 22 liters of blood per minute. On the other hand, maximum cardiac outputs of 35 to 40 liters per minute have been recorded for world-class endurance athletes.[3]

Although the average maximum cardiac output is greater for a trained person than for an untrained person, the trained person has a somewhat lower maximum heart rate for a given exercise intensity than the sedentary person of a similar age. (The lower heart rate results from a heart made stronger and more efficient through endurance training.) However, the trained individual has a much higher stroke volume at maximal workloads than an untrained counterpart of the same age, hence the higher cardiac output. The increase in stroke volume occurs mainly during the period between resting and moderate exercise. Maximum stroke volume is reached at 40 to 50 percent of maximum oxygen consumption.[4] Maximum values of stroke volume during exercise range from an average of 100 to 120 milliliters per beat in untrained individuals and 150 to 170 milliliters per beat for trained subjects. In a world-class endurance athlete, a stroke volume of over 200 milliliters per beat may be produced.

"Athlete's Heart."   Cardiorespiratory endurance training will cause the heart to increase in size (cardiac hypertrophy). Such an enlarged heart is sometimes called "athlete's heart" because athletes are associated with enlarged musculature. This hypertrophy of the heart muscle is a normal adaptation of this muscle to increased workloads.

The Vascular Bed

The vascular bed refers to the network of blood vessels through which blood is carried from the heart, transported to the tissues of the body, and then returned to the heart. This network includes arteries, arterioles, capillaries, venules, and veins.

The aorta and other large *arteries* are called elastic or conducting arteries. These large arteries divide into medium-sized muscular arteries. Arteries contain walls constructed of three layers and a hollow core, called a *lumen*. The middle layer, or tunica media, is the thickest layer, and it consists of elastic fibers and smooth muscles. The structure of the middle layer is particularly responsible for the elasticity and contractility of the arteries. (See Figure 3.6 for structural aspects of an artery, a capillary, and a vein).

Arterioles are small arteries that deliver blood to capillaries. The arterioles next to the arteries from which they extend have the same three layers or tunica as the arteries, but with fewer elastic fibers. Arterioles closest to the capillaries consist mainly of a layer of endothelium surrounded by smooth muscle cells.

Capillaries are located near almost every cell in the body. They

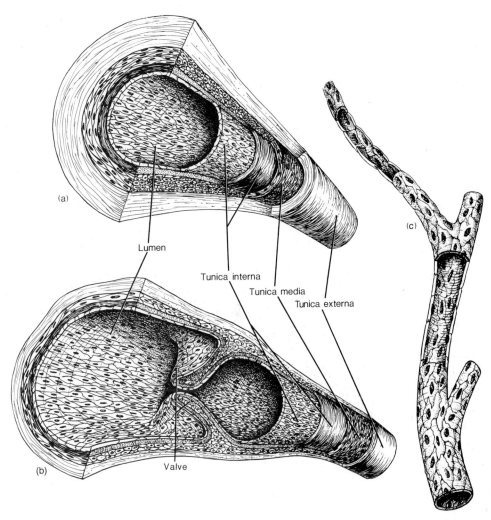

Lumen

Tunica interna

Tunica media

Tunica externa

Valve

Figure 3.6
Comparative structure of (a) an artery, (b) a vein, and (c) a capillary. The relative size of the capillary is enlarged for emphasis.

Source: Illustrations (a), (b), and (c) on page 488 of Principles of Anatomy and Physiology, *5th edition by Gerard J. Tortora and Nicholas P. Anagnostakos. Copyright © 1987 by Biological Sciences Textbooks, Inc., A & P Textbooks, Inc. and Elia-Sparta Inc. Reprinted by permission of Harper & Row, Publishers, Inc.*

permit the exchange of nutrients and wastes between the blood and the tissue cells. To carry out this function, the walls of the capillaries are composed of only a single layer of endothelium (cells).

Venules are small veins. They are extensions of capillaries, from which they collect blood and carry it to the veins. Venules closest to the capillaries consist only of an inner and outer coat. Venules closest to veins contain the middle layer or coat (tunica media) characteristic of veins.

Veins are comprised of the same three layers as arteries. However, they have much less elastic tissue and smooth muscle and more white fibrous tissue. The walls of the veins are not as strong as those of the arteries. To prevent backflow of blood and to help deliver blood to the heart, many veins, particularly those in arms and legs, contain one-way valves. These valves help to propel blood to the heart from these low-pressure areas during the "milking" action of the muscles in the veins. The "milking" action results from the alternate contraction and relaxation of the veins and the one-way action of their valves. This type of muscular contraction is a major factor in the venous return of blood to the heart. Veins are also important blood storage chambers.

Routes of Blood Flow

Oxygenated blood is carried from the left heart via the aorta to the arteries, then to the arterioles to be exchanged through the walls of the capillaries to the body tissues. Deoxygenated blood is exchanged between the capillaries and venules, which merge into veins in the body tissues. This blood travels through the veins back to the right heart via the venae cavae to be pumped to the lungs for more oxygen. Blood vessels, called *vasa vasora*, are also in the walls of blood vessels of the vascular bed to provide oxygen and nutrients to these vessels. (It should be noted that blood always flows from higher-pressure areas to lower-pressure areas.)

The Lungs and Respiration

The respiratory system and the cardiovascular system work together to deliver a constant supply of oxygen to the cells of all tissues and to remove carbon dioxide and waste materials. This is a most important function since cells can survive for only a few minutes without oxygen. Moreover, although a certain amount of carbon dioxide is necessary to help maintain the internal equilibrium of gases, an excessive amount of carbon dioxide will produce an acidic environment that is detrimental to the cells.

The organs of respiration include the nose, pharynx, larynx, trachea, bronchi, and lungs (Figure 3.7). The structure of these organs will not be discussed. For purposes of this text it is sufficient to indicate that all the organs except the lungs act collectively as a passageway for the conduct of air into the alveoli of the lungs.

Respiratory Processes

There are three basic respiratory processes: pulmonary ventilation or breathing, external respiration, and internal respiration.

Pulmonary Ventilation (Breathing).   Breathing is the process by which gases are exchanged between the atmosphere and the alveoli of the lungs. The actual act of breathing, or inhaling and exhaling, is an involuntary process and may be affected by several factors. Among these are the atmospheric pressure and the condition of the muscles responsible for pulmonary ventilation (the muscles mostly responsible for quiet breathing are the diaphragm and intercostals), height, age, temperature, and humidity.

The air in the atmosphere contains 79.04 percent nitrogen, 20.93 percent oxygen, and 0.03 percent carbon dioxide. Although these percentages are the same at all altitudes, the atmospheric pressure differs at different locations in relation to sea level. Air flows according to pressure gradients—from a high-pressure area to a low-pressure area. Thus it is more difficult to breathe in air at high altitudes where the air pressure is low.

The diaphragm and intercostal muscles, those primarily responsible for breathing, determine to a great extent the efficiency of breathing. For example, strong diaphragm and intercostals are required to expand the lungs to increase the volume and decrease the pressure in the lungs. This is important when breathing in areas where the atmospheric pressure is low.

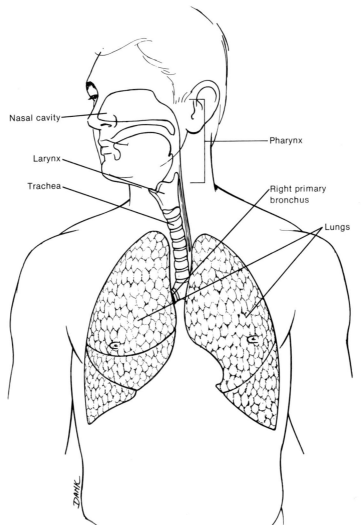

Figure 3.7
Diagram of the organs of the respiratory system.

Source: Principles of Anatomy and Physiology, *5th Edition by Gerard J. Tortora and Nicholas P. Anagnostakos. Reprinted by permission of Leonard D. Dank.*

The expiration phase of breathing is more of a passive process than the inspiration phase. However, the muscles of respiration also play an important role in regulating expiration during activities requiring cardio-respiratory endurance and when air movement from the lungs is impeded. During these instances, the diaphragm and intercostal muscles must contract to force air out into the air passageway.

Pulmonary Volume and Capacities.   About 500 milliliters of air is taken in with each inhalation. The same amount of air is released with each exhalation. *Tidal volume* is the name given to this volume of air inspired or expired with each breath. Only about 350 milliliters of this air reaches the alveoli. An *alveolus* is an elastic, thin-walled membranous air sac that, when magnified, resembles a grape. The other 150 milliliters, called *dead air volume,* remains in the air spaces of the nose, pharynx, larynx, trachea, and bronchi. Humans normally breathe approximately 12 times per minute at rest (a range of 12 to 20 has been reported.)[5] The amount of air taken in during one minute is called the *minute volume.* Calculation of the average minute volume is a simple process of multiplying the number of breaths per minute (12) times the tidal volume (500 ml), which would yield 6000 milliliters, or 6 liters per minute. Allowing for the 150 milliliters of dead air volume, approximately 4.2 liters of air will reach the alveoli (12 × 350 = 4200). In strenuous exercise the amount of air reaching the alveoli can be increased to as much as 100 liters per minute in adult males and can reach values of 200 liters per minute in well-trained athletes of large stature. However, large increases in minute volumes have very little effect on tidal volume, which rarely exceeds 55 percent of the vital capacity.[6]

Lung capacities can be calculated by combining various lung volumes. Two important lung capacities for the purposes of this text are vital capacity and total lung capacity. *Vital capacity*—the sum of inspiratory reserve volume (maximal amount of gas inspired from end-inspiration), tidal volume, and expiratory reserve volume (maximal amount of gas expired from end-expiration)—is the maximal volume of air that can be forcefully expired after one maximal inspiration. Although vital capacities vary according to body size, body position, and age at the time of measurement, values average about 4 to 5 liters in young men and 3 to 4 liters in young women. *Total lung capacity,* the sum of all volumes, is the volume of air in the lungs at the end of a maximal inspiration. This value ranges from about 4 to 5 liters in young women to about 5 to 6 liters in young men. Figure 3.8 illustrates pulmonary lung volumes and capacities.

External Respiration.   The exchange of oxygen and carbon dioxide between the alveoli of the lungs and pulmonary blood capillaries is called external respiration. The oxygen is transported from the atmosphere to the lungs through the inspiratory phase of breathing. Blood needing oxygen is pumped from the right ventricle through the pulmonary arteries into the pulmonary capillaries, which overlay the alveoli.

Through the process of diffusion approximately 250 milliliters of oxy-

Figure 3.8
Spirogram of
pulmonary lung
volumes and
capacities.

Source: Principles of
Anatomy and
Physiology, *5th edition
by Gerard J. Tortora
and Nicholas P.
Anagnostakos.
Reprinted by
permission of Harper &
Row, Publishers, Inc.*

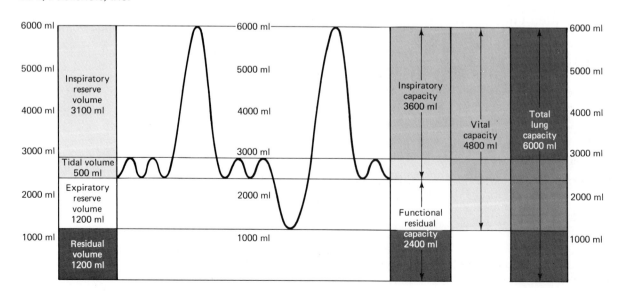

TABLE 3.1   Partial Pressures (in mm Hg) of Respiratory Gases and Nitrogen in Atmospheric Air, Alveolar Air, Blood, and Tissue Cells

	Atmospheric Air (sea level)	Alveolar Air	Deoxygenated Blood	Oxygenated Blood	Tissue Cells
pO_2	160	105	40	105	40
pCO_2	0.3	40	45	40	45
pN_2	597	569	569	569	569

Source: Gerard J. Tortora and Nicholas P. Anagnostakos, Principles of Anatomy and Physiology, *4th ed. (New York: Harper & Row, 1984), p. 562. Used by permission of the publisher.*

gen permeates the alveoli and enters the blood and about 200 milliliters of carbon dioxide travels in the reverse direction into the alveoli while the organism is at rest. This exchange of gases takes place through more than 600 million alveoli in the lungs and the pulmonary capillary cells that juxtapose them.

The diffusion of gases in external respiration operates according to Dalton's law of partial pressure and other gas laws. The direction of diffusion is from a high-pressure-gradient area to a low-pressure area. The partial pressures of the respiratory gases and nitrogen in the atmosphere, alveoli, blood, and tissue cells are shown in Table 3.1* It can be seen that the partial pressure of the oxygen of alveolar air, written as pO_2, is 105 millimeters of mercury (mm Hg). The pO_2 of the deoxygenated blood entering the pulmonary capillaries is only 40 mm Hg. This difference in pO_2 results in oxygen being diffused from the alveoli into the blood in need of more oxygen until a homeostatic condition exists whereby pO_2 of the now oxygenated blood is 105 mm Hg. During this diffusion of oxygen from the alveoli into deoxygenated blood, carbon dioxide is traveling in the opposite direction, that is, from the deoxygenated blood in the pulmonary capillaries into the alveoli. (See Figure 3.9 for partial pressure differences and direction of the movement of gases in both external and internal respiration.) The carbon dioxide that diffuses into the alveoli is eliminated from the lungs during expiration.

The actual amount of oxygen that diffuses into blood at the pulmonary capillary level is approximately 25 percent of the air breathed in quiet breathing. (This is called ventilatory equivalent and is symbolized V-1vO$_2$.) Because the air is 20.93 percent oxygen, of the 6000 milliliters of air breathed per minute in quiet breathing, only about 300 ml per minute of oxygen (.25 $\times$ 1250) diffuses into the blood. This ratio of 25 to 1 (25 liters of air breathed per liter of oxygen consumed) is for light to moderate steady-state exercise bouts. In strenuous submaximal exercise bouts, the ratio of air breathed to oxygen consumed increases tremendously, sometimes to 35 or 40 liters of air per liter of oxygen consumed.[7]

* The atmospheric pressure is the sum of the pressures of all the gases in the atmosphere, calculated to be 760 mm Hg. This includes several gases that appear in such small quantities in the atmosphere that they are not included in Table 3.1.

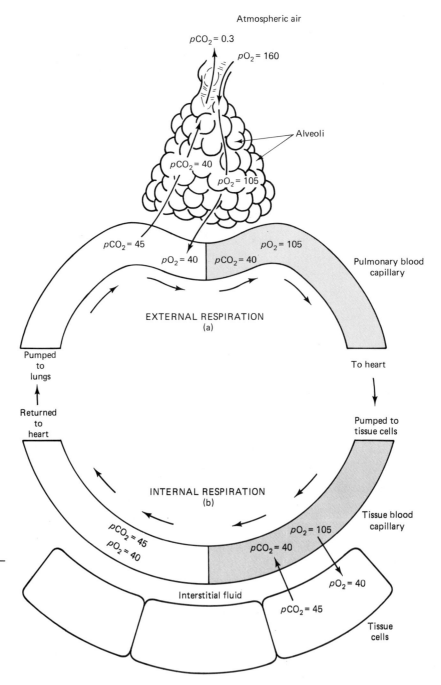

Figure 3.9
Partial pressures
involved in respiration.
(a) External.
(b) Internal. All
pressures are in
mm Hg.

Besides the influence of partial pressure gradients, the efficiency of external respiration can also be affected by such factors as altitude and surface area of alveoli available for O_2-CO_2 exchange. The effect of breathing at high altitudes has been indicated. Altitude also affects the efficiency of external respiration because at higher elevations the barometric pressure is lower, resulting in a lower partial pressure of atmospheric oxygen (pO_2) and a corresponding decrease in the alveolar pO_2. Consequently, the quantity of oxygen that is available to diffuse into the blood is progressively reduced at increasingly higher altitudes.

The cross-sectional area of the functional alveolar-capillary membrane has a direct bearing on external respiration. Pulmonary disorders such as asthma, bronchitis, and emphysema, which decrease the surface area for O_2-CO_2 exchange, also decrease the efficiency and extent of external respiration.

Smoking indirectly reduces the area of the alveoli for diffusion of respiratory gases since it is implicated in the development of bronchitis and emphysema. Chronic cigarette smoking greatly increases the airway resistance, thus increasing the oxygen cost of breathing. This increased oxygen cost is an added burden when participating in endurance activities.

Internal Respiration. Internal respiration is the exchange of oxygen and carbon dioxide between tissue capillaries and tissue cells. Remember that oxygenated blood is pumped from the left ventricle through the aorta to the tissue cells for use by the body. Carbon dioxide is taken by the veins back to the heart via the venae cavae and then to the lungs to be exchanged for oxygen. The drop-off of oxygen at the tissue cells for use by the working muscles and the pickup of carbon dioxide by the blood capillaries to be taken back to the right heart to be reoxygenated are regulated by partial pressure gradients, the same as external respiration. See Figure 3.9 for the partial pressures of oxygen and carbon dioxide and the direction of gas flow.

Cardio-respiratory Phenomena

Several important phenomena concerning cardiorespiratory functioning directly affect persons attempting to develop cardiorespiratory endurance. These include the "stitch" in the side, steady state, second wind, and oxygen debt.

The *"stitch" in the side* is a feeling of discomfort (characterized by a sharp, stabbing pain in the lower chest cavity) that may be experienced by individuals who engage in aerobic activity for several minutes continuously. This "stitch" will appear earlier in sedentary persons than in persons who have engaged in physical activities of an aerobic nature.

Although the exact cause has not been scientifically discovered, it is hypothesized that the pain results from a deficiency of blood (ischemia) and thus oxygen (anoxia) in the area of the intercostal muscles and a subsequent buildup of lactic acid, which acts on the nerve receptors for pain in that area. When the pain occurs on the left side of the body, the deficiency of blood is thought to be in the area of the spleen.[8]

Steady state is a physiological condition in which the body receives the amount of oxygen that is required for the completion of a particular activity. In other words, when the oxygen consumption equals the oxygen requirement for a particular task, the body is said to be in a steady state. The steady state is usually thought of in relation to aerobic activities that last for more than a few minutes.

The body must make several physiological adjustments to reach a steady state. The longer and more strenuous the activity, the greater the adjustments that must be made to reach the steady state. For example,

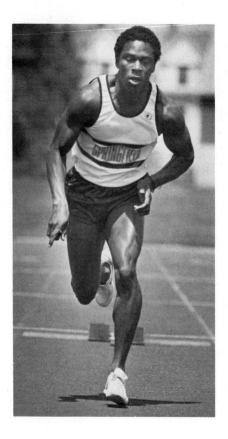

An oxygen debt is often incurred in sprinting short distances.

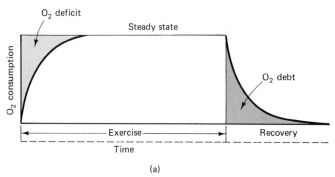

(a)

Figure 3.10
Oxygen deficit, oxygen debt, and recovery during aerobic and anaerobic exercise. (a) Small oxygen debt repaid during short recovery period following aerobic exercise in which steady state has been reached. (b) Large oxygen debt paid during long recovery period following high-intensity anaerobic exercise.

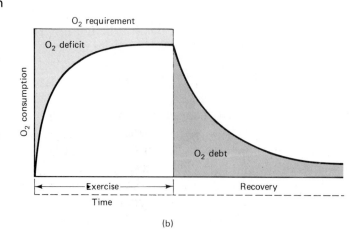

(b)

the person who runs a marathon at a five-minute-per-mile pace must make several physiological adjustments; he or she must increase the oxygen intake and the volume of blood pumped by the heart each minute and efficiently use the energy stores in the body, among other things. Engaging in an endurance fitness program on a regular basis and following sound principles of training as outlined in this textbook will enable one to reach a steady state sooner and maintain it longer.

The physiological phenomenon of *second wind* is characterized by a feeling of relief from the distress of breathlessness and the stabbing pain in the side that are usually experienced by persons engaged in endurance-type activities. Second wind occurs as the body makes the necessary physiological adjustments to strenuous aerobic activities. Although other systems are involved in the adjustments associated with second wind, it is included under cardiorespiratory functioning because it is manifested during endurance-type activities.

Oxygen debt is a physiological concept in which the oxygen consumed in excess of the amount that would normally be provided during recovery is used to replenish the energy reserves used during the exercise bout. An oxygen debt is normally incurred when a person engages in an activity of such an intensity level that a steady state cannot be achieved. In fact, oxygen debts are typically incurred in anaerobic activities such as running the 100-yard dash in track or running two blocks to catch a bus. In such cases a person can continue the activity without oxygen but must go into an oxygen debt by borrowing from the energy reserves in the body. This debt must be repaid during the recovery period after the exercise or during the rest intervals between exercise bouts in interval training.

A small oxygen debt is also incurred in aerobic activities of low to moderate intensity and relatively long duration. The oxygen debt results from the small deficit in the amount of oxygen needed by the working muscles and the amount of oxygen supplied by the body before the steady state is reached. See Figure 3.10 for an illustration of the relative oxygen deficit, oxygen debt, and recovery period for both aerobic and anaerobic exercise bouts.

Notes

1. Gerard J. Tortora and Nicholas P. Anagnostakos, *Principles of Anatomy and Physiology,* 5th ed. (New York: Harper & Row, 1987), p. 18.
2. William D. McArdle, Frank I. Katch, and Victor L. Katch, *Exercise Physiology: Energy, Nutrition, and Weight Control,* 2nd ed. (Philadelphia: Lea & Febiger, 1986), p. 271.
3. Ibid., p. 272.
4. Ibid.
5. Larry G. Shaver, *Essentials of Exercise Physiology* (Minneapolis: Burgess, 1981), p. 59.
6. McArdle et al., *Exercise Physiology: Energy, Nutrition, and Human Performance,* 2nd ed., p. 201
7. Ibid., p. 231.
8. Peter V. Karpovich, *Physiology of Muscular Activity* (Philadelphia: Saunders, 1965), p. 116.

CHAPTER 4

Nutrition, Exercise, and Weight Control

Calorie	obesity
MET	overweight
nutrient	vegetarian
nutrition	

After reading this chapter, you should be able to:
1. Define and/or explain the key words listed above.
2. State the three basic functions of nutrients.
3. Identify the three primary sources of Calories (or principal food groups) and discuss the functions of each.
4. Discuss the role of vitamins, minerals, and water in the nutritive process.
5. Identify the food categories of the basic four food groups and indicate the primary nutrient(s) in each group.
6. Indicate the recommended percentages of protein, fats, and carbohydrates needed by the healthy, active adult.
7. List the seven recommendations for achieving good health as contained in *Dietary Guidelines for Americans*.
8. Distinguish between a Calorie and a kilocalorie.
9. Describe the MET system of determining energy requirements.
10. Use the MET system to determine your daily energy requirements.
11. Compare and contrast overweight and obesity.
12. Define *anorexia nervosa* and *bulimia* and describe the symptoms of each condition.

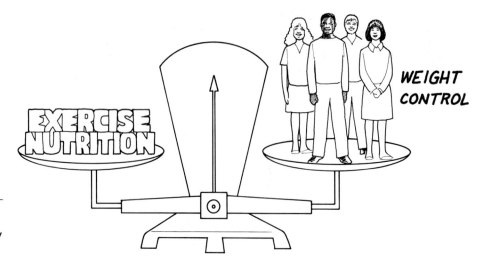

WEIGHT
CONTROL

Proper nutrition and
exercise are necessary
for weight control.

13. List and describe three pathways to weight control and
    indicate the advantages and/or limitations of each.
14. Identify the model pathway or approach to weight control
    and describe the positive features of such an approach.
15. Identify and give examples of three fad diets and state the
    hazards of each.
16. Describe the setpoint theory and use it to develop an
    argument against dieting alone as a pathway to weight
    control.
17. State the misconception regarding dieting for weight control
    and state the facts to dispel it.
18. State two misconceptions regarding exercise and weight
    control and state the facts to dispel them.
19. Compare and contrast the nutritional requirements for active
    and sedentary people.
20. Describe carbohydrate loading and state the advantages
    and/or negative effects of this procedure.
21. Identify three classes of vegetarians and summarize the
    advantages and/or hazards of vegetarian diets.
22. List and describe the special nutritional considerations for
    older people.

Achieving and maintaining an acceptable level of weight is one pathway
to physical fitness and thus to overall good health. Proper weight management seems to be a simple matter of balancing the amount of Calories
consumed with the amount of Calories expended.* In other words, one
should consume no more Calories than one burns up through physical

* What is commonly called a "calorie" is in fact a *kilocalorie* (1000 calories); to differentiate "large"
from "small" calories, nutritionists capitalize the name of the larger unit.

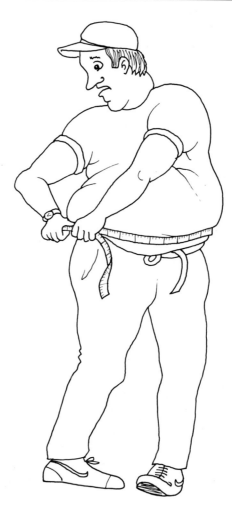

This person needs to practice "girth" control. (*After drawing by Troy Frank.*)

activity. The failure to balance caloric intake (food) with energy output (physical activity) may lead to either overweight (an excess in body weight) or obesity (too much fat tissue) or to underweight (not weighing enough).

The inability of many individuals to control their weight is a growing problem in the United States. Specifically, the problem of obesity—having too much body fat—is cause for concern. Data collected as part of the 1971–1974 National Health and Nutrition Examination Survey (NHANES I) show that some 20 percent (13.9 million) of American men and 24 percent (16.7 million) of American women between 20 and 74 years of age were obese. The prevalence of those in the same age range who were overweight was even greater: 22.8 percent of American men (14.5 million) and 25.8 percent of American women (18.1 million).[1] Further, about 13 percent of adult men and 21 percent of adult women were both overweight and obese.[2] Although no figures are yet available on the prevalence of obesity from 1976 to 1980, data from NHANES II reveal that about 34 million (26 percent) adult Americans were overweight during this period.[3]

Foundations of Nutrition

The kinds and amounts of food consumed not only play an important role in weight management but also help to determine overall health. If nutrition is thought of as the food one eats and the manner in which the body uses it, individuals should be concerned with the kind and amount of food consumed. Understanding nutrition as it relates to energy production and weight management will permit you to make intelligent nutritional decisions.

What are nutrients? They are the actual chemicals obtained from food to permit the proper functioning of the body. Nutrients fulfill three basic functions: (1) to provide energy for body processes, including exercise; (2) to provide structural material for body systems such as the skeletal and muscular systems; and (3) to aid in the regulation of body processes.

Essential Nutrients and Their Functions

By consuming the recommended amount of foods from the primary sources of protein, fats, and carbohydrates, a person will get the necessary nutrients and energy (Calories) to satisfy the body's needs. Vitamins, minerals, and water are contained in the primary food groups.

Protein

Protein is critical in the diet because it builds, maintains, and repairs tissue. In fact, protein is the primary component of the cells of the body and serves to regulate cell functions. Protein is composed of 22 different amino acids, called the "building blocks" of the body. Eight of these amino acids must be obtained through food intake; the body cannot manufacture them the way it can the other amino acids. All the essential amino acids must be available in the body at the same time to be useful. Food sources containing all the essential amino acids are known as *complete* proteins. Animal products such as meat, eggs, milk, and cheese are complete proteins. In addition, these food sources contain the essential amino acids in the proper proportions.

When consuming food sources of protein that do not contain adequate amounts of all the essential amino acids, the practice of "protein complementing" is recommended. The process of complementing protein involves combining foods that have opposite strengths and weaknesses in essential amino acid content. In other words, eat food from one group high in a particular amino acid and another food low in that amino acid but high in another essential amino acid. Combining peanut butter with whole-wheat bread or a legume with a grain illustrates the principle of protein complementing.

The recommended amount of protein for young men and young women on a daily basis is 56 and 44 grams, respectively.[4] Of one's total diet approximately 10 to 15 percent of the Calories should come from protein. Foods that have protein value include meat, fish, eggs, dairy products, and legumes (peas, beans, etc.).

Fats

Fats, also called simple lipids, are a paradox: They are vitally necessary, yet the wrong kind in great amounts can be detrimental. Fats are necessary because of the functions they perform: They act as an additional energy source, insulate the body, cushion vital organs to protect them from injury, act as carriers for fat-soluble vitamins, and aid in the prevention of heat loss. Although on an absolute weight basis fats provide twice as much energy as either carbohydrates or protein, fats not used by the body are stored as fat tissue. The fact that fat is such a concentrated source of Calories is one reason it should be limited in the diet. Another is that high levels of blood lipids (cholesterol) are associated with cardiovascular disease.

There are the two basic types of fats, saturated and unsaturated, identified according to their hydrogen components. Saturated fats are contained in meats, whole milk, butter, and cheese; they are solid at room temperature. Unsaturated fats, on the other hand, tend to be liquid at room temperature and are sometimes called "soft" fats. Unsaturated fats are either polyunsaturated (liquid vegetable oils such as corn, soybean, sunflower, and safflower oil) or monosaturated (peanut and olive oils). Saturated fats help to raise the level of cholesterol in the blood and thus should be used sparingly in the diet. Approximately 30 percent of the Calories in the diet should be supplied by fats, about two-thirds unsaturated.

Carbohydrates

The primary energy source for the body is carbohydrates (starches and sugars). Approximately 50 percent of the body's energy needs are supplied by carbohydrates. Food sources of carbohydrates include potatoes, bread, fruit, candy, spaghetti, rice, cakes and pies, and refined sugar made from cane or beets. About 50 to 60 percent of the diet should be carbohydrates.

Use of sugar as a carbohydrate source should be limited. In fact, the Senate Select Committee on Nutrition and Human Needs, which recommends a total carbohydrate consumption of 58 percent, advocates limiting your sugar intake to 10 percent of the total Calories consumed.[5] Refined sugar provides empty Calories (a high number of Calories combined with low nutritional value) and contributes to tooth decay. Nevertheless, refined sugars are used in large quantities as flavoring and sweetening agents.

Complex carbohydrates in the form of starches and sugars found in milk should be emphasized in the diet. These carbohydrates provide a continuing supply of energy through glucose. Up to a certain limit, glucose (sugar) is converted by the liver into glycogen and stored for future use. Beyond that limit, glucose is converted to fatty acids and is stored in the body as fat tissue. One type of fat is triglycerides, formed by the union of glycerol and fatty acids. Since triglycerides are linked to atherosclerosis (a condition in which fatty deposits accumulate on the walls of the arteries), it is important to keep the carbohydrate intake to a level where it can be used as fuel or stored as glycogen. Increasing the level of physical activity, emphasizing aerobic conditioning, is an excellent means of burning up carbohydrates. It is essential for marathon runners and others who participate in strenous endurance-type activities to eat a diet high in carbohydrates.

Vitamins

Vitamins, contained in extremely small quantities in foods and in body tissues, are organic compounds that are essential to the normal physiological functioning and enzyme activity of the human organism. Vitamins are required in small amounts to aid in the growth, maintenance, and repair of body tissue. They are generally grouped according to their solubility, in fat or water. Vitamins A, D, E, and K are fat-soluble; vitamin B complex and vitamin C are water-soluble.

Fat-soluble vitamins can be stored in the body and thus need not be ingested on a daily basis. Water-soluble vitamins need to be consumed daily since they are not stored in the body.

Vitamin A is essential for the proper development of healthy eyes and night vision, for normal bone and tooth development, for maintaining normal skin and lining membranes of the body, and for growth. Vitamin D is important in the regulation of calcium and phosphorus metabolism and in the maintenance of proper levels of these minerals in bone. Vitamin E is responsible for maintaining the normal stability of red blood cells, among other functions. Vitamin K is necessary to help control blood coagulation.

The water-soluble vitamins are important agents in the energy metabolism process, cell respiration, utilization of protein, and growth.

All the necessary vitamins can be obtained by eating a well-balanced and nutritious diet. In case the diet does not contain the necessary amounts of vitamins, they may be secured in vitamin supplements. However, one should consume vitamin supplements only on recommendation of a physician.

Minerals

Many essential body functions are performed by minerals. Some of the minerals present in the body in large amounts are calcium, phosphorus, magnesium, sodium, potassium, and chloride. Calcium and phosphorus are primarily responsible for bone and teeth development and repair. Calcium is also important in muscle contraction and nerve impulse transmission. Phosphorus also has a role in cell metabolism. Magnesium is an important component of cells; it contributes to enzyme activity and aids in the process of nerve impulse and conduction. Sodium and potassium are important minerals in the regulation of kidney functioning and the fluid balance in the body. Iron is an essential component of hemoglobin and is important in providing the oxygen supply to the tissues. Women need almost twice as much iron as men during the childbearing years. Besides iron, other so-called trace elements such as zinc, iodine, copper, chromium, and fluoride play important roles in the proper functioning of the body and should be part of the diet.

Food sources of various minerals are indicated in the following chart.

Mineral	Food Source
Calcium	Dairy products (milk, cheese), green leafy vegetables (cooked collard greens and turnip greens)
Phosphorus	Meat, fish, poultry, eggs, beef liver, cheese, all-bran cereal
Sodium	Milk, beef liver, lobster, shrimp, salt
Potassium	Bran and germ grains, dried and raw fruit (especially bananas and raisins), milk
Chloride	The foods high in sodium are also high in chloride.
Iron	Beef liver, clams, oysters, beef, veal, pork, prune juice
Magnesium	Dark green vegetables, nuts, whole-grain cereals, peanuts and peanut butter, milk, dry beans
Iodine	Shellfish, iodized salt
Zinc	Shellfish (especially Atlantic oysters), poultry, whole-grain cereals, dry beans
Copper	Brewer's yeast, meat, cheese, whole-grain products

Water

Although water does not supply energy, it is an important nutrient because it plays a crucial role in the chemical reactions of the body. It is the solvent in which most of the chemical reactions take place. Approximately 60 to 80 percent of the body's weight is water. The fluid properties of water allow it to serve as a medium of transportation for vital substances throughout the body and the elimination of body wastes. Water also aids in the regulation of normal body temperature. Water is available in most of the foods we consume. Furthermore, water can be ingested directly into the body. The amount of water needed by the body varies according to body metabolism, activity level, and environmental conditions (temperature, humidity, altitude, etc.). A normal, healthy adult should drink a minimum of six to eight glasses of water a day. Infants and persons who are reducing their caloric intake should consume more than eight glasses a day.

Pathways to a Nutritious Diet

The necessary nutrients for proper functioning of the body can be obtained by consuming a well-balanced and nutritious diet. With all the controversy surrounding which foods should and should not be eaten, one might well ask, "What should I eat?" Various groups and individuals have made recommendations; I believe that the guidelines that follow represent a sensible approach to nutrition.

The Basic Four Food Groups

The National Dairy Council has produced "A Guide to Good Eating" that contains the recommended daily number of servings from food groups that make similar nutritional contributions. There are four basic food groups: milk, meat, fruit and vegetable, and grain. After the initial guide was produced, another category identified as "others" was added. This group contains high-Calorie, low-nutrient foods. Table 4.1 contains

TABLE 4.1   **Guide to Good Eating: A Recommended Daily Pattern**[a]

Food Group	Recommended Number of Servings[b]			
	Child	Teenager	Adult	Pregnant Woman

MILK
1 cup milk, yogurt, or calcium equivalent:
   1½ slices (1½ oz) cheddar cheese
   1 cup pudding
   1¾ cups ice cream
   2 cups cottage cheese
	3	4	2	4

MEAT
2 oz cooked lean meat, fish, poultry, or protein
   equivalent:
   2 eggs
   2 slices (2 oz) cheddar cheese
   1 cup dried beans, peas
   4 tbsp peanut butter
	2	2	2	3[c]

FRUIT/VEGETABLE ½ cup cooked or juice 1 cup raw Portion commonly served, such as medium-size apple or banana	4	4	4	4
GRAIN Whole grain, fortified, enriched 1 slice bread 1 cup ready-to-eat cereal ½ cup cooked cereal, pasta, grits	4	4	4	4

[a]The recommended daily pattern provides the foundation for a nutritious, healthful diet.

[b]The recommended servings from the Basic Four Food Groups for adults supply about 1200 calories.

[c]The woman who is lactating needs the same number of servings as the pregnant woman, with the exception of meat, of which two servings are recommended.

Source: National Dairy Council, "A Guide to Good Eating" (Rosemont, Ill. 1977).

a summary of the recommended number of servings of the various foods in the four food groups. It should be noted that the recommended amounts of food will supply approximately 1200 Calories. People with extreme weight problems or those who engage in strenuous activities should modify their food intake accordingly.

Government Goals and Guidelines

Being primarily concerned with the problem of hunger, the United States government established the Senate Select Committee on Nutrition and Human Needs in 1968. This committee was responsible for all matters concerning the nutrition of Americans. After numerous investigations, hearings, reports, debates, and testimony by authorities on nutrition, the committee published a report titled *Dietary Goals for the United States* in February 1977 and a second edition in November 1977, putting forth specific goals and suggested changes in food selection and preparation to assist individual consumers in making wise choices in matters of nutrition (see Table 4.2).

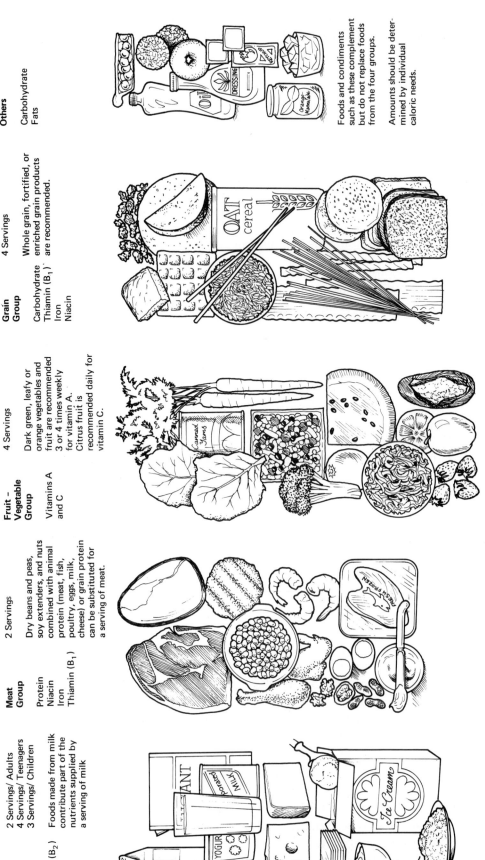

Milk Group

2 Servings/ Adults
4 Servings/ Teenagers
3 Servings/ Children

Foods made from milk contribute part of the nutrients supplied by a serving of milk

Calcium
Riboflavin (B₂)
Protein

Meat Group

2 Servings

Dry beans and peas, soy extenders, and nuts combined with animal protein (meat, fish, poultry, eggs, milk, cheese) or grain protein can be substituted for a serving of meat.

Protein
Niacin
Iron
Thiamin (B₁)

Fruit – Vegetable Group

4 Servings

Dark green, leafy or orange vegetables and fruit are recommended 3 or 4 times weekly for vitamin A. Citrus fruit is recommended daily for vitamin C.

Vitamins A and C

Grain Group

4 Servings

Whole grain, fortified, or enriched grain products are recommended.

Carbohydrate
Thiamin (B₁)
Iron
Niacin

Others

Carbohydrate
Fats

Foods and condiments such as these complement but do not replace foods from the four groups.

Amounts should be determined by individual caloric needs.

The Four Basic Food Groups. (Courtesy of the National Dairy Council.)

TABLE 4.2   **U.S. Dietary Goals**

1. To avoid overweight, consume only as much energy (calories) as is expended; if overweight, decrease energy intake and increase energy expenditure.
2. Increase the consumption of complex carbohydrates and "naturally occurring" sugars from about 28 percent of energy intake to about 48 percent of energy intake.
3. Reduce the consumption of refined and processed sugars by about 45 percent to account for about 10 percent of total energy intake.
4. Reduce overall fat consumption from approximately 40 percent to about 30 percent of energy intake.
5. Reduce saturated fat consumption to account for about 10 percent of total energy intake; and balance that with polyunsaturated and monosaturated fats, which should account for about 10 percent of energy intake each.
6. Reduce cholesterol consumption to about 300 mg a day.
7. Limit the intake of sodium by reducing the intake of salt to about 5 g per day.

The goals suggest the following changes in food selection and preparation:
1. Increase consumption of fruits and vegetables and whole grains.
2. Decrease consumption of refined and other processed sugars and foods high in such sugars.
3. Decrease consumption of foods high in total fat, and partially replace saturated fats, whether obtained from animal or vegetable sources, with polyunsaturated fats.
4. Decrease consumption of animal fat and choose meats, poultry, and fish, which will reduce saturated fat intake.
5. Except for young children, substitute low-fat and nonfat milk for whole milk and low-fat dairy products for high-fat dairy products.
6. Decrease consumption of butterfat, eggs, and other high cholesterol sources. Some consideration should be given to easing the cholesterol goal for premenopausal women, young children, and the elderly in order to obtain the nutritional benefits of eggs in the diet.
7. Decrease consumption of salt and foods high in salt content.

Source: U.S. Senate Select Committee on Nutrition and Human Needs, Dietary Goals for the United States, *2d ed. (Washington: U.S. Government Printing Office, 1977), p. 4.*

The problem of proper nutrition for Americans remained a heated topic of research, discussion, and debate. To provide further direction regarding the proper diet for individual Americans, the U.S. Department of Agriculture and the U.S. Department of Health, Education and Welfare (now the Department of Health and Human Services) published a pamphlet, *Nutrition and Your Health: Dietary Guidelines for Americans,* containing the following seven recommendations:

1. Eat a variety of foods.
2. Maintain ideal weight.
3. Avoid too much fat, saturated fat, and cholesterol.
4. Eat foods with adequate starch and fiber.
5. Avoid too much sugar.
6. Avoid too much sodium.
7. If you drink alcohol, do so in moderation.[6]

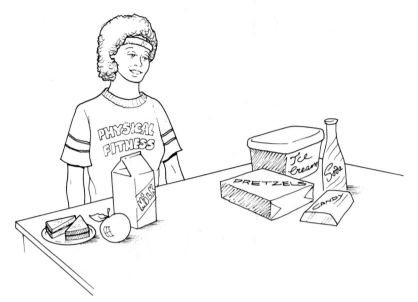

Which foods would you choose?

It is emphasized that these guidelines are not for all Americans. They are addressed to people who are already healthy. Individuals who need special diets because of diseases or health conditions should consult with their physicians or trained dietitians in consultation with a physician. Further, it is noted that following these guidelines will not guarantee health or well-being. However, adopting sensible eating habits, along with other positive lifestyle activities, will promote good health and well-being.

Some people might feel that the guidelines are too broad. While each recommendation is broad, more detailed information and suggestions for achieving each recommendation are included in the pamphlet. Besides these guidelines, Tables 4.1 and 4.2 provide more specific information on the types and amounts of foods to eat for a nutritious diet. The specific nutritive value of 730 foods commonly used is contained in *Nutritive Value of Foods.*[7] This publication compares kinds and amounts of nutrients in different foods and sometimes compares different forms of the same food. The various information and recommendations can be used to guide everyone in developing a well-balanced and nutritious diet.

Energy Requirements at Rest and During Physical Activity

Everyone needs the amount of energy necessary to maintain basic life processes (respiration, pumping of blood by the heart and circulation throughout the body, glandular activity, and so forth). The energy to enable one to perform the various biological functions is derived from the major food sources of carbohydrates, fats, and protein.

A *Calorie* (the nutritionists' kilocalorie) is the unit of measure for expressing the heat or energy value of food and physical activity. One Calorie represents the amount of heat required to raise the temperature of one kilogram of water one degree Celsius.

Energy is liberated when food is broken down through the process of metabolism. The majority of the energy for use by the body is supplied through aerobic metabolism, whereby ATP is released from the food to produce energy, as explained in Chapter 3.

Energy Requirements at Rest

The minimal rate at which energy is required to carry out essential body processes during the resting state is known as the *basal metabolic rate* (BMR). The BMR as well as the energy expenditure during various physical activities can be measured through procedures known as direct and indirect calorimetry. The direct method of calorimetry is more accurate, but it is impracticable for many studies of physical activity and sports. Moreover, the sophisticated and expensive equipment required to conduct direct calorimetry are not readily available to the average person.

Indirect calorimetry is a method by which the amount of oxygen consumed is measured under specified conditions, and then this figure is used to determine the body's energy or heat production. In calculating the BMR, oxygen consumption is measured after a person has been in a reclining, relaxed position, and without food for a minimum of 12 hours. The amount of energy (or number of Calories) required during the resting state will vary according to the individual's size, age, sex, and hormone production. Generally, females require fewer Calories than males (the BMR in women is estimated to be 10 percent lower than in men) because females have more body fat than males, and fat metabolizes more slowly than lean body mass.

The MET System.   MET (metabolic cost of activities) is a system for determining energy requirements. A MET is a unit of energy expended, with one MET being the rate of energy needed while the body is in a resting or basal state. The MET system also allows one to measure the energy expenditure during varying levels of physical activity. The metabolic rate increases in accordance with an increase in energy expenditure.

The actual calculation of the MET is based on the amount of oxygen that is used to burn Calories provided in food. Research has demonstrated that one liter of oxygen is equal to approximately 4.8 Calories used in the body. The MET system is based on the assumption that the average person in a basal state requires approximately 3.5 milliliters of oxygen per kilogram of body weight per minute. These figures can be used to determine the energy expenditure at rest.

Let's use Ann, a 155-pound female, as the example in making the computations for determining her energy expenditure at rest. Her weight of 155 pounds is 70 kilograms (155 ÷ 2.2). At 70 kilograms of weight, Ann uses approximately 245 milliliters of oxygen (70 × 3.5) per minute, or 14,700 milliliters per hour (245 × 60). This means that Ann has an estimated basal metabolic rate of 14.7 liters of oxygen per hour (14,700 ÷ 1,000). The energy expenditure for Ann for one hour can then be calculated by multiplying 14.7 (basal metabolic rate of oxygen per hour) by the energy equivalent of one liter of oxygen (4.825 Calories). For Ann this is 70 Calories minus the 10 percent reduction in BMR for a female (if the O_2 values were measured, the 10 percent reduction would not be necessary), which is 63 Calories. Thus her energy expenditure estimate for the day would be 1512 Calories (63 × 24).

The energy requirements for a man can be estimated by using the figure of one Calorie per hour being burned for each kilogram of body weight. The basal metabolic rate for 24 hours can be estimated by multiplying the body weight in kilograms by 24. For a male who weighs 70 kilograms, for example, the resting energy requirement would be 1680 Calories (70 × 24).

Each person can determine his or her basal energy requirements by following the steps used in calculating the energy expenditure for Ann. However, to expedite one's determination of individual energy expenditure, calculations for the number of Calories burned for men and women of various weights for one-half hour, one hour, and one day have been computed and are presented in Table 4.3.

To determine your resting energy expenditure, locate your weight (or the weight nearest to your actual weight) in the left-hand column under "Weight," and look at the figure in the last column under "Calories per day." To determine the resting energy expenditure for Ann, who weighs 155 pounds (70 kg), one would find her weight and read across the chart to the appropriate time period. Looking at the women's column under "Calories per day" for a 70-kilogram person, one can see that Ann would expend 1512 Calories while at rest. Remember that the BMR for women is 10 percent less than that for men. Therefore, a man weighing 70 kilograms would have a resting energy expenditure of 1680 Calories per day.

Energy Requirements During Physical Activity

To perform physical activities of increased intensity levels, the body must increase its physiological functioning; that is, heart rate and stroke volume must be increased to pump more blood to the working muscle tissue, and more oxygen must be taken in and used by the body. The degree of increase in these physiological processes will depend on the amount of energy that is necessary to complete the various physical activities. This in turn depends on several factors, including the intensity of the activity, the length of time engaged in the activity and the rate of work, and the sex, weight, skill, and physical fitness of the person performing the activity. With everything else being equal, the longer the time spent at an activity, the more energy will be used.

If the variable of weight is added, a heavier person will use more energy (burn more Calories) than a lighter person to complete the same

TABLE 4.3   Calories Burned per Half Hour, per Hour, and per Day, According to Weight and Sex

Weight		Calories per ½ hour		Calories per hour		Calories per day	
Pounds	Kilograms	Men	Women	Men	Women	Men	Women
90[a]	41	21	19	41	37	984	888
92	42	21	19	42	38	1008	912
94	43	22	20	43	39	1032	936
96	44	22	20	44	40	1056	960
98	45	23	21	45	41	1080	984
101	46	23	21	46	41	1104	984
103	47	24	21	47	42	1128	1008
105	48	24	22	48	43	1152	1032
107	49	25	22	49	44	1176	1056
109	50	25	23	50	45	1200	1080
112	51	26	23	51	46	1224	1104
114	52	26	24	52	47	1248	1128
116	53	27	24	53	48	1272	1152
118	54	27	25	54	49	1296	1176
120	55	28	25	55	50	1320	1200
123	56	28	25	56	50	1344	1200
125	57	29	26	57	51	1368	1224
127	58	29	26	58	52	1392	1248
129	59	30	27	59	53	1416	1272
131	60	30	27	60	54	1440	1296
134	61	31	28	61	55	1464	1320
136	62	31	28	62	56	1488	1344
138	63	32	29	63	57	1512	1368
140	64	32	29	64	58	1536	1392
142	65	33	30	65	59	1560	1404
145	66	33	30	66	59	1584	1416
147	67	34	30	67	60	1608	1440
149	68	34	31	68	61	1632	1464
151	69	35	31	69	62	1656	1488
153	70	35	32	70	63	1680	1512
156	71	36	32	71	64	1704	1536
158	72	36	33	72	65	1728	1560
160	73	37	33	73	66	1752	1584

task (especially when engaged in weight-bearing activities like walking and jogging). For example, let's compare the energy requirements for two men, weighing 120 and 200 pounds, respectively, who walk for 30 minutes at 3 miles per hour. The man who weighs 120 pounds (55 kg) will use approximately 112 Calories, since it requires 4 METs a minute to walk at a rate of 3 miles per hour (see Table 4.4) and his half-hour MET value is 28 (28 × 4 = 112). The person who weighs 200 pounds (91 kg) will burn approximately 184 Calories for the same 30-minute walk, since his half-hour MET value is 46 and it requires the same 4 METs (46 × 4 = 184).

The energy expenditure can be increased by increasing the time

TABLE 4.3 (*Continued*)

Weight		Calories per ½ hour		Calories per hour		Calories per day	
Pounds	Kilograms	Men	Women	Men	Women	Men	Women
162	74	37	34	74	67	1776	1608
164	75	38	34	75	68	1800	1632
167	76	38	34	76	68	1824	1632
170	77	39	35	77	69	1848	1656
171	78	39	35	78	70	1872	1680
173	79	40	36	79	71	1896	1704
175	80	40	36	80	72	1920	1728
178	81	41	37	81	73	1944	1752
180	82	42	37	82	74	1968	1776
182	83	42	38	83	75	1992	1800
184	84	42	38	84	76	2016	1824
186	85	43	39	85	77	2040	1848
189	86	43	39	86	77	2064	1848
191	87	44	39	87	78	2088	1872
193	88	44	40	88	79	2112	1896
195	89	45	40	89	80	2136	1920
197	90	45	41	90	81	2160	1944
200	91	46	41	91	82	2184	1968
202	92	46	42	92	83	2208	1992
204	93	47	42	93	84	2232	2016
206	94	47	43	94	85	2256	2040
208	95	48	43	95	86	2280	2064
211	96	48	43	96	86	2304	2064
213	97	49	44	97	87	2328	2088
215	98	49	44	98	88	2352	2112
217	99	50	45	99	89	2376	2136
219	100	50	45	100	90	2400	2160
222[b]	101	51	46	101	91	2424	2184

[a]If you weigh less than 90 pounds, multiply your weight by 2 (double your weight), find that weight in the table, then divide the caloric figure by 2.

[b]If your weight is more than 222 pounds, divide it by 2 and find that weight in the table, then double the caloric figure for that weight.

spent in the activity. Let's consider the same two persons to clarify this point. Suppose that the heavier person decided to continue walking for another hour and the lighter person sat down to rest after the 30-minute walk. The 200-pound person would use an additional 364 Calories (91 × 4). On the other hand, the 120-pound man would burn only about 83 additional Calories (55 × 1.5), assuming he averaged about 1.5 METs over the 60-minute cool-down period, since it costs one MET to sit quietly. (See Table 4.4 for these values.) By walking for an additional hour, the person who weighs 200 pounds would burn up about 353 more Calories than the 120-pound person (548 to 195 Calories).

Metabolic costs of many occupational and recreational activities in

TABLE 4.4   **Common Activities Grouped According to Relative Metabolic Cost**

MET Cost	Activity
0.85 MET[a]	Sleeping
1 MET	Awake, resting quietly, reading, watching TV
1.5 METs	Any moving, sitting activity such as eating, writing, sewing, typing, knitting, desk work, driving; also, stationary standing such as showering, dressing
2 METs	Light moving, standing activity, such as cooking, strolling, and light housework
3 METs	Level walking (2.5 mph), cycling (5.5 mph), social dancing, archery, sailing, bowling, golf (using cart), heavy housework
4 METs	Walking (3 mph), cycling (8 mph), badminton singles, tennis doubles, raking leaves, many calisthenics
5 METs	Walking (4 mph), cycling (10 mph), ice or roller skating, digging in garden, shoveling light earth
6 METs	Walking (5 mph), cycling (11 mph), tennis singles, splitting wood, shoveling snow, square dancing
7 METs	Jogging (5 mph), cycling (12 mph), basketball, mountain climbing, canoeing (5 mph), touch football, paddleball
8 METs	Running (5.5 mph), cycling (13 mph), basketball (vigorous), fencing, handball (social), squash (social)
9 METs	Competitive handball or racquetball, ski touring (4.5 mph)
10 METs	Running (6 mph), shoveling 10 shovelfuls per minute (15 lb)

[a]One MET is the energy expenditure at rest while awake and is equivalent to approximately 3.5 milliliters of O_2 per kilogram of body weight per minute; therefore, 0.85 MET, the energy expenditure while asleep, is about 3 milliliters of O_2 per kilogram of body weight per minute.

Source: Adapted from Samuel M. Fox et al., "Physical Activity and Cardiovascular Health," in Modern Concepts of Cardiovascular Disease *(New York: American Heart Association, 1972), pp. 27–28. Used by permission.*

the form of METs have been determined by Samuel Fox and colleagues,[8] and this information is presented in Tables 4.4 and 4.5. Information from these tables can be used to determine the energy requirements for various activities. One MET represents the energy expenditure when one is at rest but awake. Two METs would represent double the resting metabolic rate, 3 METs would be triple the resting rate, and so on. The number of Calories used each minute is indicated for the various MET values. For example, a person would use 2 to 3 METs and 2.5 to 4 Calories per minute to perform activities such as bowling, riding a lawn mower, and janitorial work (Table 4.5).

To use the MET system for determining your energy requirements, you should use the Activity Record Form (a blank one appears in Appendix I) to record your MET values for each half hour. All the MET values for a 24-hour period should be totaled to get the values for the day. This figure should be multiplied by the half-hour MET value (caloric expenditure) for your weight (from Table 4.3), which will indicate the total Calories burned that day.

Ann's completed Activity Record Form (Figure 4.1) shows a total caloric expenditure of 2128 for the day, determined by multiplying the total MET (66.5) by the half-hour MET value (caloric expenditure) of 32. Figure 8.3 in Chapter 8 shows an Activity Record Form for Ann when she was heavier. Comparing the two, note that Ann burned 207 more Calories on a typical day (2335 to 2128) when she was heavier. However, note that the difference in energy expenditure above the basal metabolic rate was only 39 Calories (655 to 616).

Another Method for Determining Energy Requirements. The MET system is not the only method that can be used to determine the energy cost of various physical activities. Another approach involves determining your energy expenditure from activities that have been classified according to the number of Calories expended per kilogram of body weight per minute. A list of energy expenditures for a variety of common household activities, selected industrial tasks, and popular recreational and sports activities is presented in Appendix F.

In the list of activities in Appendix F, values in the various columns corresponding to particular body weights represent the caloric costs of the activities for one minute. To estimate the total cost of participating in an activity, multiply the value listed in the table (under your weight) by the number of minutes of participation. For example, a 157-pound person sitting quietly would burn 1.5 Calories per minute. If this person were engaged in this activity for two hours (120 min), the total caloric cost of 180 Calories would be determined by multiplying the value of 1.5 Calories per minute by 120 (the total time engaged in the activity). On the other hand, if the same person were engaged in a more strenuous activity such as climbing a hill for one hour, the energy expenditure would be 552 Calories. This value would be calculated by multiplying the caloric value of climbing a hill with a 5-kilogram load (9.2) by 60, the time spent in the activity.

The values for activities in Appendix F include the resting values (the energy expended while at rest, known as the resting metabolic rate or RMR) as well as the energy values associated with performing the activities. (The RMR is slightly higher than the basal metabolic rate, which represents the energy required for basic life functions.) Remember that the caloric values represent averages that might vary with a person's age, skill, sex, and general physical condition. These values should be used as guides rather than as absolutes in planning a physical activity program.

TABLE 4.5   **Approximate Metabolic Cost of Activities**

MET Value[a]	Kcal/min[a] (per kg body wt)	Occupational Activities	Recreational Activities
0.85 MET	1	Sleep	
1 MET	1.2		Sitting reading, watching TV
1½–2 METs	2–2.5	Desk work Auto driving Typing (electric) Using electric calculating machine	Standing Walking (strolling 1 mph) Flying an airplane Riding a motorcycle Playing cards Sewing, knitting
2–3 METs	2.5–4	Auto repair Radio, TV repair Janitorial work Typing (manual) Bartending	Level walking (2 mph) Level bicycling (5 mph) Riding lawn mower Billards, bowling Skeet shooting, shuffleboard Woodworking (light) Powerboat driving Golf with power cart Canoeing (2.5 mph) Horseback riding (at walk) Playing piano and many other instruments
3–4 METs	4–5	Bricklaying, plastering Pushing wheelbarrow (100-lb load) Machine assembly Driving trailer truck in traffic Welding (moderate load) Cleaning windows	Walking (3 mph) Cycling (6 mph) Horseshoe pitching Volleyball (6-person noncompetitive) Golf (using cart) Archery Sailing (small boat) Fly fishing (standing) Horseback riding (sitting to trot) Badminton (social doubles) Pushing light power mower Playing a musical instrument energetically
4–5 METs	5–6	Painting, masonry Paperhanging Light carpentry	Walking (3.5 mph) Cycling (8 mph) Table tennis Golf (carrying clubs) Dancing (foxtrot) Badminton (singles) Tennis (doubles) Raking leaves Hoeing Many calisthenics

TABLE 4.5 (*Continued*)

MET Value[a]	Kcal/min[a] (per kg body wt)	Occupational Activities	Recreational Activities
5–6 METs	6–7	Digging in garden Shoveling light earth	Walking (4 mph) Cycling (10 mph) Canoeing (4 mph) Horseback riding ("posting" to trot) Walking in a stream with a light current Ice or roller skating (9 mph)
6–7 METs	7–8	Shoveling 10 shovelfuls/min (10 lb)	Walking (5 mph) Cycling (11 mph) Badminton (competitive) Tennis (singles) Splitting wood Shoveling snow Mowing lawn (manual) Square dancing Light downhill skiing Ski touring (2.5 mph in loose snow) Water skiing
7–8 METs	8–10	Digging ditches Carrying 80 lb Sawing hardwood	Jogging (5 mph) Cycling (12 mph) Horseback riding (gallop) Vigorous downhill skiing Basketball Mountain climbing Ice hockey Canoeing (5 mph) Touch football Paddleball
8–9 METs	10–11	Shoveling 10 shovelfuls/min (14 lb)	Running (5.5 mph) Cycling (13 mph) Ski touring (4 mph in loose snow) Squash (social) Handball (social) Fencing Basketball (vigorous)
10 or more METs	11–12	Shoveling 10 shovelfuls/min (16 lb)	Running: 6 mph = 10 METS 7 mph = 11.5 METS 8 mph = 13.5 METS 9 mph = 15 METS 10 mph = 17 METS Ski touring (5+ mph in loose snow) Handball (competitive) Squash (competitive)

[a]Values are for a 154-pound (70-kg) person.

Source: Adapted from Samuel M. Fox et al., "Physical Activity and Cardiovascular Health," in Modern Concepts of Cardiovascular Disease *(New York: American Heart Association, 1972), pp. 27–28. Used by permission.*

Activity Record Chart

Name ANN		Wt. 155 1/2-hr MET 32 Date		7/19/87
	1/2 MET		1/2 MET	Total METS per hr
A.M. 6:00 SLEEP	.85	6:30 SLEEP	.85	1.7
7:00 "	.85	7:30 "	.85	1.7
8:00 "	.85	8:30 "	.85	1.7
9:00 "	.85	9:30 "	.85	1.7
10:00 "	.85	10:30 GET UP / MAKE BED	1.5	2.4
11:00 SEWING	1.3	11:30 LIGHT CALISTHENICS	2.5	3.8
1200 BRUSH TEETH	2	12:30 SHOWER / COMB HAIR	1.5	3.5
P.M. 1:00 GET DRESSED	1.5	1:30 DRIVE TO MOVIE	1.5	3.0
2:00 SITTING (MOVIE)	1	2:30 SITTING (MOVIE)	1	2.0
3:00 "	1	3:30 "	1	2.0
4:00 RIDING IN CAR	1	4:30 WATCHING T.V.	1	2.0
5:00 WATCHING T.V.	1	5:30 COOKING DINNER	2	3.0
6:00 COOKING / EATING	2	6:30 EATING / SITTING	1.5	3.5
7:00 PREPARE TO JOG	2	7:30 JOGGING / COOL DOWN	7	9.0
8:00 WATCHING T.V.	1	8:30 WATCHING T.V.	1	2.0
9:00 WASHING DISHES	2	9:30 LIGHT HOUSE CLEANING	2	4.0
10:00 WATCHING T.V.	1	10:30 WATCHING T.V.	1	2.0
11:00 SHOWER/DRESS FOR BED	1.5	11:30 WASH CLOTHES	3	4.5
12:00 WASH CLOTHES/VACUUM	3	12:30 GET READY FOR BED	1.5	4.5
A.M. 1:00 SLEEP	.85	1:30 SLEEP	.85	1.7
2:00 "	.85	2:30 "	.85	1.7
3:00 "	.85	3:30 "	.85	1.7
4:00 "	.85	4:30 "	.85	1.7
5:00 "	.85	5:30 "	.85	1.7
		Total METS per day (add down)		66.5
		Multiply by your 1/2-hr MET value		32
		Total calories burned this day		2,128

Figure 4.1
Daily Activity Record
Form.

Caloric Intake Versus Energy Expenditure and Associated Problems

Proper weight management involves balancing caloric intake with caloric (energy) expenditure. To maintain a stable weight, individuals must ingest no more Calories than they expend. When one takes in more

Calories than one burns up, one gains weight (3500 Calories equal approximately one pound of fat). When one consumes fewer Calories than one burns up, one loses weight. Problems resulting from an inability to balance caloric intake with energy expenditure include being overweight, being obese, and being underweight. Anorexia nervosa and bulimia are two eating disorders associated with the desire to be thin or the fear of becoming fat.

A distinction should be made between overweight and obesity. Overweight means that the body has too much weight in relation to one's height, build, and sex. According to the Metropolitan Life Insurance Company's table of ideal weights for young women, for example, a woman who is 5 feet 3 inches tall and of medium build should weigh between 121 and 135 pounds (see Table 5.1). A woman of this height and body frame who weighed 145 pounds would be considered overweight.

Overweight and Obesity

Would a woman who is 10 pounds overweight be considered obese? The answer could be yes or no. It depends on the amount of fat that the person has. A person could be considered overweight without being *obese,* which is having a greater percentage of body fat than normal for one's total body weight. The actual percentage of body fat that is considered normal varies from expert to expert. In this text, the figures of 25 and 30 percent are used to determine obesity for men and women, respectively.*

An individual can be overweight without being obese. Many professional athletes who engage in strenuous weight training, for instance, develop muscle mass to the extent that they weigh more than they should according to height-weight charts. However, their percentage of body fat is often in the "very low" category. Being a little overweight is not a problem if the extra weight does not contribute to other health problems.

The problem of obesity—too much fat—is cause for concern, however, since it is associated with chronic diseases such as cardiovascular disease, diabetes, and high blood pressure, among others. The topic of weight control is recognized by the U. S. Public Health Service (USPHS) as a national health priority.

Although a complete knowledge of the causes and effective treatments of obesity remain elusive, efforts to help prevent obesity and to treat people who are obese must not be waived. A first step in this direction is to understand that there are several types of obesity. Suitor and Crowley divide obesity into the following categories:[9]

1. Obesity secondary to another condition. Some metabolic disorders (such as hypothyroidism and Praeder-Willi syndrome) lead to obesity. However, obesity arising from serious physical disorders is rare.
2. Recent obesity (adult onset). This type may be due to failure to adjust eating habits with age. It may be responsive to treatment.
3. Long-term obesity (juvenile onset or developmental obesity). When seen in adults, this type of obesity tends to be resistant to treatment. Juvenile-onset obesity may often be characterized by an overabundance of fat cells (hyperplastic obesity).

* These figures are based on formulas developed by Sloan and are discussed in Chapter 5.

4. Reactive obesity (weight gain following a traumatic emotional experience). This may appear at any time of life. If reactive obesity is detected in an early stage, counseling may help the person find a more appropriate means of coping with the problem.

What these authors categorize as "recent obesity" might also be described as "creeping obesity" since the weight gain accumulates over a period of years. This type of weight gain is a slow process and becomes noticeable after many years. For instance, some people gain one or two pounds each year during their adult years. All of a sudden, at age 40, they realize that they are obese. It might appear to be recent, but the slow accumulation of fat weight over the years is the essence of "creeping obesity." A normal reduction in the basal metabolic rate, an increase in caloric intake, and a sedentary lifestyle combine to cause "creeping obesity." Consequently, a comprehensive program of activities aimed at altering these variables is the proper mode of treatment for this condition.

Underweight

Although the condition of being underweight has received scant attention in both the popular press and professional publications, it is a problem of concern for many individuals. A person is considered underweight when his or her body weight falls more than 10 percent below the normal range as indicated by height-weight tables. For females, McArdle, Katch, and Katch list the following three criteria for underweight: (1) body weight lower than minimal weight calculated from skeletal measurements, (2) body weight lower than the 20th percentile by height for age, and (3) percent body fat lower than 17 percent.[10]

Underweight individuals should undergo a complete medical examination to determine their health status. If the results of the examination indicate that they are otherwise healthy, underweight persons should monitor their food intake and activity patterns for at least two weeks. Based on the results of these analyses, a suitable exercise program should be instituted and a well-balanced diet with an increased number of Calories should be consumed (a pound of lean weight is equivalent to approximately 2500 Calories). The increased caloric intake should consist mainly of complex carbohydrates to build muscle mass (and to provide fuel for the Calories burned through exercise), with some additional protein (1 to 1.5 grams per kilogram of body weight daily is recommended) for growth and maintenance of muscle tissue. The additional Calories should be consumed via four or five small meals with nutritious high-Calorie snacks between meals. The exercise program should be vigorous enough to develop muscle mass. This type of program can consist of weight training with barbells, dumbbells, weight machines, and body resistance exercises such as pull-ups and push-ups. It is recommended that these progressive resistance exercises be alternated with moderate aerobic activities such as jogging, swimming, and aerobic dance.

Associated with obesity as an abnormal fear of fatness and a preoccupation with body size, both anorexia nervosa and bulimia are considered extreme eating disorders. These disorders are thought to be reaching epidemic levels, according to some sources. For example, Jean Hall, science and medicine editor for Gannett Westchester newspapers, reports that there is an estimated incidence of from 1 in 100 to 1 in 250 anorexic adolescent girls and 1 to 3 million bulimics in America today.[11]

Anorexia nervosa is most prominent among preteen and teenage girls and young women. Most anorexics come from middle-class or upper-middle-class backgrounds, and they may have been considered well adjusted before the eating disorder developed. The pattern of symptoms usually begins when a young girl unexpectedly becomes obsessed with the idea that she is fat. She begins a diet regimen, often involving a fad diet. Even after a substantial amount of weight has been lost, she still perceives herself as fat and continues to restrict her caloric intake. In severe cases the person suffering from anorexia nervosa becomes emaciated to the point of death. The expected death rate of anorexic cases is around 10 percent.[12]

Bulimia, the "binge-purge" eating disorder that is predominant among college-age women, is also common among high school girls. The disorder involves eating binges followed by vomiting or using other purging methods such as laxatives or diuretics (or both) to cleanse the body. Because of the self-induced vomiting or use of laxatives following eating binges, the bulimic is usually of normal weight. Diagnostic criteria

Anorexia Nervosa and Bulimia

TABLE 4.6 **Symptoms of Anorexia Nervosa and Bulimia**

Anorexia Nervosa Symptoms	Bulimia Symptoms
Intense fear of becoming obese, which does not diminish as weight loss progresses.	Recurrent episodes of binge eating (rapid consumption of a large amount of food in less than two hours).
Disturbance of body image, e.g. claiming to "feel fat" even when emaciated.	At least three of the following: Consumption of high-calorie, easily ingested food during a binge.
Weight loss of at least 25 percent of original body weight; or, if under 18 years of age, weight loss from original body weight plus projected weight gain expected from growth charts may be combined to make the 25 percent.	Termination of such eating episodes by abdominal pain, sleep, social interruption, or self-induced vomiting. Repeated attempts to lose weight by severely restrictive diets, self-induced vomiting, or use of cathartics or diuretics.
Refusal to maintain body weight over a minimal normal weight for age and height.	Frequent weight fluctuations greater than 10 pounds due to alternating binges and fasts. Awareness that the eating pattern is abnormal and fear of not being able to stop eating voluntarily.
No known physical illness that would account for the weight loss.	Depressed mood and self-depreciating thoughts following eating binges.

Source: Janet B. W. Williams, ed., Diagnostic and Statistical Manual of Mental Disorders, 3d ed. (Washington D.C.: American Psychiatric Association, 1980), pp. 67–69.

for anorexia and bulimia have been developed by the American Psychiatric Association and are presented in Table 4.6.[13]

Pathways to Weight Control

Many methods of weight control have been and continue to be used by some individuals to help them reach their "normal" weight. Some of these approaches are outright gimmicks that have no lasting beneficial effects. These include using steam and sauna baths, wearing rubberized suits and other approaches designed to lose body water through dehydration, and spot reducing. I do not recommend these methods and will not discuss them here; however, persons interested in reading more about these gimmicks can consult several sources.[14]

Other methods of weight management that might be recommended in limited cases but have serious disadvantages are discussed. The use of drugs and surgery are examples of methods that might be recommended for the grossly obese person. Other methods for weight control are dieting, increasing physical activity levels, and behavior modification. The pathway to weight control that seems to be most successful is one that combines caloric reduction with increased physical activity and is supplemented by behavior modification techniques aimed at changing undesirable eating and exercise habits.

Drugs and Weight Control

Both prescription and over-the-counter drugs are marketed as effective weight reduction products. Though a variety of drugs are used, appetite suppressants or anorectic drugs are the most common. Based on a thorough review of the research on weight control, it was reported in the *Dairy Council Digest* that there are no long-term beneficial effects of using drugs to reduce or control weight. Furthermore, these drugs produce such side effects as nervousness, irritability, euphoria, insomnia, and elevated blood pressure as well as possible dependence on the drugs.[15]

Not so widely used but equally as ineffective are such other drugs as thyroid hormones and starch blockers. Both are also considered unsafe as weight reducing products. (The FDA has ruled that it is false advertising to proclaim starch blockers as weight loss products.) The weight loss produced by thyroid hormones is due mainly to a decrease in lean body mass, not fat tissue. The assumption underlying the use of starch blockers is that they inhibit the intestinal enzyme necessary for starch digestion, thus permitting persons to eat large amounts of carbohydrates without gaining weight. However, research cited by the National Dairy Council has failed to support the use of starch blockers as an effective weight reduction method.[16] A study on the use of starch blockers by a team of investigators from Stanford University School of Medicine and the Veterans Administration Medical Center of Palo Alto, California, also showed that starch blockers did not work in preventing the body from getting Calories, since the starch blockers failed to "block" the carbohydrates from absorbing into the digestive tract.[17]

Surgical procedures (including gastric bypass to reduce the stomach's volume to limit food intake, intestinal bypass surgery to reduce the intestinal absorption area, and jaw wiring) may be indicated in a few cases with grossly obese patients more than 100 percent overweight who meet other stringent requirements. These requirements are that the obese individuals have not benefited from nonsurgical procedures and are at increased risk of death or other debilitating health problems. The final justification for using surgical procedures for the grossly obese should be a determination that the risks associated with the surgery are less than those of remaining morbidly obese.

Although the majority of patients who have had surgical treatment for obesity indicated an improved quality of life despite their still being overweight, it is not known whether these procedures reduced morbidity and mortality. Furthermore, there are several side effects associated with surgery for obese patients, including weakness, lethargy, nausea, vomiting, and liver failure.[18]

Surgery

It might be an understatement to say that dieting as a weight control modality has been unsuccessful for a vast majority of the 30 to 50 million obese persons in America. This conclusion is reached despite the billions of dollars spent on diet books and diet programs each year. Diet plans range from the starvation diet (consuming no Calories) to the nutritionally balanced diet in which the total caloric intake is slightly reduced. Diets that reduce caloric intake below energy expenditure will result in weight loss. Therefore, diets that greatly restrict caloric intake will cause the greatest weight loss. However, such weight loss is short-lived, and the side effects can be severe (sometimes fatal).

For this discussion diets are separated into two broad categories: fad diets and reduced-Calorie diets. Fad diets (such as high-protein, low-carbohydrate diets; high-carbohydrate, low-protein diets; and starvation diets) should not be used because they are nutritionally unbalanced and produce unhealthy side effects. For example, the high-protein, low-carbohydrate diet is usually high in fat and cholesterol and produces such side effects as nausea, dizziness, low blood pressure, and stress on the kidneys.

Jane Brody, science editor for the *New York Times,* has summarized the conclusions reached on diets by several experts in the area of weight control (see Table 4.7). It can be observed that diets that stress a reduced caloric intake are to be recommended over diets that require an extreme reduction in any one food group. However, it should be pointed out that while some diets are advised and others are not, the effectiveness of diets in general is questionable. Many of the diets are lacking in nutritional value, and some are hazardous to health and life. Moreover, most popular diets are monotonous and often too difficult to follow for any length of time.[19] Dieters usually resume their old ways of eating and gain more weight.

Besides emphasizing the unattractiveness and lack of long-term ben-

Dieting for Weight Control

TABLE 4.7 **Principles of Popular Diets**

Examples	Rationale	Hazards
High-protein, Low-carbohydrate		
Atkins Diet Revolution, Scarsdale, Calories Don't Count, Drinking Man's, Stillman Quick Weight Loss Diet	Rapid initial loss due to water excreted when body must get rid of extra protein; protein and fat hold less water in body than carbohydrates; untrue that ketones formed from fats can depress appetite.	Nutritionally unbalanced; some are high in fat and cholesterol; toxic ketones from fats cause nausea, dizziness, low blood pressure, fatigue, apathy; excess protein stresses kidneys and promotes bone loss; lack of roughage results in constipation; vitamin and mineral deficiencies.
Low-protein (nearly all carbohydrates)		
Rice, Stillman Quick-Inches-Off, Macrobiotic, Banana Diet	No Calorie counting; rapid initial weight loss.	Nutritionally unbalanced; body loses needed protein; vitamin and mineral deficiencies.
Protein-sparing		
Liquid or powdered protein, meat and fish only, Linn Last Chance	Not tempted by real food; no decisions to make; rapid weight loss.	Nutritionally very unbalanced; excess ketone hazard (see above); several deaths caused by abnormal heart rhythms; sluggishness; headaches; bad breath. Close medical supervision essential.
Starvation		
Total fast	Decreased hunger after first day or two; rapid weight loss; no decisions about what to eat.	Same as for protein-sparing diets; gout; depression; sudden death; body loses needed protein.
Reduced-Calorie (no food type overemphasized)		
Weight Watchers, Rechtschaffen, Redbook Wise Woman Diet	Establishes good nutritional habits; gradual weight loss is better maintained.	Safe because nutritionally balanced; can be continued indefinitely.

Source: Copyright © 1981 by the New York Times Company. Reprinted by permission.

efits of most diets, Bennett and Gurin have presented evidence in support of a "setpoint" theory that supports the futility of dieting to lose weight.[20] These authors argue that every person has a "setpoint" for body fat: a level of fatness that the body strives to maintain. This setpoint seems to be predetermined for each person. According to the setpoint theory, your body, at the request of your body cells, will maintain a certain level of stored fat.

The cells send messages to the brain indicating how much fat they contain and, when necessary, requesting more. The brain decides what the setpoint should be after analyzing much data about the state of the body and the environment. Sensory stimuli (particularly the taste and smell of food), drugs such as amphetamine and nicotine, and physical activity affect the setpoint. The quantity of fat that the body wants is maintained by regulating food intake, physical activity, and metabolic efficiency.

The authors cite many studies in animal research to support the setpoint theory, but little research on humans, and those studies were inconclusive. Especially lacking is an explanation for some people's having more fat cells than others. The authors explore some theories to explain why some people have a greater amount of fat cells than others but reject them as unconvincing. The authors agree that heredity is responsible, in part, for the body makeup of individuals. The degree of such hereditary influence is uncertain. The only genetic fact in this regard is that women have more fat than men.

Although the setpoint theory does not provide all the answers to the many questions concerning obesity, it is a plausible explanation for the perpetual fatness of a large percentage of the American population. However, the setpoint theory does not help to explain why many people do not lose weight by dieting. In fact, except for a certain amount of weight loss through exercise, Bennett and Gurin feel that there is not much one can do to lower one's setpoint safely.

For those who plan to use a diet to lose weight despite the evidence against the effectiveness of diets, the following guidelines should be adhered to:[21]

1. Provide a caloric intake of not less than 1200 kilocalories per day for normal adults to get a proper blend of foods to meet nutritional requirements. (This requirement may change for children, older individuals, athletes, and others with special needs.)
2. Include foods acceptable to yourself from viewpoints of sociocultural background, usual habits, taste, cost, and ease of preparation.
3. Provide a negative caloric balance (Calories consumed less than those used by the body) not to exceed 500 to 1000 kilocalories per day. This will result in gradual weight loss without metabolic derangements. Maximal weight loss should be one kilogram (2 pounds) per week.

Many people think dieting is the best way to lose weight because they believe the fallacy that obese people eat more than people of normal weight. The research evidence does not support this notion. In fact, research studies show that in general fat people eat no more than thin individuals, and sometimes eat less.[22] Dieting on the basis of this misconception is inappropriate.

Misconception Regarding Dieting for Weight Control

Exercise for Weight Control.   Based on the assumption that weight will be lost if the caloric intake is less than the energy expenditure, physical activity can be recommended as a modality for weight control. It should be mentioned from the outset, however, that weight loss through increased physical activity alone will be small. For example, in one review by Epstein and Wing, it was found that weight losses from exercise programs averaged about 0.3 pounds per week for obese subjects and 0.11 pounds per week for subjects of normal weight.[23] These are not to be taken as absolute weight losses, since the type of activity and its intensity, duration, and frequency will ultimately determine the amount of weight that will be lost.

Aerobic activities such as walking, running, and bicycle riding provide the best means for weight control. The activity should be engaged in on a long-term basis for best results. Unlike the intensity level for the development of cardiorespiratory endurance, which should be from 70 to 85 percent of the age-adjusted heart rate maximum,* the intensity level for weight control does not have to be as high. It is more important to continue the activity for a longer period of time.

The computation of the caloric expenditure of a 200-pound male who would like to institute a walking program to lose weight is used to illustrate the importance of duration with this weight loss method. The resting energy expenditure for this person is 2184 Calories per day (Table 4.3). He would burn up an additional 364 Calories by walking for an hour at a rate of 3 miles per hour. If this person were to walk for an hour each day of the week, he would expend a total of 2548 Calories a week, or 10,192 Calories a month. Since body fat contains about 3500 Calories per pound, almost 3 pounds could be lost in a month (assuming that caloric intake remains constant). Extending these figures over a year, a person could lose approximately 30 to 35 pounds by walking one hour per day.

Obviously, if one were to run the same length of time at an increased intensity level, the caloric expenditure would be greater. For instance, the 200-pound male would expend 910 Calories an hour by running at 6 miles per hour (10-minute miles). If the person runs only four days a week, he would burn 3400 Calories per week, 14,560 Calories per month, and 174,720 Calories a year. At this rate, a 200-pound male would theoretically lose about 50 pounds in a year by running an hour a day, four days a week.

The temptation to advise individuals to use running or an equally strenuous activity for weight reduction is great. However, the realization that many people drop out of exercise programs after a few months militates against suggesting a strenuous activity. Walking seems to be an activity that the majority of obese individuals will like to do, despite the small weight loss in comparison to more strenuous activities.

Grant Gwinup reached this conclusion in a study of the effects of exercise on obese women. In his study, 11 obese women progressively increased periods of walking each day for one year or longer without any dietary restriction. Greater weight loss occurred when walking was increased, and weight stabilized at a lower level. The average weight loss was 22 pounds for the year. Most of the weight loss was accounted for

---

* The concept of "age-adjusted heart rate maximum" is discussed in Chapter 9. It is based on the assumption that the maximum heart rate any person can attain is 220 beats per minute minus the person's age.

by a loss in fat tissue.[24] Subjects in Gwinup's study also reported that they felt stronger and more relaxed.

Misconceptions Regarding Exercise and Weight Control

1. Since most activities require little caloric expenditure, it would take too much time in an activity to burn enough Calories to reduce one's weight significantly. For example, the 200-pound male would have to walk for approximately 10 hours to lose one pound.
2. An increase in physical activity causes a corresponding increase in appetite. Therefore, the increased food intake will negate any weight loss through the additional exercise and may actually cause a gain in weight.

You are being misled if you are not exercising because you believe either of these misconceptions. Both are inaccurate. Research by Dr. Jean Mayer,[25] an internationally recognized nutritionist, and information in this chapter refute these misconceptions.

Although exercise alone does not provide the best means of weight control, it can be used as one modality in a multifaceted program that also includes dietary management and behavior modification. The caloric costs for a variety of physical activities are presented in Tables 4.4 and 4.5 in this chapter and in Appendix F.

Diet, Exercise, and Behavior Modification

Increasing the activity level and lowering caloric intake to the point where caloric expenditure is greater than caloric intake will theoretically cause a reduction in weight (if the caloric imbalance is 3500 calories or more). Several research studies[26] have confirmed this theoretical construct. However, the poor adherence to exercise programs by the obese and overweight is a persistent problem and reduces the effectiveness of this approach for those who drop out of the program before full benefits are realized. Behavior modification, along with sound dietary management and increased physical activity, is proposed as the model approach to weight control.

Before indicating how behavior modification should be integrated into the program, the effectiveness of a program combining exercise and caloric reduction for weight reduction is shown by revising the figures for the 200-pound male. Using dieting alone, the person would have to consume 500 fewer Calories each day to lose one pound in one week (500 × 7 = 3500). With the exercise program alone, the person would have to walk more than an hour each day (approximately 364 Calories are burned per hour by walking at 3 mph). Using both exercise and caloric restriction, the person could lose a pound each week by reducing his caloric intake by only 240 Calories a day and by walking a mile a day, five days a week.

$$240 \times 7 = 1680 \text{ Calories by dieting}$$
$$364 \times 5 = \underline{1820} \text{ Calories by walking}$$
$$3500 \text{ total Calories}$$

The fact that a person could lose a pound of weight each week with such little energy expenditure and caloric reduction and the knowledge that obesity is a risk factor in cardiovascular disease and that both obesity and overweight are associated with health hazards such as increased risk of high blood pressure, gout, kidney stones, and arthritis may prompt one to ask, Why is a majority of the American population failing to participate in regular aerobic-type physical activities?

Despite the demonstrated benefits of strenuous physical activity and the relationship of inactivity to obesity, some 31 million Americans are obese. The use of behavior modification techniques with exercise programs and dietary management seeks to help people focus on their behaviors regarding weight control. This approach applies the principles of the laws of learning and emphasizes relevant reinforcement strategies to enhance positive behavior change. In fact, a self-modification of behavior plan is included in Chapter 8, since I believe that each person must take responsibility for designing and executing his or her own program. The specifics of the plan are presented in Chapter 8, with the necessary instructions and guidelines for each person to develop a successful weight control program using both exercise and dietary management.

The modification-of-behavior technique (especially in plans for self-modification of behavior) has been used successfully in some cases and is advocated as an adjunct to a program of dietary management and increased physical activity by the American College of Sports Medicine and the eminent researcher and writer on obesity, George Bray, among others.[27] However, this approach should not be viewed as a panacea. If behavior modification were the final answer to the problem of obesity, there would not be the ever-increasing proliferation of fad diets and other gimmicks for weight control being sold to the American public. Individuals who have tried dieting or an exercise program in attempts to lose weight and have failed are urged to consider the self-modification-of-behavior plan presented in this text. The objective of the plan is to help people change their lifestyles from inactive to active by following valid learning principles that stress positive reinforcement.

I am currently using the self-modification-of-behavior plan with dietary management and increased physical activity with two individuals. The results to date are encouraging. Both Ann and Iola weighed 170 pounds at the start of the program on November 11, 1986. As of August 4, 1987, Ann weighed 153 pounds and Iola 155 pounds. Besides the loss in weight for both individuals, the percentage of body fat for each was reduced. Ann's body fat went from 27 percent to 20 percent.

Your Proper Weight

An "ideal" weight for each person is difficult to determine. The determination of whether someone is overweight or underweight is most often made by comparing that person's weight with recommended weights for a particular height, sex, and body frame in height-weight charts.

You should compare your weight with the recommended weight

range for your height and body frame published by the Metropolitan Life Insurance Company (see Tables 5.3 and 5.4) to determine if you are overweight. Weight information from these tables should be used with an assessment of overall body composition, the procedures and techniques for which are presented in Chapter 5.

You should not be too concerned if you are a few pounds overweight or a little on the "plump" side according to the results of your body composition evaluation. Since the public's view of the desired body size changes from time to time, each person should strive to maintain a weight that is comfortable to live with. This is not to suggest that one should ignore proper nutritional and exercise habits; quite the contrary. However, it is acknowledged that some people who eat nutritious, well-balanced meals and get proper physical exercise are still overweight according to height-weight charts. Yet some of these people are far from obese. The suggestion is that you practice sound eating and exercise habits to keep your weight and body fat at a level that will not predispose you to diseases or illnesses. Beyond that, do not let the so-called "normal" weight syndrome become an obsession.

Special Nutritional Considerations

A balanced diet consisting of food from the Basic Four Food Groups (milk, meat, fruit and vegetables, and grains) that contain sufficient Calories to meet the energy requirements will satisfy the nutritional needs of most healthy persons. However, athletes and other individuals who are engaged in strenuous physical activities, older adults, and vegetarians, among others, have special dietary needs.

Athletes and Other Active People

The only nutritional requirement for athletes and other active people is to consume an adequate amount of Calories in foods from the Basic Four Food Groups—dairy products, protein-rich foods, fruits and vegetables, and breads and cereals—to meet their increased energy requirements. In general, athletes and other active people can get the proper nutrients by eating a diet that is 10 to 15 percent protein, 30 percent fats, and 55 to 60 percent carbohydrates.

One possible exception to this general rule is the need to modify the recommended percentage of protein and carbohydrates for persons engaged in body building and power lifting on a daily basis; they might need to increase their protein intake beyond the recommended 15 percent. Young athletes whose muscles are still developing also need more protein in the diet than the average active person. This added protein is needed to build and repair tissue rather than to produce extra energy, which should be supplied by increased carbohydrates.

The amount of added protein will depend on the intensity and duration of the activity as well as the frequency at which it is performed. One study of the energy expenditure and protein needs of weight lifters concluded that the protein requirement of athletes was 2.2 to 2.6 grams per kilogram of body weight.[28] Excessive protein intake should be avoided because it produces large amounts of nitrogen, which must be excreted, and this places extra work on the liver and kidneys. A high-protein diet may lead to dehydration, loss of appetite, and diarrhea. In summary, one needs to balance the benefits to be gained from an increased intake of protein with the possible side effects of consuming too much protein.

The greatest difference in nutritional requirements of active individuals in comparison with sedentary persons is the increased need for carbohydrates. People who engage in prolonged, strenuous endurance-type activities need considerably more carbohydrates than the recommended percentage for the average healthy adult. A diet containing more than 70 percent carbohydrates was said to have enhanced the performance of some athletes engaged in prolonged endurance events. As was indicated for protein, the intensity, duration, and frequency of the activity should be the factors used to determine how much to increase the carbohydrate intake. The increase should be gotten through an increase in Calories from the four food groups rather than from diet supplements.

Carbohydrate Loading.   Some individuals who perform endurance-type activities such as marathon running may benefit from "carbohydrate" or "glycogen" loading. This is a procedure designed to saturate the muscles with glycogen stores before an endurance activity. The basic plan, which lasts for a week, involves two steps:

1. An exhausting exercise on the first day to deplete or significantly reduce muscle glycogen levels.
2. Consumption of a high-carbohydrate (75 to 90 percent) diet for the next three days, with a drastic reduction in training to keep glycogen stores high for the race.

The carbohydrate loading regimen is usually divided into two phases: the *depletion phase,* which starts seven days before the activity and lasts until four days before the activity, and the *loading phase,* which comprises the three days of ingesting the high-carbohydrate diet. Suggested food plans for carbohydrate loading have been developed by M. T. Forgac and appear in Table 4.8.

Dr. David Costill, exercise physiologist at Ball State University, questions the validity of the depletion phase of the carbohydrate loading plan. Based on his research, Dr. Costill advises marathon runners to maintain a normal diet until three days before the event, then load up with foods high in carbohydrates. He argues against the use of carbohydrate loading for runs shorter than the marathon. For such runs the normal diet should be eaten (with an increase in total caloric intake and a corresponding increase in carbohydrates).

For those who use carbohydrate loading as a strategy to increase glycogen stores, Dr. Costill recommends the consumption of about 500 to 600 grams of carbohydrates per day during the three days before the race, eating the bulk of the food in two large meals. This would translate to about 2000 to 2450 Calories for a person who consumes a total of 3500 Calories per day and uses between 58 and 70 percent of the diet for

TABLE 4.8 **Carbohydrate Loading Food Plans**

Food	Depletion Phase (days 7 to 4 before event)	Loading Phase (days 3 to 1 before event)
Meat, fish, poultry, eggs, cheese	12–18 oz kcal: 900–1350	6–8 oz kcal: 450–600
Breads and cereals	4 servings kcal: 280	8–16 servings kcal: 560–1120
Vegetables	2 servings kcal: 50	4 servings kcal: 100
Fruits and juices	2 servings kcal: 80	4 servings kcal: 160
Fats and oils	4–12 tbsp. kcal: 540–1620	2–4 tbsp. kcal: 270–540
Milk (whole)	2 servings kcal: 300	2 servings kcal: 300
Desserts	1 or 2 servings, unsweetened kcal: 400	2 servings, sweetened kcal: 800
Beverages	Unsweetened, unlimited kcal: 0	Sweetened, unlimited to kcal level kcal: 0–360
Water	8 or more servings kcal: 0	8 or more servings kcal: 0
Total	kcal: 2550–4080	kcal: 2640–3980

Source: Adapted from M. T. Forgac, "Carbohydrate Loading: A Review." Copyright The American Dietic Association. Reprinted by permission from Journal of the American Dietetic Association *75 (1979): 43.*

carbohydrates. The last meal should be eaten 15 to 17 hours before the race. A light carbohydrate snack is permitted before retiring for the night. Those who feel that they can tolerate it may eat a light carbohydrate breakfast three to four hours before the race.

Negative Effects? Dr. Jack M. Cooperman, director of nutrition education at New York Medical College, says that carbohydrate loading affects cellular mineral balance and may result in dehydration. He advises the unskilled person to avoid carbohydrate loading, except under a physician's instructions. It should be noted that dehydration is a possibility in all prolonged endurance activities, especially under hot and humid environmental conditions. At the 1984 Olympic Games in Los Angeles, Gabriela Anderson-Schiess, who finished the marathon in 37th place, literally staggered the last 400 meters to the finish line. It was reported after the race that she had suffered from dehydration but that her body temperature was only 100 degrees after over two hours in the 75 percent humidity and near-90-degree heat.[29]

A review of the research leads to the conclusion that persons engaged in prolonged endurance-type activities lasting two hours or more who are healthy can safely engage in the practice of carbohydrate loading. However, the practice should be restricted to once or twice a year.

People with health problems such as heart disease and diabetes should consult their doctor before attempting carbohydrate loading.

The Physically Active Vegetarian

The recent emphasis on physical fitness has encouraged many people to change lifestyles. Some have adopted different dietary practices. For example, more and more people are altering their diets to include foods low in fat and cholesterol. Some have become vegetarians, including many young people.

There are several categories of vegetarians. The *vegan* or true vegetarian eats only plant foods; the *lacto-ovo-vegetarian* consumes dairy products and eggs as well. The *lacto-vegetarian* uses only dairy products and plant foods.

Individuals on all three types of vegetarians diets can get the required nutrients by eating a variety of foods from groups their diets allow. The true vegan, however, will have a problem because vitamin B_{12} cannot be gotten through an all-plant diet. Lacto-vegetarians can get vitamin B_{12} through milk and eggs, but the vegan would have to consume fortified soybean milk or a vitamin B_{12} supplement.

Individuals on extreme vegetarian diets, such as those who eat only fruits, juices, and nuts, will have a low level of many essential nutrients. This type of diet is not recommended as a permanent practice.

To help ensure a nutritionally balanced diet for vegetarians, the following guidelines are offered:[30]

1. Use foods that contain complementing proteins (one food high in a particular amino acid and the other food low in that same amino acid but high in another amino acid). In other words, use food combinations that have opposite strengths and weaknesses in essential amino acid content.
2. Eat generous portions of animal protein sources such as eggs, cheese, and milk to get the essential amino acids. (Vegans should follow the guidelines in Table 4.9).
3. Use whole grain as the basic food of the diet, especially in the form of yeast-leavened bread. This involves increasing the number of servings from the grain group. Vary the types of grain used. Nuts and seeds are grouped with grains.
4. Be sure to use the recommended number of servings of milk or milk equivalents for the age group. Fortified skim milk and fortified low-fat milk products are recommended. Milk products will be the only source of vitamin B_{12} unless eggs are eaten.
5. Use servings of legumes, lentils, meat analogs, eggs, or an additional milk product daily. Vary the choice.
6. Use a wide variety of vegetables and fruits, including at least one serving of a dark leafy vegetable daily.
7. Severely limit the use of foods that are primarily a source of "empty" Calories.

Table 4.9 contains daily requirements of the Basic Four Food Groups for the adult vegan. However, lacto-ovo-vegetarians and lacto-vegetarians can also use this guide as well as the Basic Four Food Groups as a food guide for meal planning. Information in Table 4.9 and a good cook-

TABLE 4.9   **Daily Requirements of the Four Food Groups
for the Adult Vegan**[a]

Grains

4 slices of whole-grain yeast-leavened bread; 3 to 5 servings of grain
(number based on normal body size) plus 1 serving of nuts or seeds (ground
or thoroughly chewed). This provides a total of about 30 g grain protein for
men, 28 g for women.

Legumes

2 cups fortified soybean milk; ⅓ cup cooked dried peas or beans or 1¼ cups
cooked dried peas or beans; Other sources of vitamin B_{12}, calcium, and
riboflavin.

Vegetables

4 or more servings, including 2 large servings of dark green leafy vegetables:
Mustard, turnip, and collard greens, kale, broccoli, bok choy, and romaine
and other dark loose-leafed lettuce provide calcium in usable form; 2
additional servings, emphasizing variety

Fruit

1 to 4 servings, according to caloric needs; Include a source of vitamin C.

Extras Necessary for Adequate Nutrition

Supplemental vitamin B_{12}, unless enough fortified soy milk is used to provide
2 to 3 μg daily; Supplemental calcium, unless soy milk fortified with this
mineral or 1½ cups of cooked calcium-rich vegetables are used; Riboflavin,
as from 1 tbsp. brewer's yeast or the equivalent; Supplemental vitamin D for
children and pregnant and lactating women.

[a]Pregnant and lactating women need more good nutrient sources to meet their higher RDAs.

Source: Carol J. W. Suitor and Merrily F. Crowley, Nutrition: Principles and Application in Health
Promotion, *2d ed. (Philadelphia: Lippincott, 1984), p. 73. Reprinted by permission of the publisher.*

book will aid in the preparation of palatable food. Two sample menus,
one for a lacto-ovo-vegetarian and one for an adult vegan are presented
in Table 4.10.

Health Advantages and Hazards.   The literature reveals that the diets
of vegetarians of all three types produce no health hazards, provided
they respect established nutritional principles. (The guidelines in this
chapter should assist vegetarians in such nutrition planning. Furthermore, in Appendix E is a table of food composition that contains the
nutritive values of the 49 foods on the vegetarian Exchange List and 18
additional nonmeat foods.)

Although adherence to a vegetarian diet that has been planned according to sound nutritional principles can be problem-free, such a diet
without careful planning can result in serious nutritional deficiencies,
especially in certain amino acids, iron, zinc, calcium, vitamin B_{12}, and
riboflavin (vitamin B_2). Such deficiencies have resulted in cases of
scurvy, anemia, hypoproteinemia (an abnormal decrease in protein in
the blood), hypocalcemia (low blood calcium), emaciation due to starvation, and other forms of malnutrition, besides loss of kidney function due

TABLE 4.10   **Two Sample Vegetarian Menus**

Breakfast	Lunch	Dinner[a]
	For a Lacto-ovo-vegetarian	
Whole-grain toast with peanut butter	Homemade bean soup	Meatless lasagna with whole-grain pasta
Yogurt with fresh fruit and nuts	Corn sticks	Sautéed zucchini or collard greens
Herb tea	Romaine and tomato salad with cheese dressing	Spinach and mushroom salad
		Milk
	For an Adult Vegan[b]	
Orange	Split pea soup	Soybeans
Bulgur with brewer's yeast	Peanut butter sandwich:	Brown rice cooked fried in oil
Toasted wheat-soy bread with honey	peanut butter	with chestnuts
	whole-wheat	and sesame seeds
	bread	Collards
	honey	Pear
	Fruit–sunflower seed salad:	
	apple	
	banana	
	sunflower seeds	
	lettuce	

[a]Seventh-day Adventists might substitute a meat analog such as vegetarian wieners, turkeylike loaf, or breakfast slices for one of the main dishes.

[b]Milk and eggs are not included. A source of vitamin B_{12} and possibly one of iodine are needed. This menu also allows for a snack after breakfast, lunch, and dinner.

Sources: Carol J. W. Suitor and Merrily F. Crowley, Nutrition: Principles and Application in Health Promotion, *2d ed. (Philadelphia: Lippincott, 1984), p. 73; Nancy R. Raper and Mary M. Hill, "Vegetarian Diets,"* Nutrition Reviews/Supplement *32 (1974): 32. Reprinted by permission of the publisher.*

to restricted fluid intake. Some of these deficiencies have resulted in death.[31]

There is a greater probability for nutritional deficiencies in vegetarians who eat only plant foods than in those with fewer dietary restrictions. One prevalent problem for vegans is the deficiency in vitamin B_{12} (not contained in plant food), which can cause disturbances in the functioning of the nervous system. And the limited caloric intake may predispose pure vegetarians who are underweight to other health problems as well.

Children raised as vegans are particularly susceptible to the health problems just identified. In a study of the nutritional status of four infants from a new vegan community, for example, it was discovered that all the infants had profound protein-caloric malnutrition, severe rickets, osteoporosis, and vitamin B_{12} and other deficiencies. One infant even died.[32]

The following health benefits have been ascribed to vegetarian eating:

1. A reduced risk of coronary heart disease due to the lower intake of foods that are high in saturated fats and cholesterol. One of several studies reviewed by Register and Sonnenberg compared the dietary habits and serum cholesterol of vegetarians and nonvegetarians, and the conclusion was that as the degree of nonvegetarianism increased, the serum cholesterol increased.[33] A similar conclusion was reached in a study of the dietary status of Seventh-day Adventists and nonvegetarians.[34]
2. A positive factor in weight management programs because of foods in the diet that are nutritious yet low in caloric content. A vegetarian is consequently able to consume more Calories while getting the proper nutrients.
3. Such diets promote increased gastrointestinal functioning due to increased fiber consumption.

In summary, the evidence indicates that by adhering to a diet based on sound nutritional principles, vegetarians can get well-balanced and nutritious meals. Such a diet enables vegetarians to participate in sports and other physical activities without diminished physical energy or productivity. It is recommended that individuals planning to change from a nonvegetarian to a vegetarian diet should consult a dietitian or nutritionist for advice. A good vegetarian cookbook and a short course in food preparation would also be helpful.

The Older Adult

There has been a dramatic increase in the number of older persons in America during the past few decades, and this trend is expected to continue. By the year 2000 it is estimated that more than 15 percent of the population will be over 65 years old.

With the ever-increasing number of elderly persons and the higher incidence of chronic diseases associated with advancing age, it is critical that increased attention be paid to potential problems encountered by members of this age group. The problem of poor nutrition among the older population is receiving more attention by health care professionals.

One could simply exhort older adults to eat a well-balanced and nutritious diet. They could even be informed of the recommended daily dietary allowances that have been published by the Research Council of the National Academy of Sciences (these appear in Appendix B of this text). These actions are unrealistic, however, because of the special life situations that might interfere with sound nutritional health planning by persons 60 years old and over.

Some of the changes among older adults are a reduced basal metabolic rate, bone loss in the jaw resulting in loose alveolar bone, a decrease in the sense of taste, and a reduced ability of the intestine to operate properly. In addition, psychosocial problems such as depression and isolation among people in this age group may adversely affect nutritional habits. Also, because many older adults operate on fixed budgets and others are homebound, they might not be able to afford certain foods, and the health status of the homebound might make it difficult for them to purchase their food.

Based on this information, the following guidelines for the older adult are offered:

1. Reduce total caloric intake to be consistent with energy expenditure (don't take in more Calories than you burn up).
2. Greatly reduce the intake of foods high in saturated fats.
3. Increase the intake of foods high in complex carbohydrates and reduce the consumption of simple refined sugars.
4. Pay careful attention to menu planning so that the required minerals and vitamins will be provided in the diet.
5. Do not be afraid or ashamed to apply for food stamps under the USDA food stamp program if you qualify and are on a fixed budget that requires supplemental help.
6. Adjust food preparation methods to account for aging problems such as bone loss in the jaw or the use of dentures. Some suggestions are to cook meats until they are tender, prepare more cooked vegetables, and cut meats into small pieces before eating.
7. Drink six to eight glasses of liquids each day: juices, diet soda, unsweetened coffee and tea, and consomme.
8. Consume two or more cups of milk or the equivalent in a milk alternate every day. Milk alternates include cheddar cheese, cream cheese, cottage cheese, ice cream, and ice milk.

TABLE 4.11   **Nutrient Recommendations for Older Persons**[a]

Nutrient	Men	Women
Calories[b]	2400/day	2000/day
Protein	56 g/day	45 g/day
Fat	25% of total daily Calories (67 g/day)	25% of total daily Calories (56 g/day)
Carbohydrates	60% of total daily Calories (360 g/day)	60% of total daily Calories (300 g/day)
Fiber	Increase to 10 g	Increase to 10 g
Vitamins	Increase B_{12} to more than 0.003 mg/day	Increase B_{12} to more than 0.003 mg/day
Calcium	950 mg/day	950 mg/day
Phosphorus	800 mg/day	800 mg/day
Iron	10–20 mg/day	10–20 mg/day

[a]These requirements are for most average healthy older adults. Persons who are extremely active, who are unusually sedentary, or who have a medical problem should adjust their caloric intake accordingly.

[b]After age 75, the average energy requirement is 2050 Calories for males and 1600 Calories for females.

Source: Adapted from National Academy of Sciences—National Research Council, Recommended Dietary Allowances, 9th ed. (Washington, D.C., 1980).

TABLE 4.12 **Sources of Iron**

Food	Weight	Serving[a]
Calf's liver	42 g	1½ oz
Beef liver	70 g	2½ oz
Chicken liver	70 g	2½ oz
Chicken (fresh only)	364 g	13 oz
Beef (lean only)	168 g	6 oz
Sardines, Atlantic	168 g	6 oz
Pork, loin (lean only)	170 g	6 oz
Whole-wheat bread (soft and firm crumb)	196 g	7 slices
White bread (soft crumb)	280 g	10 slices
White bread (firm crumb)	243 g	9 slices
Lima beans, cooked	238 g	⅓ cups
Kidney beans, cooked	240 g	1¼ cups
Tofu (soybean curd)	340 g	2½ pieces

[a]Each serving provides approximately 6 mg of iron.

Source: S. Jamie Rozovski, "Nutrition for Older Americans," in Aging (Washington, D.C.: U.S. Government Printing Office, 1984), p. 55.

TABLE 4.13 **Distribution of Fats in Common Foods**

High in Polyunsaturated Fats

Safflower oil; Corn oil; Soft margarine made of corn oil; Walnuts; Soybeans; Sunflower seeds; Sesame seeds; Sunflower and sesame oils.

Moderately High in Polyunsaturated Fats

Soybean oil; Cottonseed oil; Soft margarines other than corn oil margarine; Commercial salad dressings; Mayonnaise.

High in Mono-unsaturated Fats

Peanut oil; Peanuts and peanut butter; Olive oil; Olives; Almonds; Pecans; Cashews; Brazil nuts; Avocados.

High in Saturated Fats

Meats: sausages, cold cuts, prime cuts, etc.; Chicken fat; Meat drippings; Lard; Hydrogenated shortening; Stick margarine; Coconut oil; Butter and other products with dairy fat: cheese, cream, whole milk, ice cream, chocolate, baked goods

High in Cholesterol

Egg yolks; Liver; Kidney; Sweetbreads; Brains; Heart; Pâté; Caviar; Dairy fats; Products made with the above: cakes, pies, pastries, gravies, etc.

Source: S. Jamie Rozovski, "Nutrition for Older Americans," in Aging (Washington, D.C.: U.S. Government Printing Office, 1984), p. 55.

To aid in meeting these guidelines, nutrient recommendations for the elderly (Table 4.11), sources of iron (Table 4.12), foods of different fat content (Table 4.13), and three sample menus (Table 4.14) are presented. Planning and consuming a well-balanced, nutritious diet and getting adequate exercise will help the older adult to live a longer and more satisfying life.

TABLE 4.14   Sample Three-Day Menu for the Older Adult[a]

Day 1	Day 2	Day 3
This menu is planned to use today's leftovers for the meal on the next day.	*Leftovers are starred.*	*A meatless day can provide the proper nutrients.*

Breakfast

Day 1	Day 2	Day 3
Prune juice French toast with powdered sugar Coffee	Orange juice Cheese omelet *Toasted cornbread Coffee	Tangerine Scrambled eggs Toast with spread Coffee

Midday Meal

Day 1	Day 2	Day 3

Meat loaf
Potatoes au gratin
Broccoli
Cornbread with
   spread
Instant butterscotch
   pudding
Tea
	Ham divan
	   (*broccoli, ham,
	   cream of chicken
	   soup)
	Roll with spread
	*Butterscotch pudding
	Tea
		Macaroni and cheese
		Brussels sprouts,
		French dressing
		Orange-grapefruit
		   salad
		Tapioca pudding

Evening Meal

Day 1	Day 2	Day 3

Salmon salad
Tomato–green pepper
   salad
Bread with spread
Apricots
Milk
	*Meat loaf sandwich
	Dill pickle
	Tossed salad
	*Apricots with
	   custard sauce
	Tea
		Fish chowder
		Carrot and raisin
		   salad
		Bread with spread
		Apple crisp
		Milk

Snack

Day 1	Day 2	Day 3
Toast Tea	Hot chocolate	Toast Tea

[a]These menus contain food that satisfies the nutrient requirements for adults as recommended in the National Dairy Council's "Guide to Good Eating."

Source: U.S. Department of Agriculture, Food Guide for Older Folks, *Home and Garden Bulletin No. 17 (Washington, D.C.: U.S. Government Printing Office, 1973), pp. 4–6.*

This booklet also contains, in summary form, some very valuable information on foods to prepare to satisfy the nutrient requirements, tips on buying food and using simple food-preparation equipment, and recipes.

Notes

1. Sidney Abraham et al., *Obese and Overweight Adults in the United States,* National Center for Health Statistics, Data from the National Health Survey Series II, No. 230. DHHS Publication No. (PHS) 83-1680 (Hyattsville, Md.: Public Health Service, U.S. Department of Health and Human Services, February 1983).
2. Ibid., p. 5.
3. National Center for Health Statistics, Unpublished data from the second National Health and Nutrition Examination Survey, 1976–1980.

4. National Academy of Sciences—National Research Council, *Recommended Dietary Allowances*, 9th ed. (Washington D.C., 1980).

5. U.S. Senate Select Committee on Nutrition and Human Needs, *Dietary Goals for the United States*, 2d ed. (Washington D.C.: U. S. Government Printing Office, 1977), p. 4.

6. U.S. Department of Health and Human Services, *Nutrition and Your Health: Dietary Guidelines for Americans* (Washington, D.C.: Home and Garden Bulletin No. 232, 1980), pp. 19.

7. U.S. Department of Agriculture, Science and Education Administration, *Nutritive Value of Foods* (Washington D.C.: U.S. Government Printing Office, 1981), 40 pp.

8. Samuel M. Fox et al., "Physical Activity and Cardiovascular Health," in *Modern Concepts of Cardiovascular Disease* (New York: American Heart Association, 1972), pp. 27–28.

9. Carol J. W. Suitor and Merrily F. Crowley, *Nutrition: Principles and Application in Health Promotion*, 2d ed. (Philadelphia: Lippincott, 1984), p. 466.

10. William D. McArdle, Frank I. Katch, and Victor L. Katch, *Exercise Physiology: Energy, Nutrition, and Human Performance*, 2d ed. (Philadelphia: Lea & Febiger, 1986), p. 489.

11. Jean Hall, "Anorexia Reaching Epidemic Levels," (Westchester Co., N.Y.) *Reporter Dispatch*, July 19, 1984, p. B1.

12. "Anorexia, the 'Starving Disease' Epidemic," *U.S. News and World Report*, August 30, 1982, p. 47.

13. Janet B. W. Williams, ed., *Diagnostic and Statistical Manual of Mental Disorders*, 3d ed. (Washington, D.C.: American Psychiatric Association, 1980), pp. 67–69.

14. Joseph Di Gennaro, *The New Physical Fitness: Exercise for Everybody* (Englewood, Colo., 1983); Bud Getchell, *Physical Fitness: A Way of Life*, 3d ed. (New York: Wiley, 1983); William P. Marley, *Health and Physical Fitness: Taking Charge of Your Health* (Philadelphia: CBS College Publishing, 1982).

15. "Weight Control," *Dairy Council Digest* 22 (1984):13.

16. Ibid.

17. "Starch Blockers Fail the Test Again," *Tufts University Diet & Nutrition Letter* 2 (May 1984):2.

18. M. M. Cegielski and J. A. Saporta, "Surgical Treatment of Massive Obesity: Current Status of the Art," *Obesity and Bariatric Medicine* 7 (1978):156.

19. Jane Brody, "Dieting," *Columbia* (S.C.) *Record*, March 25, 1981, p. B1.

20. William Bennett and Joel Gurin, *The Dieter's Dilemma* (New York: Basic Books, 1982), pp. 142–167.

21. American College of Sports Medicine, "Proper and Improper Weight Loss Programs," *Medicine and Science in Sports and Exercise* 15 (1983):10.

22. Bennett and Gurin, p. 61.

22. L. H. Epstein and R. R. Wing, "Aerobic Exercise and Weight," *Addictive Behaviors* 5 (1980):371–388.

24. Grant Gwinup, "Effect of Exercise Alone on the Weight of Obese Women," *Archives of Internal Medicine* 135 (1975):676–680.

25. Jean Mayer, "Exercise and Weight Control," in Warren R. Johnson, ed., *Science and Medicine of Exercise and Sports* (New York: Harper & Row, 1960), pp. 301–309.

26. American College of Sports Medicine, 9–10; E. R. Buskirk et al., "Energy Balance in Obese Patients During Weight Reduction: Influence of Diet Restriction and Exercise," *Annals of the New York Academy of Science* 110 (1963):918–940; M. M. Kenrick, M. F. Ball, and J. J. Canary, "Exercise and

Weight Reduction in Obesity," *Archives of Physical and Medical Rehabilitation* 61 (1976):323–327; J. E. Martin and P. M. Dubbert, "Exercise Applications and Promotion in Behavioral Medicine: Current Status and Future Directions," *Journal of Consulting and Clinical Psychology* 50 (1982):1004–1014; W. B. Zuti and L. A. Golding, "Comparing Diet and Exercise as Weight Reduction Tools," *Physician and Sports Medicine* 4 (1976): 49–53.

27. Robert J. Presbie and Paul Brown, *Physical Education: The Behavior Modification Approach* (Washington, D.C.: National Education Association, 1977); American College of Sports Medicine, 9–13; George A. Bray, "Energetics of Obesity," *Medicine and Science in Sports and Exercise* 15 (1983):39.

28. K. A. Laritcheva et al., "Study of Energy Expenditure and Protein Needs of Top Weight Lifters," in Jane Parikova and V. A. Rogoszkin, eds., *Nutrition, Physical Fitness, and Health* (Baltimore: University Park Press, 1978), p. 162.

29. George Vecsey, "First Gasps, Then Cheers," *New York Times,* August 6, 1984, p. C1.

30. Carol J. W. Suitor and Merrily F. Crowley, *Nutrition: Principles and Application in Health Promotion,* 2d ed. (Philadelphia: Lippincott, 1984), pp. 71–75.

31. U. D. Register and L. M. Sonnenberg, "The Vegetarian Diet," *Journal of the American Dietetic Association* 62 (1973):253.

32. Ehud Zmora, R. Gordischer, and J. Bar-Ziv, "Multiple Nutritional Deficiencies in Infants from a Strict Vegetarian Community," *American Journal of Diseased Children,* 133 (1979):141.

33. Register and Sonnenberg, 58–59.

34. Terry D. Shultz and James E. Leklem, "Dietary Status of Seventh-day Adventists and Nonvegetarians," *Journal of the American Dietetic Association* 83 (1983):27–33.

Evaluation of Physical Fitness

anthropometric measurements
assessment
body composition
bicycle ergometer
evaluation
fat weight
lean body weight

mean
norm
recovery index
resting heart rate
standard deviation
stress test
t score

After reading this chapter, you should be able to:
1. Define and/or explain the key words listed above.
2. State three purposes of fitness testing.
3. Evaluate test data using *t* scores.
4. Administer each of the fitness tests in this chapter.
5. Determine whether you are overweight or underweight.
6. Estimate your percentage of body fat by using skinfold calipers and the relevant nomograms.
7. Identify your resting pulse rate (or heart rate).
8. Evaluate your overall fitness status, using appropriate tests in this chapter.

If you have not begun a systematic physical fitness program during the reading of the first four chapters, plan to begin one now. First, evaluate your present physical fitness level to provide a sound basis for the development of an individualized physical fitness program. Such an examination will provide valuable information about the physical state of your body and the intensity of exercise that its various systems can tolerate safely.

Preliminary Evaluation

An evaluation of an individual's present fitness level can provide much useful information. First, it enables one to determine where one is now in terms of the condition of the important health-related fitness components and thereby aid in the planning of a realistic fitness program. Second, it provides baseline data against which to measure future progress. And the assessment of one's present level of fitness can provide information to motivate one to engage in a program of physical activities that will improve the level of fitness. Even discouraging results do not mean that it is hopeless to begin a fitness program; it is important to begin such a program regardless of one's present physical condition. Adherence to the principles and procedures of program development discussed in Chapter 9 should enable all individuals to become fit and enjoy life to the utmost.

There are several ways to evaluate one's present fitness level. Let's begin by recalling our definition of physical fitness, which is the condition of the systems of the body that enables them to function at their optimal efficiency. These body systems include the cardiorespiratory system, the skeletal system, and the muscular system. To evaluate one's fitness level, therefore, one must assess the functioning of the heart, lungs, blood vessels, muscles, and bones. Sophisticated laboratory tests can be used to evaluate these fitness components; however, such testing is not accessible to the average person. Therefore, so-called field tests which have been positively correlated with the more precise laboratory tests, may be used.

A battery of inexpensive, accurate, and easy-to-administer tests (see Table 5.1) has been chosen for use in this text. These tests are designed to measure the basic fitness components of body composition, strength, muscular endurance, flexibility, and cardiorespiratory endurance. Unlike the highly technical tests used in exercise physiology laboratories, which require trained individuals to perform the testing, the tests in this book can be administered by the teacher or by students. Moreover, the tests have been correlated with laboratory tests and have been found to be highly accurate in measuring the selected fitness components.

Time of Testing

When an evaluation of physical fitness status should be undertaken depends on the purpose of the evaluation. If testing is to determine the progress of a fitness program, for example, it should be done both before and after the program. On the other hand, if the goal is simply to assign students to a particular program based on their present level of fitness, only a test at the beginning of the program is necessary.

Regardless of the time of testing, it is recommended that a few sessions be devoted to general movement activities to get the subjects ready for the tests. If the individuals to be tested have been sedentary for a

TABLE 5.1   **Physical Fitness Test Battery Profile Chart**

Name_____   Age_____   Sex_____   Date_____

Body weight_____   Height_____   Percent body fat_____

Resting heart rate_____

ANTHROPOMETRIC MEASUREMENTS

Chest/bust_____in.

Waist_____in.

Hips_____in.

Thighs (R)_____in.   (L)_____in.

Upper arm (R)_____in.   (L)_____in.

STRENGTH	Raw score	*t* Score
Dominant-hand grip strength	_____kg	_____
Nondominant-hand grip strength	_____kg	_____
Bench press	_____lb	_____

MUSCULAR ENDURANCE	Raw score	*t* Score
Sit-ups (bent-knee)	_____no.	_____
Pull-ups	_____no.	_____
Flexed-arm hang	_____sec.	_____
Push-ups	_____no.	_____
Modified push-ups	_____no.	_____
Squat thrusts	_____no.	_____

FLEXIBILITY		
Sit-and-reach	_____in.	_____
Back arch	_____in.	_____

CARDIORESPIRATORY ENDURANCE (Use one of the two tests.)		*t* Score
12-minute run-walk	_____mi.	
Step test_____	Recovery Index_____	

period of time, it is advisable to increase the activity level gradually during the first several class periods before testing.

Making Sense of the Test Results

John, a 25-year-old college junior, performed 30 sit-ups at the testing session at the beginning of the semester of his fitness class. Mary, a 17-year-old freshman, performed 35 sit-ups on the same test. What is the level of muscular endurance of these two students? This question cannot be answered with only the one score for each student. The sit-up test is designed to measure muscular endurance of the abdominal muscles. The raw scores would have to be converted to some standard score scale before an interpretation of the value of obtained scores could be made.

To evaluate the results of the physical fitness assessment test data properly, the raw scores should be converted to standard scores, and norms should be established. The t score is the standard score used in this text. A t score provides an expression of any score in a distribution as it deviates from the mean of a normal distribution in standard deviation units. (A standard deviation is a measure of variability that indicates the scatter or spread of approximately two-thirds of a distribution of scores about the mean. In the t scale the mean is 50 and the standard deviation is 10.) Conversion of raw scores to standard scores permits the comparison of scores of dissimilar test items. For example, scores of 10 pull-ups, 30 sit-ups, and 40 seconds for the flexed-arm hang are almost meaningless by themselves. However, when converted to standard scores they can be used to indicate the relative fitness level of the participants on these test items. (A procedure for computing t scores appears in Appendix G.)*

Establishing Norms

Norms are standards against which raw scores may be compared. Norms can be developed by recording the results of test scores for a large representative sample of the population for which the norms are to be developed. It is important to know the characteristics of the population (that is, age and sex) from which the test norms were developed. Other important information to consider when using test norms developed by others include the time that the test was administered (before or after the fitness program), the general condition of the subjects, and the instructions for test administration. It is advisable to develop your own local norms when possible. Norms for some test items are given in this text. You may use these norms to compare your scores on the various test items. Please keep in mind the characteristics of the population from which the norms were developed when comparing your scores with the norms.

The Medical Examination

Obtaining medical clearance based on the results of a complete medical examination should be a first step before participating in any physical fitness testing program. The objectives of the medical examination should be (1) to determine the level of health in freedom from injury,

---

* Tables for converting raw scores to t scores for men and women appear at the end of this chapter (Tables 5.16 and 5.17). A t score classification scale appears in Table 5.18.

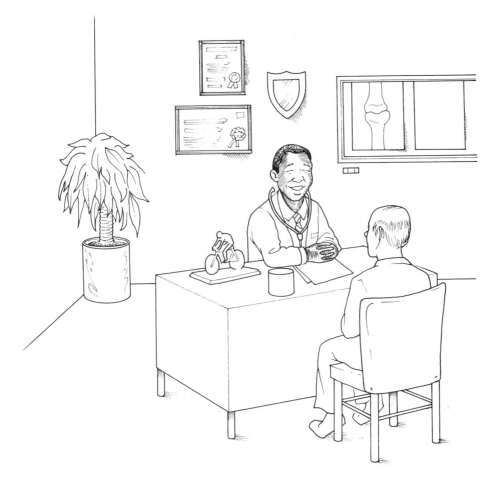

Reviewing the medical
history is an important
part of a thorough
medical examination.

disease, or abnormality and (2) to evaluate the person's physical and
functional state to determine his or her aptitude for taking part in stressful performance tests. The physician will determine the extensiveness of
the examination.

For persons over 35 years of age and those with symptoms of cardiovascular disease, the medical examination should include an exercise
stress test—a work test on either a bicycle ergometer or treadmill while
a physician monitors heart rate, blood pressure, and electrocardio-
graphic pattern. The stress test is designed to reveal possible latent
ischemic disease and to determine the person's cardiovascular functional capacity to ensure that the person does not engage in a testing
program that exceeds his or her capacity. (Consult a physician for additional information regarding stress tests.)

It should be mentioned that not everyone needs to have a medical
examination before initiating an exercise program or taking a fitness
test. For instance, healthy college students in their late teens and early
twenties without any coronary heart disease risk factors would probably
not need medical clearance before participating in a testing program.
However, a person who has any of the risk factors identified in Chapter
6 should have a medical examination before engaging in a physical
fitness testing program.

Evaluating Body Composition

The objective of body composition evaluation is to determine the relative percentages of body fat and lean body mass or weight. The first step in assessing body composition is to determine the individual's weight and compare it to the desirable weight for persons of similar sex, age, height, and body frame. Next, measurements of selected body parts (anthropometric measurements) are taken to reveal the individual's general physique and how it compares with desirable physiques. Finally, the percentage of body fat is determined.

Measurement of Body Weight

Overweight has been defined as weighing more than what is recommended in height-weight tables for a person of the same age, sex, height, and body frame. Individuals weighing less than the recommended weight would be considered underweight. How do you rate? You may make this determination by following these instructions:

1. Have a partner determine your height and body frame. Most medical scales have height indicators. Frame size can be determined by following the instructions in Table 5.2.
2. Determine your weight in pounds while wearing indoor clothing and shoes.

TABLE 5.2 Determination of Frame Size

Instructions

Extend your arm and bend the forearm upward at a 90 degree angle. Keep fingers straight and turn the inside of your wrist toward your body. If you have calipers, use them to measure the space between the two prominent bones on either side of your elbow. Without calipers, place thumb and index finger of the other hand on these two bones. Measure the space between your fingers against a ruler or tape measure. Compare it with the measurements in this table, which are elbow measurements for *medium-framed* men and women. Measurements lower than those listed indicate you have a small frame, and higher measurements indicate a large frame.

Measurements			
Height in 1″ Heels	Elbow Breadth	Height in 1″ Heels	Elbow Breadth
Men		Women	
5′2″–5′3″	2½″–2⅞″	4′10″–4′11″	2¼″–2½″
5′4″–5′7″	2⅝″–2⅞″	5′0″–5′3″	2¼″–2½″
5′8″–5′11″	2¾″–3″	5′4″–5′7″	2⅜″–2⅝″
6′0″–6′3″	2¾″–3⅛″	5′8″–5′11″	2⅜″–2⅝″
6′4″	2⅞″–3¼″	6′0″	2½″–2¾″

Source: Courtesy of the Metropolitan Life Insurance Company.

TABLE 5.3   **Desirable Weights for Men**[a]

Height	Small Frame	Medium Frame	Large Frame
5′2″	128–134	131–141	138–150
5′3″	130–136	133–143	140–153
5′4″	132–138	135–145	142–156
5′5″	134–140	137–148	144–160
5′6″	136–142	139–151	146–164
5′7″	138–145	142–154	149–168
5′8″	140–148	145–157	152–172
5′9″	142–151	148–160	155–176
5′10″	144–154	151–163	158–180
5′11″	146–157	154–166	161–184
6′0″	149–160	157–170	164–188
6′1″	152–164	160–174	168–192
6′2″	155–168	164–178	172–197
6′3″	158–172	167–182	176–202
6′4″	162–176	171–187	181–207

[a]Weights at ages 25–59 based on lowest mortality. Weight in pounds according to frame (in indoor clothing weighing 5 lb and shoes with 1″ heels).

Source: Courtesy of the Metropolitan Life Insurance Company.

TABLE 5.4   **Desirable Weights for Women**[a]

Height	Small Frame	Medium Frame	Large Frame
4′10″	102–111	109–121	118–131
4′11″	103–113	111–123	120–134
5′0″	104–115	113–126	122–137
5′1″	106–118	115–129	125–140
5′2″	108–121	118–132	128–143
5′3″	111–124	121–135	131–147
5′4″	114–127	124–138	134–151
5′5″	117–130	127–141	137–155
5′6″	120–133	130–144	140–159
5′7″	123–136	133–147	143–163
5′8″	126–139	136–150	146–167
5′9″	129–142	139–153	149–170
5′10″	132–145	142–156	152–173
5′11″	135–148	145–159	155–176
6′0″	138–151	148–162	158–179

[a]Weights at ages 25–59 based on lowest mortality. Weight in pounds according to frame (in indoor clothing weighing 3 lb and shoes with 1″ heels).

Source: Courtesy of the Metropolitan Life Insurance Company.

3. Compare your weight with the desired weight for your sex, height, and body frame (see Table 5.3 or 5.4).
4. Record these data in the Physical Fitness Test Battery Profile Chart (Table 5.1) and wherever else this information is needed.

The importance of maintaining a desirable weight was discussed in Chapter 4. It is imperative to reiterate here that the weight ranges indicated in this chapter should be viewed as guides rather than absolute weights that each person must attain. One might weigh more than the weight indicated for one's height in the height-weight chart and be in perfectly good health. Muscular football players are examples of individuals who weigh more than deemed desirable by height-weight charts but who are able to function at an optimal level. These individuals have a high percentage of lean body mass rather than fat tissue.

Measurement of Selected Body Parts

One can get an idea of body proportions or general physique by measuring the circumference or girth of certain body parts. All that is needed is someone to take the measurements and a tape measure. Either an anthropometric steel flexible tape or clothed fiberglass tape is recommended.

Measurements should be taken at the following sites, as described:

Chest/bust. In the horizontal plane (at the nipple line), at the end of a normal expiration.

Waist. At the minimal abdominal girth, below the rib cage and just above the top of the hipbone.

Hips. At the symphysis pubis (between the anterior surfaces of the pubic bones) in front and at the outermost protrusion of the buttocks in back. The feet should be together when this measurement is taken.

Thigh. At a point midway between the hip and knee joints. The subject should be standing with both feet slightly apart and with legs straight.

Upper arm. At a point midway between the shoulder and elbow joints (at the maximum circumference of the upper arm). The subject's arm should hang slightly and should be slightly away from the body.

One or two persons should be instructed in the techniques of taking girth measurements, and these individuals should perform all the measurements. The persons who are measuring should be careful not to pull the tape so tightly that the underlying tissue and fat shift under the tape. The tape should be applied lightly but firmly with no indentation of the skin. All measurements should be taken at the exact sites indicated in the instructions. Persons being measured should be instructed to relax when measurements are being taken.

Here are recommended girth proportions for men and women, proposed by Bud Getchell.[1]

Proportions for Men

Chest. Should measure same as hips.

Waist. Should measure 5 to 7 inches less than chest or hips.

Hips. Should measure same as chest.

Thighs. Should measure 8 to 10 inches less than waist.

Upper arm. Should measure twice the size of the wrist.

Proportions for Women

Bust. Should measure same as hips.
Waist. Should measure 10 inches less than bust or hips.
Hips. Should measure same as bust.
Thighs. Should measure 6 inches less than waist.
Upper arm. Should measure twice the size of the wrist.

The underwater weighing technique for measuring body fatness is one of the most accurate indirect measurement procedures. However, this method requires elaborate and expensive equipment, entails complicated testing procedures, and is time-consuming to administer. Consequently, our recommended technique for measuring percentage of body fat will be skinfold calipers.

First, however, two simple methods of determining obesity are indicated: the mirror test and the pinch test. Though simple, these two methods can be used successfully even by people who are extremely overweight. The mirror test simply requires the person to disrobe and look at his or her nude body in a full-length mirror. If it looks like there's too much fat, there probably is.

The pinch test is a little more objective and reliable than the mirror test. It should be conducted according to the following instructions:

1. Stand in a relaxed position with the arms at the sides.
2. For women, have someone pinch the skin and underlying fat tissue at the triceps (midway between the elbow and the shoulder) and at the suprailiac skinfold site. The subscapular and thigh skinfold sites should be pinched for men. (See Figure 5.1 for the locations of these body sites.)

Evaluating Body Fatness and Body Leanness

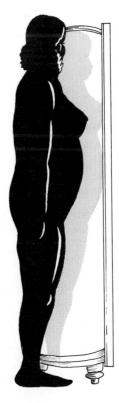

The mirror test. (*After drawing by Troy Frank.*)

3. The tester should pinch the skin with the thumb and index finger of one hand and measure the fat tissue with a ruler held in the other hand.

Scoring: Take the average of three measurements. An inch or more of fat tissue indicates too much fat. A little less than an inch of fat tissue for men would indicate too much fat.

Using Skinfold Calipers.   A practical and accurate method of assessing the percentage of body fat is taking measurements with skinfold calipers and converting these measurements to percentages by means of nomograms. Users of skinfold calipers to evaluate body fat should be aware of the probable errors inherent in such a technique. For example, Sloan and his coworkers reported an error variance of ± 3 percent of body fat for the prediction equations they used.[2] This means that percent body fat can be 3 percent below or above the value one gets when using the nomograms developed by Sloan and his coworkers.

The accuracy of using skinfold calipers to estimate body fat percent-

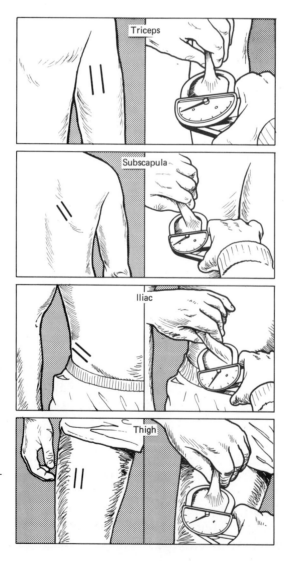

Figure 5.1
Anatomic locations of skinfold measurement sites.

ages also depends on the quality and accuracy of the calipers and the accuracy of the person taking the measurements. Therefore, only skinfold calipers that have been proven accurate should be used. Also, the person taking skinfold measurements should practice the technique several times before actual measurements are recorded to ensure that he or she can correctly identify the measurement sites and obtain consistent results.

The following recommendations are offered to help ensure valid and reliable measurements:

1. Only the persons who are trained to use the calipers should be allowed to take the measurements.
2. All measurements are taken on the right side of the body.
3. Grasp the skinfold between the thumb and forefinger and pull the skin and subcutaneous fat away from the underlying muscle.
4. Apply the calipers approximately ½ inch from the tips of the fingers. The skinfolds at the triceps and the thigh are measured in the vertical plane, and the measurements at the subscapula and the suprailiac are taken in the oblique plane (at a slant that runs in the natural fold of the skin). See Figure 5.1 for an illustration of the sites to be measured.
5. Allow the reading on the calipers to "settle" for three seconds, and then read the measurement to the nearest 0.5 mm. Take a third measurement if the first two are more than 0.5 mm apart. Record the average of the three measurements.
6. Measure different skinfold sites in succession; then repeat the procedure (e.g., triceps, suprailiac, triceps, suprailiac).
7. Descriptions of the locations for skinfold measurements are as follows:
   a. Triceps—the back of the arm midway between the shoulder and the elbow joint.
   b. Suprailiac—above the top of the hipbone (crest of the ilium) at the middle of the side of the body.
   c. Subscapula—just below the shoulder blade (scapula).
   d. Thigh—the front of the thigh midway between the hip and the knee.

Using Nomograms.   The percentage of body fat and body density can be evaluated quickly and accurately for men and women using graphs developed by Sloan and Weir (see Figures 5.2 and 5.3).[3] Skinfold measurements can be converted to percent body fat by using a straight edge (an index card will do) to draw a straight line connecting the skinfold values; this line will intersect the corresponding percentage of body fat and body density values. Suppose, for example, that a female has a skinfold measure of 24 for the triceps and 20 for the suprailiac site. The straight edge would be aligned with the suprailiac measurement (20 mm) and rotated to connect with the triceps measurements (24 mm). The percent body fat would be 25.5 percent (where the line connecting the two values crosses). The percentage of body fat should be determined and the number recorded in the chart in Table 5.1.

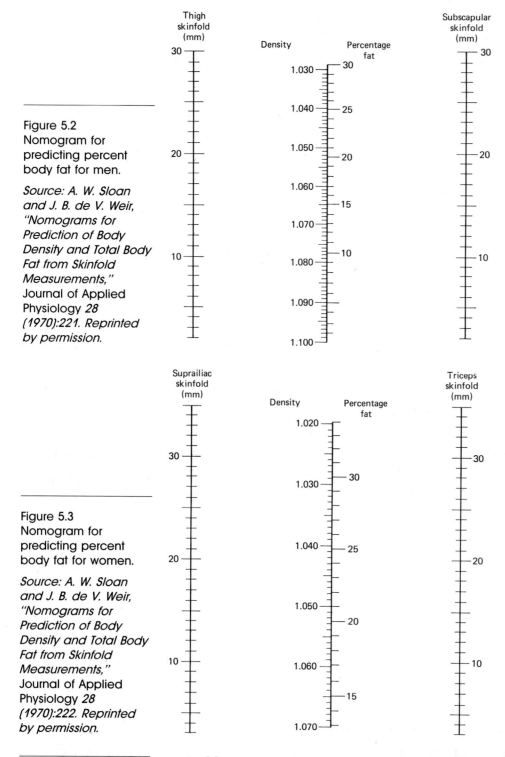

Figure 5.2
Nomogram for predicting percent body fat for men.

Source: A. W. Sloan and J. B. de V. Weir, "Nomograms for Prediction of Body Density and Total Body Fat from Skinfold Measurements," Journal of Applied Physiology *28 (1970):221. Reprinted by permission.*

Figure 5.3
Nomogram for predicting percent body fat for women.

Source: A. W. Sloan and J. B. de V. Weir, "Nomograms for Prediction of Body Density and Total Body Fat from Skinfold Measurements," Journal of Applied Physiology *28 (1970):222. Reprinted by permission.*

Body Fat Norms

Table 5.5 contains a rating scale with the various percentages of body fatness for college-age men and women. These norms were based on the average of ratings for a large group of subjects and may not be the most desired rating for each person. Furthermore, the norms were derived from measurements made on young Caucasian adults only. They do not reflect the body makeup of various racial and ethnic groups.

What is the proper percentage of body fat? While there is no one

TABLE 5.5   **Body Fat Norms**[a]

Rating	Women (%)	Men (%)
Very low fat: thin	14.0–16.9	7.0–9.9
Low fat: trim	17.0–19.9	10.0–12.9
Average fat: normal	20.0–23.9	13.0–16.9
Above normal fat: plump	24.0–26.9	17.0–19.9
Very high fat: fat	27.0–29.9	20.0–24.9
Obese: too fat	30.0+	25.0+

[a]Based on the Sloan formulas for young adult Caucasian men and women.

definitive answer, there are some guidelines that will aid in making this determination. The first guideline is to avoid becoming obese. Also, with the possible exception of jockeys and others whose occupation requires them to be light, one should strive not to be in the thin category. For the other ratings, some people might function better with above-normal fat and others might be more productive if they are trim. For instance, long-distance swimmers will benefit from a little more adipose tissue than normal because it helps to insulate them from the cold water. On the other hand, being trim will probably be advantageous to gymnasts. For them, any extra body fat is dead weight. Other than avoiding the extremes, the percentage of body fat a person carries should be influenced by his or her body frame, activity level, personal preferences, and occupation.

Determining Body Leanness

It cannot be emphasized too strongly that lean body mass should constitute most (80 to 85 percent) of total body weight. The lean body weight (LBW) can be calculated by subtracting the fat body weight (FBW) from the total body weight (TBW), where FBW is calculated by multiplying the percentage of body fat times the total body weight. Here are the formulas for these calculations:

$$FBW \text{ (lb)} = \% \text{ body fat} \times TBW \text{ (lb)}$$
$$LBW \text{ (lb)} = TBW - FBW$$

Here is an example of the calculation of body leanness using a female who weighs 150 pounds and whose percentage of body fat is 25.

$$FBW = .25 \times 150 = 37.5 \text{ lb (17 kg)}$$
$$LBW = 150 - 37.5 = 112.5 \text{ lb (51 kg)}$$

The 150-pound female with 25 percent body fat has 37.5 pounds of body fat and 112.5 pounds of lean body mass.

Evaluating Strength*

Strength is defined in this text as the ability of a muscle or muscle group to exert one maximal force against a resistance. It is impractical to

* General instructions and scoring instructions for testing large groups are in Appendix J.

evaluate the strength of every muscle or group of muscles in the body. However, the tests chosen will provide an indication of a person's overall strength. These include the grip strength for both dominant and nondominant hand and the bench press.

Grip Strength (Figure 5.4)

Purpose:	To test the strength of the flexor muscles of the forearm, hand, and fingers.
Description:	In a standing position, the person holds the hand dynamometer in one hand and exerts one maximum gripping force on the dynamometer. (See Table 5.6 for norms.)

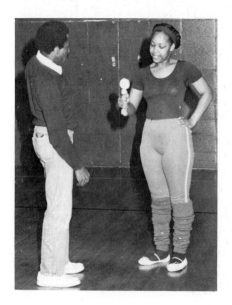

Figure 5.4
Assessing grip strength with a hand dynamometer.

TABLE 5.6 **Grip Strength Norms for Men and Women**

Fitness Category	Men—Grip (kg)		Women—Grip (kg)	
	Dominant Hand	Non-dominant Hand	Dominant Hand	Non-dominant Hand
Superior	70+	68+	40+	38+
Excellent	63–69	61–67	37–39	36–37
Good	58–62	56–60	35–36	34–35
Average	47–57	45–55	30–34	29–33
Fair	43–46	41–44	28–29	27–28
Poor	42 or fewer	40 or fewer	27 or fewer	26 or fewer

Bench Press (Figure 5.5)

Purpose: To test the strength of the pectoral muscles of the chest, the shoulder muscles, and the extensor muscles of the forearm.

Description: Lie flat on your back on a bench with the knees bent and the feet flat on the floor. Grip the bar with a palms-up grip, and keep the hands shoulder width apart. Extend the arms fully, pressing the bar upward. (Inhale as you prepare to lift the weight and exhale as you execute the lift.)

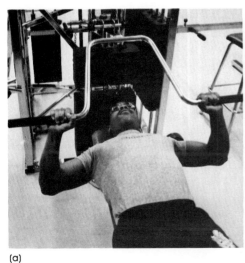
(a)

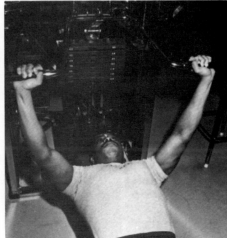
(b)

Figure 5.5
Bench press or chest press. (a) Start. (b) Finish.

Evaluating Muscular Endurance

Muscular endurance is the ability of a muscle or muscle group to exert repeated contractions against a resistance for an extended period of time or to maintain an isometric contraction for an extended time period. Tests chosen to measure muscular endurance are bent-knee sit-ups, pull-ups for men and flexed-arm hang for women, push-ups for men and modified push-ups for women, and squat thrusts.

Bent-knee Sit-ups (Figure 5.6)

Purpose: To evaluate the endurance of the abdominal muscles.

Description: Lie on your back with your hands on top of your head. Place both feet flat on the floor and flex the knees, forming an angle of approximately 90°. With a partner grasping your ankles to hold your feet down,* curl your

---

* The most difficult sit-ups are the ones performed without the feet being anchored down. Performing bent-knee sit-ups without assistance requires the abdominal muscles to do all the work. Some instructors might wish to have students perform such sit-ups.

back and raise your trunk off the floor until your elbows touch your knees. Return to the starting position and repeat the procedure as many times as possible in two minutes (or the time period set by the instructor). (Resting is permitted only when the subject is on his or her back with hands interlocked on top of the head.) (See Table 5.7 for norms.)

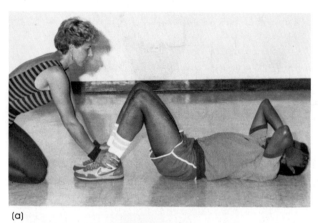

(a)

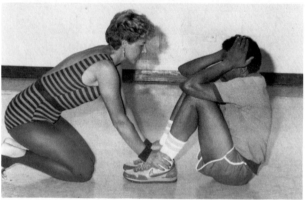

(b)

Figure 5.6
Bent-knee sit-ups.
(a) Start. (b) Finish.

TABLE 5.7   Sit-up Norms for Men and Women

Fitness Category	Men (no.)	Women (no.)
Superior	75+	57+
Excellent	69–74	54–56
Good	53–68	45–53
Average	36–52	33–44
Fair	21–35	20–32
Poor	20 or fewer	19 or fewer

Pull-ups (Figure 5.7)*

Purpose: To evaluate the endurance of the biceps, the primary muscle of the major muscle group used in this move-

* The flexed-arm hang (Figure 5.8) should be used for anyone who cannot perform pull-ups.

ment. Muscles in the shoulder girdle and back are also used to some degree.

Description: Grasp the horizontal bar with both hands (palms facing forward) and assume a "dead hang" position with the arms fully extended and the feet off the floor. Raise the body until the chin is above the bar; then lower the body until the arms are fully extended. Repeat this procedure as many times as possible. (See Table 5.8 for norms.)

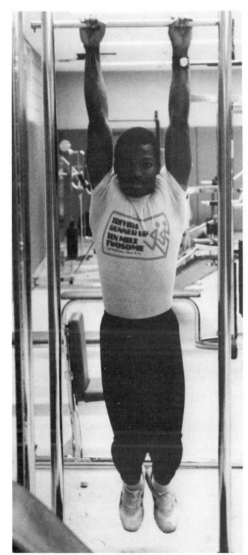
(a)

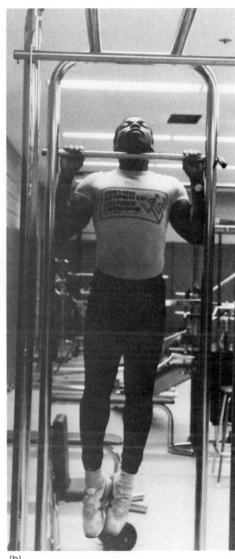
(b)

Figure 5.7
Pull-ups.
(a) Start. (b) Finish.

TABLE 5.8   **Norms for Pull-ups (Men) and Flexed-Arm Hang (Women)**

Fitness Category	Pull-ups (no.)	Flexed-Arm Hang (sec.)
Superior	20+	47+
Excellent	15–19	39–46
Good	12–14	27–38
Average	7–11	17–26
Fair	4–6	15–16
Poor	3 or fewer	14 or less

Flexed-arm Hang (Figure 5.8)

Purpose: To evaluate the endurance of the biceps, the primary muscle used in this movement. Muscles in the shoulder girdle and back are also used to some degree.

Description: Grasp the horizontal bar with both hands (palms facing forward) and assume a hanging position with the arms flexed, the chin above the bar, and the feet off the floor. Hold this position as long as possible. (See Table 5.8 for norms.)

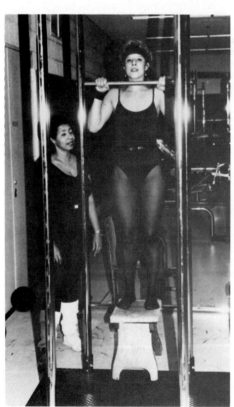 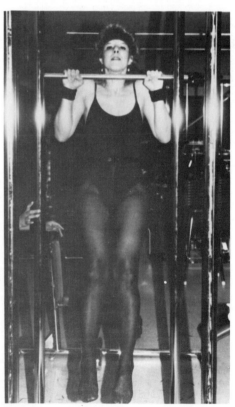

Figure 5.8
Flexed-arm hang.
(a) Start. (b) Finish.

(a)   (b)

Push-ups (Figure 5.9)

Purpose: To test the endurance of the triceps muscle, the primary muscle in the extensor muscle group of the forearm. The muscles of the shoulder girdle and wrist are also involved in this movement.

Description: Assume a prone position on the floor with the hands aligned even with the shoulder joints, the elbows fully extended, the legs straight and together, and the toes in contact with the floor. From this position, lower the body by bending the elbows until the chest touches the floor (or the spotter's hand); then return to the starting position by pushing up with the hands and extending the elbows fully. Keep the body straight throughout the push-up movement. Repeat this procedure as many times as possible in one minute without stopping or resting between push-ups. (See Table 5.9 for norms.)

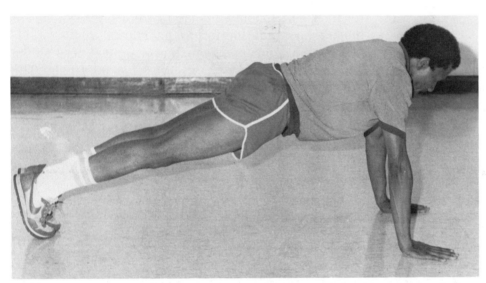

(a)

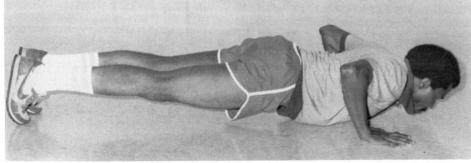

(b)

Figure 5.9
Push-ups. (a) Start.
(b) Finish.

TABLE 5.9   **Norms for Push-ups (Men) and Modified Push-ups (Women)**

Fitness Category	Push-ups (no.)	Modified Push-ups (no.)
Superior	55+	45+
Excellent	50–54	40–44
Good	45–49	35–39
Average	38–44	25–34
Fair	30–37	18–24
Poor	29 or fewer	17 or fewer

Modified Push-ups (Figure 5.10)

Purpose: This test is designed to serve the same purpose as the regular push-up, only it is modified to suit the needs of those who cannot perform regular push-ups.

Description: Assume a front support position with the knees on the floor and bent so the legs are at a 90° angle. The modified push-ups are performed as described for the regular push-ups. (See Table 5.9 for norms.)

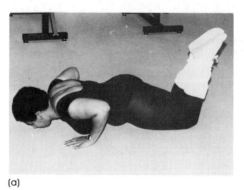 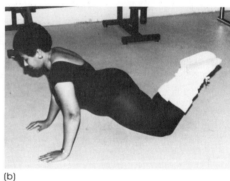

(a)   (b)

Figure 5.10
Modified Push-ups.
(a) Start. (b) Finish.

Squat Thrusts (Figure 5.11)

Purpose: To test the endurance of the flexor and extensor muscles of the legs.

Description: This test is performed in four counts or stages. To start, stand erect with the feet together and the hands at the sides. (1) Squat to assume a position on the floor with the hands in front of your feet and your knees bent. (2) Thrust your legs to the rear so the body is in a front support position (with the body straight and only the hands and toes touching the floor). (3) Return the feet back to the hands so that the body is again in the squat position. (4) Straighten up to a standing position. Repeat as many times as you can in thirty seconds.(See Table 5.10 for norms.)

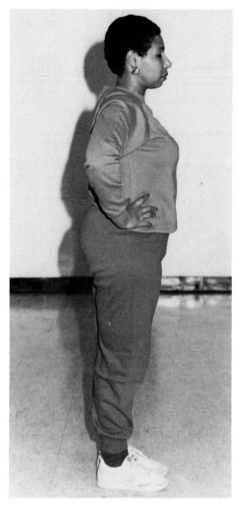

(a)

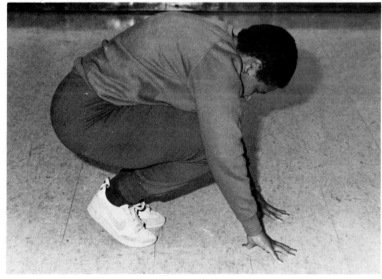

(b)

Figure 5.11
Squat thrusts.
(a) Standing.
(b) Squat position.
(c) Front leaning
position.
(d) Return to standing
position.

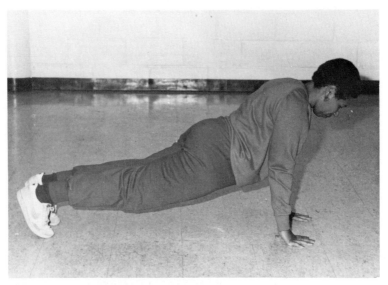

(c)

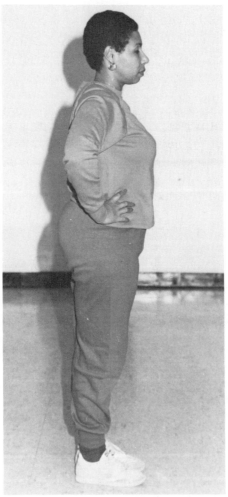

(d)

TABLE 5.10   **Squat Thrusts Norms for Men and Women**

Fitness Category	Men (no.)	Women (no.)
Superior	23+	19+
Excellent	21–22	17–18
Good	19–20	15–16
Average	17–18	13–14
Fair	15–16	11–12
Poor	14 or fewer	10 or fewer

Evaluating Flexibility

Flexibility is the ability of a muscle or muscle group to move body parts through their full range of motion. Good flexibility requires muscles that are strong yet lithe. Flexibility is important for proper execution of everyday activities such as house cleaning and dressing, which require bending, twisting, and reaching, as well as specialized sports activities such as gymnastics and dance.

It is important to engage on a regular basis in activities that require flexibility because so many jobs require sitting for long periods of time, which results in the muscles' losing their elasticity, thereby diminishing joint flexibility. This often results in shortened muscles, low-back pain, and general lack of mobility of body parts.

Developing adequate flexibility is also an important means of injury prevention, especially when engaging in activities that require a wide range of motion—gymnastics, track and field events, and racquetball are examples.

Activities chosen to evaluate flexibility are the sit-and-reach test (mainly for trunk flexion) and the back arch test (for trunk extension). These tests, designed to evaluate the flexibility of the lower back and trunk, including the hip joint, also indicate the muscle suppleness of the back of the thighs.

Flexibility is specific to a particular joint or combination of joints. Therefore, one might be flexible in one body area and lack flexibility in some other area. Engage in the exercises and activities in Chapter 11 if you discover that you need greater flexibility in some body parts.

Sit and Reach (Figure 5.12)

Purpose: To measure the flexibility of the hip and trunk areas, concentrating mainly on the degree of trunk flexion, which involves the trunk extensor muscles and the hamstring muscles (in the back of the thighs).

Description: Assume a sitting position with your legs fully extended and the soles of your feet flat against a box (or any flat surface on which a ruler can be placed). Place a ruler on top of the box so it extends 7 inches in front of the nearest edge (commercial sit-and-reach equipment can also be used; see Figure 5.12). Extend your hands and arms as far as possible and hold this position for 3 seconds. Measure the distance the fingertips reach on the ruler. (See Table 5.11 for norms.)

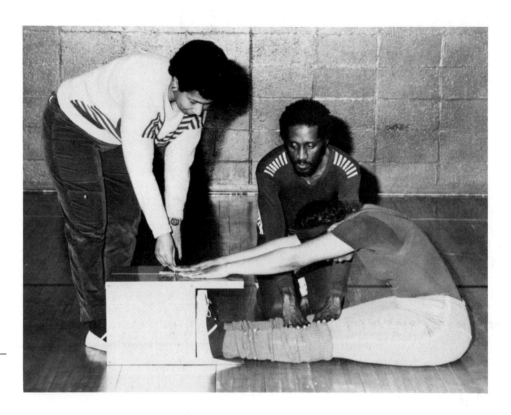

Figure 5.12
Sit and reach.

TABLE 5.11   **Sit-and-Reach Test Norms for Men and Women**[a]

Fitness Category	Men (in.)	Women (in.)
Superior	24+	28+
Excellent	22–23	24–27
Good	20–21	21–23
Average	14–19	16–20
Fair	12–13	13–15
Poor	11 or less	12 or less

[a]Adults 18 and over.

Back Arch (Figure 5.13)

Purpose:	To measure the flexibility of the lower back (trunk extension).
Description:	Assume a prone (face-down) position on the floor with

a partner kneeling astride you holding your buttocks and legs down. With your fingers interlocked behind your neck, raise your chest and head off the floor as high as possible. Hold this position for 3 seconds. Measure the distance from the floor to the chin. (See Table 5.12 for norms.)

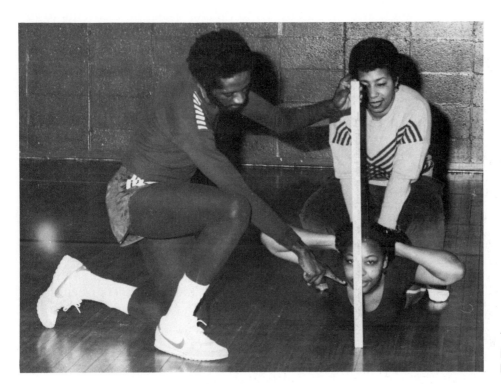

Figure 5.13
Back arch.

TABLE 5.12   **Back Arch Test Norms for Men and Women**

Fitness Category	Men (in.)	Women (in.)
Superior	20+	24+
Excellent	18–19	22–23
Good	16–17	20–21
Average	14–15	18–19
Fair	12–13	16–17
Poor	11 or less	15 or less

Evaluating Cardiorespiratory Endurance

As was stated in Chapter 2, in my opinion cardiorespiratory endurance is the single most important fitness component. It indicates the ability of the heart, lungs, and blood vessels to deliver essential nutrients to the working muscles and remove waste materials from the body.

Tests of cardiorespiratory endurance are designed to determine how the heart, lungs, and blood vessels respond to the increased demands that are placed on them during aerobic activities lasting more than a few minutes in duration. Are these body systems able to deliver oxygen to the working muscles and remove carbon dioxide from the muscles? How much of an increase in heart rate is necessary to handle the increased workload, and how quickly does the heart rate return to its resting rate? The answer to these and other questions will provide an indication of the condition of the cardiorespiratory system.

Several tests are available to measure cardiorespiratory endurance. Laboratory tests usually involve having the subjects perform a demanding work task on either a treadmill or a bicycle ergometer and measuring the maximal oxygen uptake (vO_2 max). Other tests, which have been correlated highly with the more precise laboratory tests, are more suitable for testing large groups of individuals. Two field tests of cardiorespiratory endurance are described: the 12-minute run-walk test and the step test.

A test to determine the resting heart rate is also presented. The resting heart rate is an important measure of cardiorespiratory endurance. Generally, the lower the resting heart rate, the more efficient the cardiorespiratory system. It should be stated, however, that while a low resting heart rate is a general indication of good cardiorespiratory functioning, it does not necessarily follow that a high resting heart rate means that a person has a poorly functioning cardiorespiratory system. Besides the strength and efficiency of the heart muscle, the resting heart rate is influenced by many other physiological, psychological, and environmental factors. Evaluating the resting heart rate along with the other measures of cardiorespiratory fitness should present a comprehensive evaluation of cardiorespiratory endurance.

Resting Heart Rate (Figure 5.14)

Purpose: To determine the number of times the heart beats per minute while the body is at rest.

Description: Sit quietly and relax. After 3 to 5 minutes, locate the pulse by placing your fingers (not the thumb because it has its own pulse) on the carotid artery (located on the side of the neck just under the jaw) or at the radial artery (located on the thumb side of the wrist). Press lightly at the chosen site, and when the pulse is located and the signal to begin is given, count the number of

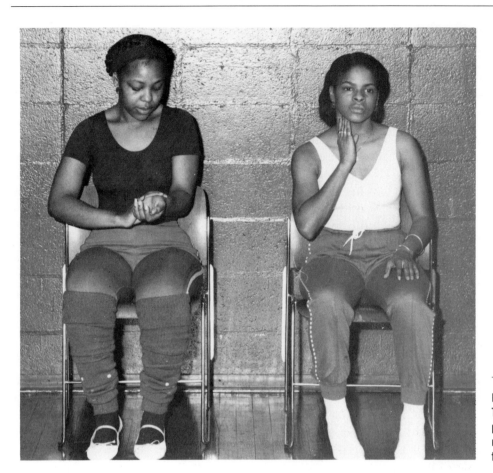

Figure 5.14
Taking the heart rate or
pulse rate at (left) the
radial artery and (right)
the carotid artery.

TABLE 5.13   **Norms for Resting Heart Rate for Men and Women**[a]

Classification	Men	Women
Excellent	49 or less	51 or less
Very Good	50–59	52–63
Good	60–68	64–75
Average	69–78	76–87
Fair	79–88	88–99
Poor	89+	100+

[a]Based on tests of men and women aged 18 to 25 years.

Source: Health and Physical Fitness: Taking Charge of Your Health *by William P. Marley. Copyright © 1982 by CBS College Publishing. Reprinted by permission of CBS College Publishing.*

times the heart beats (the "pulse" rate) for 30 seconds. Double this number to get the resting heart rate for one minute.*(See Table 5.13 for norms.)

* Subjects might be instructed to take their resting heart rate when they awaken and are still in a reclined position. This should provide the most accurate count of the resting heart rate.

12-Minute Run-Walk (Figure 5.15)

Purpose: To evaluate cardiorespiratory endurance by measuring the distance a subject is able to cover in a maximal effort run (or run-walk) of 12 minutes and comparing this distance with preestablished norms that indicate the rate and value of oxygen consumption, an important criterion of cardiorespiratory capacity.

Description: Run or run and walk as many laps or cover as great a distance as possible in a 12-minute time period. Walking is permitted; however, the more you walk, the less distance you are able to cover. (See Table 5.14 for norms.)

QUARTER-MILE TRACK   100-YARD STRAIGHTAWAY

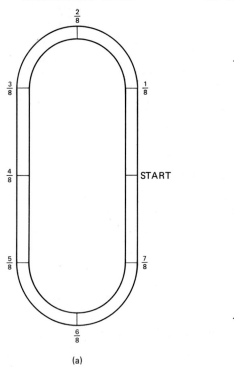
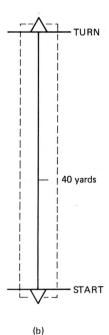

Figure 5.15
Run-walk sites.
(a) Quarter-mile track.
(b) 100-yard straightaway.

**TABLE 5.14   Norms for the 12-Minute Run-Walk Test for Men and Women
(distance covered, in miles)**

Fitness Category	Males (by age)					
	13–19	20–29	30–39	40–49	50–59	60+
Superior	> 1.87	> 1.77	> 1.70	> 1.66	> 1.59	> 1.56
Excellent	1.73–1.86	1.65–1.76	1.57–1.69	1.54–1.65	1.45–1.58	1.33–1.55
Good	1.57–1.72	1.50–1.64	1.46–1.56	1.40–1.53	1.31–1.44	1.21–1.32
Fair	1.38–1.56	1.32–1.49	1.31–1.45	1.25–1.39	1.17–1.30	1.03–1.20
Poor	1.30–1.37	1.22–1.31	1.18–1.30	1.14–1.24	1.03–1.16	.87–1.02
Very poor	< 1.30	< 1.22	< 1.18	< 1.14	< 1.03	< 0.87

Fitness Category	Females (by age)					
	13–19	20–29	30–39	40–49	50–59	60+
Superior	> 1.52	> 1.46	> 1.40	> 1.35	> 1.31	> 1.19
Excellent	1.44–1.51	1.35–1.45	1.30–1.39	1.25–1.34	1.19–1.30	1.10–1.18
Good	1.30–1.43	1.23–1.34	1.19–1.29	1.12–1.24	1.06–1.18	0.99–1.09
Fair	1.19–1.29	1.12–1.22	1.06–1.18	0.99–1.11	0.94–1.05	0.87–0.98
Poor	1.00–1.18	0.96–1.11	0.95–1.05	0.88–0.98	0.84–0.93	0.78–0.86
Very poor	< 1.00	< 0.96	< 0.95	< 0.88	< 0.84	< 0.78

Source: Kenneth H. Cooper, The Aerobics Way *(New York: Bantam Books, 1977), pp. 88–89.*

Step Test (Figure 5.16)

The step test, a heart-rate recovery test, is a modification of the Harvard Step Test developed in 1943 by Lucien Brouha and associates at the Harvard University Fatigue Laboratory. Although not as highly correlated with laboratory tests that measure maximal oxygen uptake as the 12-minute run-walk test, the step test is an acceptable alternative to the running tests. Certain features make the step test especially appealing as a test of cardiorespiratory endurance: It is easy to administer and can be administered to a large group indoors; it is not too time-consuming, it requires little equipment, and it is easy to evaluate.

The logic behind the step test is that for a submaximal work task a person with a higher level of cardiorespiratory endurances will not only have a smaller increase in exercise heart rate but that following the work task the recovery heart rate will be faster. In other words, following a submaximal work task, the heart rate for a person in good cardiorespiratory condition will return to normal much faster than a person who has a lower level of cardiorespiratory endurance.

Purpose: To evaluate the recovery rate as a measure of cardiorespiratory endurance.

Description: Step up and down on an 18-inch bench or box for 3 minutes at a rate of 30 steps per minute. Begin with either foot, but step down first with the same lead foot used to step up with (example: right, left, right, left). (See Table 5.15 for norms.)

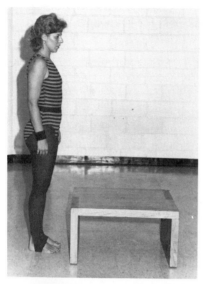

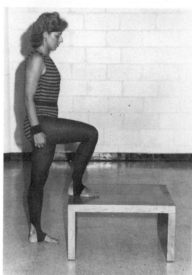

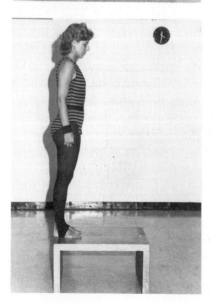

Figure 5.16
Stepping sequence for
the step test.

TABLE 5.15 **Norms for the Step Test for Men and Women**[a]

Fitness Category	Men	Women
Superior	105–97	105–95
Excellent	125–104	127–106
Good	145–124	150–128
Average	164–146	176–152
Fair	187–166	199–175
Poor	207–181	222–189
Very Poor	217–206	233–221

[a]Based on step test scores for college-aged men and women who used an 18-inch bench for the testing.

Source: Adapted from Bud Getchell, Physical Fitness: A Way of Life, *3d ed. (New York: Wiley, 1983), pp. 222–225.*

Concluding Remarks

The importance of evaluating your present level of physical fitness cannot be overemphasized. An assessment of your current state of fitness can provide the information necessary to plan intelligently a realistic physical fitness program. It will also provide you with the data to measure the progress you make when participating in a physical fitness program in a school setting or through a personally developed individualized program.

It is essential that your overall fitness status be assessed. For example, it is as important to know whether you are obese or have a normal resting heart rate as it is to know your level of cardiorespiratory endurance. The test battery in this chapter is designed to evaluate your overall fitness status. It includes tests to assess the health-related components of fitness: body composition, muscular endurance, strength, flexibility, and cardiorespiratory endurance.

Sometimes more than one test is presented for the assessment of a particular fitness component. In these cases you should use the test that is most suitable for your particular situation, considering such factors as facilities and equipment required for the test and personnel to administer the test. Remember that a medical examination should precede any involvement in a strenuous testing program.

Ultimately you should aim to develop and maintain a state of physical fitness at a level that is appropriate for your age, occupation, physical capacity, and recreational and personal interests. Therefore, you should not be compulsive about comparing your scores on the fitness tests with others. It might be helpful as a first step, however, to use the norms that

TABLE 5.16   Fitness Data for Men: Conversion of Raw Scores to *t* Scores

t Score	Grip, Dominant Hand (kg)	Grip, Nondominant Hand (kg)	Sit-ups (no. in 2 min)	Pull-ups (no.)	Squat Thrusts (no. in 30 sec)	Step Test (no.)
80	84	76	83	19	34	97
79	83	75	82			99
78	82	74	80			101
77	81	73	79	18	33	103
76	80	72	78			105
75	79	71	77	17		107
74	78	70	75		32	109
73	77	69	74			111
72	76	68	73	16	31	113
71	75	67	71			115
70	74	66	70	15		117
69	73	65	69		30	119
68	72	64	67			121
67	71	63	66	14	29	123
66	70	62	65			125
65	68	61	64	13		127
64	67	60	62		28	129
63	66	59.5	61			131
62	65	59	60	12	27	133
61	64	58.5	58			135
60	63	58	57	11		137
59	62	57	56		26	139
58	61	56	54			141
57	60	55	53	10	25	143
56	59	54.5	52			145
55	58	54	51	9		147
54	57	53	49		24	149
53	56	52	48			151
52	55	51	47	8	23	153
51	54.5	50.5	45			155
50	54	50	44	7		157
49	53	49	43		22	159

have been provided to see how you rate in comparison with others of the same age, sex, and general physical condition.

Instructors should keep a record of the test scores of all classes and compile local norms. It is essential to keep testing data for tests for which no norms are provided in this book. Besides the uses previously mentioned for evaluation data from the testing program, the test results can also be used to aid in determining student grades.

Information is presented in the chapters that follow to help motivate those who need such a stimulus. Also included are principles, procedures, techniques, and activities for developing each of the fitness components covered in this chapter. This material should provide you with the necessary information to plan and conduct an effective fitness program, based on the assessment results of your present fitness status.

TABLE 5.16 (*Continued*)

t Score	Grip, Dominant Hand (kg)	Grip, Nondominant Hand (kg)	Sit-ups (no. in 2 min)	Pull-ups (no.)	Squat Thrusts (no. in 30 sec)	Step Test (no.)
48	52	48	41			161
47	51	47	40	6	21	163
46	50	46	39			165
45	49	45	38	5		167
44	48.5	44	36		20	169
43	48	43	35			171
42	47	42	34	4	19	173
41	46	41	32			175
40	45	40	31	3		177
39	44	39	30		18	179
38	43	38	28			181
37	42	37	27	2	17	183
36	41	36	26			185
35	40	35	25	1		187
34	39	34	23		16	189
33	38	33.5	22			191
32	37	33	21		15	193
31	36	32.5	19		14	195
30	35	32	18			197
29	34	31	17		14	199
28	33	30	15			201
27	32	29	14		13	203
26	31	28	13			205
25	30	27	12			207
24	29	26	10		12	209
23	28	25	9			211
22	27	24	8		11	213
21	26.5	23.5	6			215
20	26	23	5		10	217

Source: Data for pull-ups and step test are from Bud Getchell, Physical Fitness: A Way of Life, *3d ed. (New York: Wiley, 1983).*

TABLE 5.17   Fitness Data for Women: Conversion of Raw Scores to _t_ Scores

_t_ Score	Grip, Dominant Hand (kg)	Grip, Non-dominant Hand (kg)	Sit-ups (no. in 2 min)	Flexed-Arm Hang (sec.)	Squat Thrusts (no. in 30 sec)	Step Test (no.)
80	56	50	57	47	34	95
79	55	49.5	56	46		97
78	54	49	55	45	33	100
77	53	48	54			102
76	52	47	53	44	32	105
75	51	46	52	43	31	107
74	50.5	45	51	42		109
73	50	44.5	50	41	30	111
72	49	44	49			113
71	48.5	43.5	48	40	29	116
70	48	43	47	39	28	118
69	47	42.5	46	38		120
68	46	42	45	37	27	123
67	45	41	44			125
66	44.5	40.5	43	36	26	127
65	44	40	42	35	25	130
64	43	39.5	41	34		132
63	42.5	39	40	33	24	134
62	42	38	39			136
61	41.5	37.5	38	32	23	139
60	41	37	37	31	22	141
59	40	36.5	36	30		143
58	39	36	35	29	21	146
57	38	35	34			148
56	37.5	34	33	28	20	150
55	37	33	32	27	19	153
54	36.5	32.5	31	26		155
53	36	32	30	25	18	157
52	35	31	29			159
51	34.5	30.5	28	24	17	162
50	34	30	27	23	16	164
49	33.5	29	26	22		166

TABLE 5.18   _t_ Score Classification Scale

_t_ Score	Classification
75 +	Superior
65 to 74	Excellent
55 to 64	Good
43 to 54	Average
33 to 42	Fair
32 or less	Poor

TABLE 5.17 (*Continued*)

t Score	Grip, Dominant Hand (kg)	Grip, Non-dominant Hand (kg)	Sit-ups (no. in 2 min)	Flexed-Arm Hang (sec.)	Squat Thrusts (no. in 30 sec)	Step Test (no.)
48	33	28.5	25	21	15	169
47	32	28	24			171
46	31.5	27.5	23	20	14	173
45	31	27	22	19	13	176
44	30	26	21	18		178
43	29	25.5	20	17	12	180
42	28	25	19			182
41	27.5	24.5	18	16	11	185
40	27	24	17	15	10	187
39	26	23.5	16	14		189
38	25.5	23	15		9	192
37	25	22	14	13		194
36	24.5	21.5	13	12	8	196
35	24	21	12	11	7	199
34	23	20	11	10		201
33	22	19	10		6	203
32	21	18	9	9		205
31	20.5	17.5	8	8	5	208
30	20	17	7	7	4	210
29	19	16.5	6	6		212
28	18.5	16	5		3	215
27	18	15	4	5		217
26	17.5	14.5	3	4	2	219
25	17	14	2	3	1	222
24	16.5	13.5	1	2		224
23	16	13				226
22	15	12		1		228
21	14.5	11.5				231
20	14	11				233

Source: Data for pull-ups and step test are from Bud Getchell, Physical Fitness: A Way of Life, *3d ed. (New York: Wiley, 1983).*

1. Bud Getchell, *Physical Fitness: A Way of Life,* 3d ed. (New York: Wiley, 1983), p. 62.
2. A. W. Sloan, J. J. Burt, and C. S. Blyth, "Estimation of Body Fat in Young Women," *Journal of Applied Physiology,* 17 (1962):967–970.
3. A. W. Sloan and J. B. de V. Weir, "Nomograms for Prediction of Body Density and Total Body Fat from Skinfold Measurements," *Journal of Applied Physiology,* 28 (1970):222.

Notes

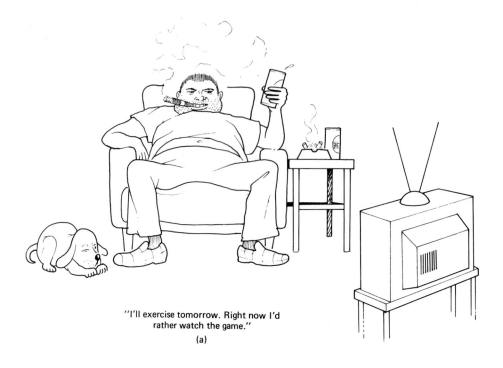

"I'll exercise tomorrow. Right now I'd rather watch the game."

(a)

Some individuals need outside motivation to exercise.

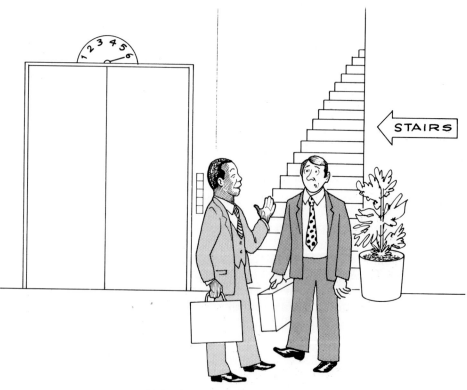

"It's only two flights. Let's walk up."

(b)

MOTIVATION FOR FITNESS

This section presents information to motivate individuals to initiate and adhere to a program of regular physical activity. The relationship of physical inactivity and other risk factors associated with cardiovascular disease is presented first. Then a chapter discusses the beneficial effects of regular participation in physical activities. Finally, specific motivational strategies and techniques are presented to aid in the initiation of and adherence to a physical fitness program.

CHAPTER 6

Risk Factors in Cardiovascular Disease

angina pectoris
arteriosclerosis
atherosclerosis
cardiac rehabilitation
cardiovascular disease
cholesterol
coronary heart disease
high-density lipoprotein

hyperlipidemia
hypertension
low-density lipoprotein
myocardial infarction
stress
triglyceride
type A personality

Key Words

After reading this chapter, you should be able to:
1. Define and/or explain the key words listed above.
2. Summarize the statistics regarding the leading causes of death in the United States in 1981 and the deaths due to cardiovascular diseases in 1980.
3. Identify the symptoms of myocardial infarction and angina pectoris.
4. Identify the normal blood pressure and the upper limit of normal blood pressure.
5. Identify the upper limits of the normal plasma lipids—cholesterol and triglycerides.
6. List three uncontrollable risk factors and seven controllable risk factors that are implicated in the development of coronary heart disease.
7. Identify the three primary risk factors and the four secondary risk factors.
8. Develop a rationale for the use of regular, aerobic exercise and a nutritional diet as a preventative measure against coronary heart disease.

Chapter Highlights

9. Describe the type A personality.
10. Determine a person's risk for heart attack or stroke.
11. Explain the role of exercise and diet in the cardiac
    rehabilitation process.

Cardiovascular (CV) disease refers to disease of the heart and blood vessels. Several cardiovascular diseases have been identified, including stroke, rheumatic heart disease, hypertension, and coronary heart disease.

Morbidity and mortality statistics regarding CV disease in the United States are both alarming and distressing. Based on 1981 provisional statistics, it was estimated that 42,750,000 Americans had one or more forms of heart or blood vessel disease. Of this number, 989,610 deaths

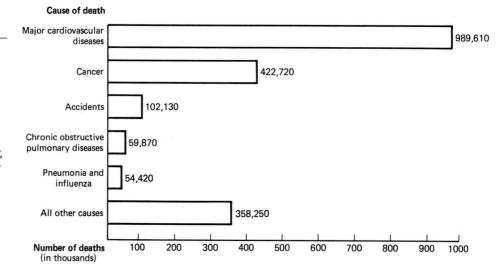

Figure 6.1
Leading causes of
death in the United
States, 1981 estimate.

*Source: American
Heart Association,
Heart Facts, (New York,
1984). (Based on data
from the National
Center for Health
Statistics, U.S. Public
Health Service,
Department of Health
and Human Services.)*

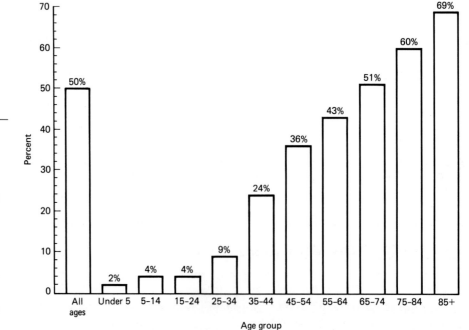

Figure 6.2
Percentage (by age)
of all deaths due to
cardiovascular
diseases in the United
States, 1980.

*Source: National
Center for Health
Statistics, "Advance
Report: Final Mortality
Statistics, 1980,"*
Monthly Vital Statistics
Report *32 (4) supp.*

TABLE 6.1   **Death Rates per 100,000 U.S. Residents in 1979**[a]

Cause of Death	Black Males	White Males	Black Females	White Females
Diseases of the heart	306.5	271.0	184.0	124.3
Cancer	223.4	125.6	124.8	104.5
Accidents	80.1	62.8	23.3	22.4
Cerebrovascular diseases	78.0	42.4	60.8	35.0
Homicide	69.2	9.9	13.8	2.9
Chronic liver diseases and cirrhosis	30.3	15.5	13.4	7.0
Influenza and pneumonia	24.0	14.2	10.8	7.5
Diabetes mellitus	17.0	9.2	20.8	7.6
All causes of death	1066.7	731.0	599.4	394.0

[a]These are age-adjusted death rates from all major causes, according to sex and race. The rates are based on population estimates rather than actual figures for 1979. These death rates are for comparative purposes only; actual death rates would vary greatly from the figures given here.

Source: Jacqueline J. Jackson, "Leading Causes of Death," Black Enterprise, May 1983, p. 36. Copyright May 1983 The Earl G. Graves Publishing Co., Inc., 130 Fifth Avenue, New York, NY 10011. All rights reserved.

resulted, making cardiovascular diseases the leading cause of death in the United States (Figure 6.1). As can be noted in Figure 6.1, other causes of death in 1981, in descending order, were cancer, accidents, chronic obstructive pulmonary diseases, and pneumonia and influenza. Clearly, CV diseases are the leading cause of death, accounting for 50 percent of all deaths in 1980 (see Figure 6.2).

Data regarding deaths due to cardiovascular disease will probably also be alarming to young persons who think that this disease only affects people in their middle or later years. While people in the 75–84 and 85+ categories have the highest incidence of death due to CV disease (60 and 69 percent, respectively), 24 percent of individuals in the 35–44 age category died from cardiovascular disease in 1980 (see Figure 6.2). It is also evident from data in Figure 6.2 that in 1980 some individuals in all age groups died as a result of CV disease.

An examination of death rates according to race and sex revealed that the black population had higher death rates than the white population for all the leading causes of death in 1979 (see Table 6.1). One can also see in Table 6.1 that the number of deaths per 100,000 United States residents was highest in the black male population for each of the leading causes of death, except diabetes mellitus, which was a little lower than the death rate for black females (17.0 versus 20.8).

Coronary Heart Disease

Coronary heart disease (CHD) is the leading single cause of death in the United States, accounting for more than a half million lives each year.

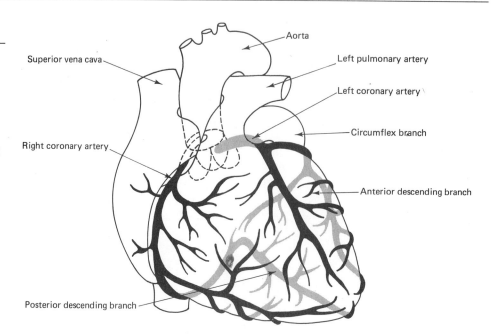

Figure 6.3
Coronary artery network in a healthy heart. The two main coronary arteries descend from the aorta, then divide and subdivide, girdling the entire heart in the manner of a crown.

Source: Redrawn from Heartbook, *copyright* © *1980 by the American Heart Association. Reprinted by permission of the publisher, E. P. Dutton, Inc.*

The heart is a muscle that pumps about 5 to 6 liters of blood each minute during regular activity and may increase its output to more than 20 liters of blood per minute during strenuous physical activity. Besides providing blood to body tissues via the general arterial circulation process, the heart must also supply itself with oxygen. Its nutrients are supplied through coronary arteries located in the heart muscle itself (see Figure 6.3).

Coronary heart disease is the result of a gradual buildup of cholesterol and other fatty substances in the inner layer of the walls of one or more of the coronary arteries in the heart. These fatty deposits cause a thickening of the inner walls of the coronary arteries and a narrowing of the vessels, resulting in a condition known as *atherosclerosis* (see Figure 6.4a). Atherosclerosis is a specific form of *arteriosclerosis* or hardening of the arteries. Arteriosclerosis occurs during the latter stages of athersclerosis when the buildup of these deposits, called *plaques,* results in a loss of pliability of the arteries, which leads to hardening of the arteries.

If the blockage of the coronary arteries results in a reduced oxygen supply that weakens the cells but does not kill them, a condition called *angina pectoris* might occur. *Myocardial infarction* results when an area of tissue in the heart dies because of prolonged deprivation of oxygen in the artery due to an interrupted blood supply.

Angina Pectoris

Angina pectoris is a chest pain caused by a temporary lack of adequate oxygen to the heart muscle. This condition usually occurs when one or more of the coronary arteries is partially closed (see Figure 6.4a). Angina can also be caused by spasm of the heart's blood vessels. In such cases angina might occur when the person is at rest. Drug therapy can be used to increase the blood supply to the coronary arteries in these cases.

The symptoms of angina pectoris (usually occurring when an individ-

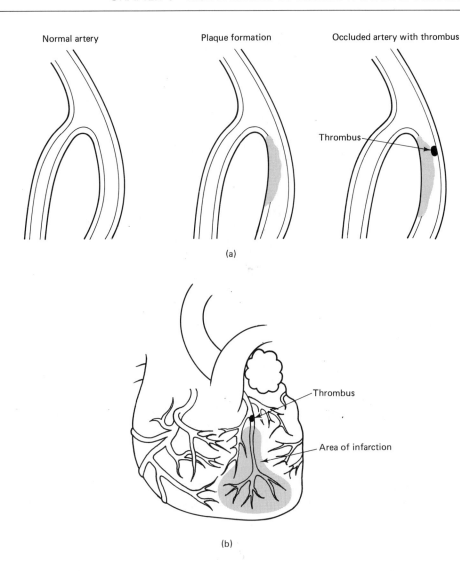

Normal artery   Plaque formation   Occluded artery with thrombus

Thrombus

(a)

Thrombus

Area of infarction

(b)

Figure 6.4
Atherosclerosis and infarction. (a) Enlarged coronary artery showing formation of fatty tissue (plaque) in the inner wall. (b) Heart with a thrombus (blood clot) obstructing the flow of blood in the coronary arteries, causing a heart attack or myocardial infarction.

Source: Redrawn from Heartbook, *copyright © 1980 by the American Heart Association. Reprinted by permission of the publisher, E. P. Dutton, Inc.*

ual is under physical or emotional stress, is engaged in strenuous exercise, or is eating a heavy meal), include discomfort in the chest area, in the left shoulder, neck, jaw and down the left arm. The pain associated with angina is transient, lasting for only a few seconds to a few minutes, and disappears if the individual stops the activity causing the discomfort or places a nitroglycerin tablet under the tongue.

Myocardial Infarction

As has been mentioned, this form of coronary heart disease occurs when one or more of the coronary arteries is closed or nearly closed so that no oxygen reaches the heart muscle, resulting in the death of muscle tissue in that area (see Figure 6.4b). Myocardial infarction is also called a "coronary" or a "heart attack."

Some of the symptoms of a myocardial infarction include a heavy pressure and dull aching pain in the chest area, which sometimes spreads to the left shoulder, down the left arm or down both arms, and into the neck and jaw. Shortness of breath, dizziness, sweating, and nausea are often associated with the severe pain. Unlike the transient pain associated with angina pectoris, the pain accompanying myocardial infarction might persist for several hours, unless relieved by drugs.[1] Acute myocardial infarction may result in immediate death.

Risk Factors in Coronary Heart Disease

Attempts to understand the causes and thus the control of coronary heart disease have resulted in many research studies on this topic. Based on the results of these studies, several risk factors have been identified as being correlated with CHD. Factors such as age, sex, race, and heredity are said to be uncontrollable. Other risk factors can be altered or controlled, including the primary factors of high blood pressure (hypertension), high levels of serum triglyceride and/or serum cholesterol (hyperlipidemia), and cigarette smoking; and the secondary factors of obesity, sedentary lifestyle, stress and personality type. This is not an exhaustive list of risk factors; these are simply the ones most often mentioned in discussions on the topic. Each will be discussed briefly.

Hypertension

Hypertension or high blood pressure means that the pressure needed to pump the blood through arteries is higher than normal. An average blood pressure is usually indicated as 120/80 for adults. The higher number represents the systolic pressure—the amount of pressure being exerted on the blood vessels during contraction of the heart. The lower number indicates the diastolic pressure—the force being exerted on the blood vessels during the rest between heartbeats.

Blood pressure varies according to age and sex. Children have somewhat lower pressure than adults, with an increase occurring about age 17. Women, most notably after age 40, normally have slightly lower blood pressure than men.

While acknowledging the difficulty of defining where normal ends and high blood pressure begins, Henry Blackburn noted that most experts set the upper limit of normal blood pressure at 140/90. He also indicated that blood pressures over this reading are potential cause for concern because of an increased risk of heart attacks, strokes, and other serious complications.[2] A reduction of salt intake, weight reduction for people who are obese, and increased physical activity for persons who lead sedentary lives are modalities used to reduce or control high blood pressure.

Hyperlipidemia

Hyperlipidemia is elevated serum triglyceride and/or serum cholesterol. Cholesterol, a soapy, waxy substance found in all body tissues, is a necessary component of the body, needed especially for cell structure and for the development of steroid hormones produced by the adrenal and sex glands. The liver is the principal producer of cholesterol in the body; cholesterol is also ingested through certain foods in the diet. Increased levels of cholesterol are produced with a diet high in saturated fats (foods such as dairy products and fatty meats). Polyunsaturated fats (those obtained from vegetable sources), however, are associated with lower blood cholesterol levels.

What is the normal level of blood cholesterol for an average American? This is a difficult question that almost defies an answer. There is a wide variation in normal plasma lipids, as indicated in Table 6.2. For instance, 95 milligrams per 100 milliliters of blood is the upper limit of normal blood cholesterol in fetuses, compared with 265 milligrams per 100 milliliters of blood in individuals 50 years old and over. The diets of children should contain even lower levels of cholesterol. Individuals who are concerned about the level of cholesterol in their blood should check with their physician. Advice for individuals with abnormally high cholesterol levels has been to reduce their dietary intake of high-cholesterol food, especially saturated fats. Some physicians and nutritionists have also advocated engaging in a vigorous exercise program as a means of lowering blood cholesterol levels.

Recent research and discussions regarding the relationship of cholesterol and certain protein "carriers" in the development of coronary heart disease have provided interesting insights into the problem. Cholesterol, which is one of several lipids in the blood, must be combined with a protein molecule to make them soluble in the blood fluid (serum). It is thus combined with protein molecules of different sizes and weights to form lipoproteins. Low-density lipoproteins (LDL) and high-density lipoproteins (HDL) are two of the carriers of cholesterol that have been studied in connection with coronary heart disease.

The low-density lipoproteins are thought to contain the largest proportion of cholesterol of any of the lipoproteins. A high ratio of LDL to total cholesterol (LDL-C) is thus implicated as a factor in the buildup of fatty lipids on the walls of the coronary arteries and is therefore significantly related to coronary heart disease. High-density lipoproteins, on the other hand, are thought to be of value in transporting fatty substances, including cholesterol, through the arteries. The higher amounts of HDL in relationship to total cholesterol (HDL-C) are believed to lower the risk of coronary heart disease.

TABLE 6.2   **Upper Limits of Normal Plasma Lipids**[a]

Age	Cholesterol	Triglycerides
Umbilical blood	95	65
1–9	200	140
10–19	205	140
20–29	210	140
30–39	240	150
40–49	265	160
50+	265	190

[a]Used to define hyperlipidemia at the Lipid Clinic, Methodist Hospital, Houston, Texas.

Source: David Kritchevsky, "Dietary Interactions," in B. Rifkind Levy et al., eds., Nutrition, Lipids, and Coronary Heart Disease, vol. 1 (New York: Raven Press, 1979), p. 249. Used by permission of Raven Press, New York.

The conclusion reached in a ten-year study of 3806 middle-aged men with high levels of cholesterol was that reducing total cholesterol levels by lowering LDL-C produced a corresponding lowering of risk of heart attack. Based on the study it was suggested that persons with moderate levels of cholesterol might use diet alone as a means of lowering the cholesterol levels. Individuals with high levels of blood cholesterol would probably be advised to use a drug such as cholestyramine to reduce LDL-C levels. It was concluded that for every percent reduction in plasma cholesterol there would be a 2 percent reduction in the incidence of coronary heart disease.[3]

Triglycerides are the other lipids in the blood that are associated with coronary heart disease. Triglycerides are contained primarily in very low density lipoproteins (VLDL). Like cholesterol, triglycerides are consumed in the diet and manufactured in the body. They are not ingested directly like cholesterol but are the end products of carbohydrate and fat metabolism. Triglycerides (carried by VLDL) are the primary means of transporting fat in the blood; they also act as storehouses for fats that are not immediately used for energy. These deposits can be seen in the unusually rotund abdomen, thighs, and arms of sedentary persons who eat diets excessively high in simple carbohydrates and saturated fats. VLDLs are converted to LDLs within a few hours after circulating in the bloodstream. These LDLs result in a buildup of fatty lipids on the arterial walls. That explains their association with CHD.

The same foods that are high in cholesterol are also high in triglycerides. As a general rule, all people should endeavor to keep their triglyceride level below 150 milligrams per 100 milliliters of blood. Current values used to define hyperlipidemia at the Lipid Clinic of the Methodist Hospital in Houston (see Table 6.2) may be used as guidelines for people of different ages. It cannot be emphasized too strongly that these values should not be considered as absolute in determining the level of blood lipids. One should not assume, for example, that if one is 21 years of age with a triglyceride level of 140 one is immune to premature death from coronary heart disease. Remember that high blood lipids is just one of many risk factors associated with coronary heart disease. It would be safe to keep your triglyceride level below the levels indicated here. Blood lipid levels can be regulated through diet and exercise.

Cigarette Smoking

Cigarette smoking is listed as a major risk factor in coronary heart disease by the American Heart Association, as well as other important groups and individuals. Cigarette smoking is also associated with lung cancer and other respiratory diseases. Because of the linkages, many national bodies concerned with preventive medicine have urged the elimination of smoking. These include the American Heart Association, the National Heart and Lung Institute, the Senate Select Committee on Nutrition and Human Needs, and the Inter-Society Commission Report for Heart Disease Resources.[4]

The number of cigarettes smoked daily and the number of years of smoking affect the degree of CHD risk from smoking. Smoking cigarettes low in tar and nicotine, taking fewer puffs, and not inhaling do not lower the health risks. Total abstinence is the only way to remove the risk of smoking as a factor in CHD. It is estimated by the American Heart Association that a person who smokes more than a pack of cigarettes a day has almost twice the risk of heart attack than a nonsmoker.

Not all the mechanisms linking smoking with CHD are fully understood. However, the harmful effects of two substances associated with cigarette smoking—carbon monoxide and nicotine—have been delineated.

Recent research has indicated that carbon monoxide in the smoke displaces oxygen from hemoglobin, forming carboxyhemoglobin (COHB). Carbon monoxide thus enhances the deposition of cholesterol in the walls of the arteries (part of the atherosclerotic process), thereby narrowing them and diminishing the supply of oxygen and other nutrients. Carbon monoxide comprises approximately 1 to 5 percent of cigarette smoke.[5]

Nicotine, the addictive element in tobacco, also acts on the cardiovascular system through the production of powerful stimulants called catecholamines. Heart rate and blood pressure are raised by the catecholamines, prompting the heart to work harder, thus requiring more oxygen. However, the volume of oxygen in the blood has been reduced by the increased carbon monoxide resulting from cigarette smoking. This combined effect of carbon monoxide and nicotine may be a predisposing factor in the development of coronary heart diseases.

Obesity and Physical Inactivity

Obesity alone is considered a secondary risk factor in the development of coronary heart disease. However, a combination of physical inactivity, consumption of a diet excessively high in saturated fats and simple carbohydrates, and obesity is associated with high blood pressure and stress on the heart and circulatory system. These conditions together are significantly implicated in coronary heart disease and deaths resulting from it.

Obesity is a condition whereby the body contains an excessive amount of fat tissue (usually expressed as a percentage). An adult male with 25 percent or more body fat or an adult female with over 30 percent body fat is considered obese.[6]

Until recently, the value of exercise as a protective measure against CHD was suggestive. For example, in 1974, Leon and Blackburn enumerated the following possible protective effects of exercise for CHD patients:[7]

1. Reduction of other coronary risk factors
2. Improved cardiovascular function and efficiency
3. Increased myocardial vascularity and coronary artery size
4. Increased resistance to ventricular fibrillation
5. Decreased tendency to thrombosis
6. Improved tolerance to stress

More recently (1985), Powell and Paffenbarger stated: "A reduced risk of coronary heart disease, desirable weight control, and the reduction of symptoms of anxiety and mild to moderate depression are established."[8] Not only are some researchers saying that habitual physical activity is associated with a reduced risk of coronary heart disease, but they also assert that "the effect of vigorous physical activity on CHD is independent of its effects on other known CHD risk factors such as hypertension, cigarette smoking, and obesity."[9]

In support of the value of vigorous physical activity in reducing coronary heart disease risk, Paffenbarger, in a study of more than 17,000 Harvard alumni between 1962 and 1978, found that habitual postcollege exercise predicts low coronary heart disease.[10] Paffenbarger indicated that favorable alterations in serum lipoprotein patterns and metabolic processes are examples of two mechanisms by which exercise influences body systems essential to cardiovascular health.[11]

Stress

Dr. Hans Selye, an internationally recognized endocrinologist who is considered by many to be the father of modern stress theory, defines stress as "the nonspecific response of the body to any demand made upon it."[12] In other words, although each demand made upon the body is unique or specific (shivering to produce heat when cold; sweating to help cool off when hot; increasing both the strength and frequency of heartbeats to get more blood to the working muscles during vigorous exercise), the response is general and predictable—to adapt to the condition or agent that causes the stress and thus reestablish internal equilibrium (homeostasis). The conditions or situations causing the body to respond and adapt are termed *stressors*.

Selye called this general response to stressors the "general adaptation syndrome" (GAS). It consists of three stages: (1) the alarm reaction, (2) the stage of resistance, and (3) the stage of exhaustion. During the alarm reaction stage, the body responds on a local level and in a general manner through actions by the nervous and glandular systems. During the stage of resistance, the body attempts to adjust to the stressor. If the body is unable to resist the stressor or if the stressful event persists for a long period of time, exhaustion (death) results.[13]

Although the body will automatically attempt to respond to stressors and adjust its actions accordingly, continual action on the body by stressors will cause the body to wear out. Thus it is necessary to learn to cope with the stressors of life. David Glass feels that our perception of the stressful event is critical in our reaction to that event. If a person views a stressor as harmful, for example, it will take a greater toll on the body than a stressor viewed as nonthreatening. This is the psychological stress reaction.[14]

Glass noted the relationship between cardiovascular function and stressors as well as between stress and serum cholesterol and catecholamines.* He also said that the physiological effects of stressors may depend on whether they are perceived as controllable or uncontrollable.

Dr. John Farquhar, director of Stanford's Heart Disease Prevention Program, believes that stress is the most pervasive of the risk factors in cardiovascular disease prevention. He indicates that people who learn stress management will be better equipped to make and maintain changes in other activities such as eating, smoking, and exercise habits.

---

* Catecholamines are hormones, including adrenaline and nonadrenaline.

TABLE 6.3   **Simplified Self-scoring Stress and Tension-Level Test**[a]

Behavior	Often	A Few Times a Week	Rarely
1. I feel tense, anxious, or have nervous indigestion.	2	1	0
2. People at work/home make me feel tense.	2	1	0
3. I eat/drink/smoke in response to tension.	2	1	0
4. I have tension or migrane headaches, or pain in the neck or shoulders, or insomnia.	2	1	0
5. I can't turn off my thoughts at night or on weekends long enough to feel relaxed and refreshed the next day.	2	1	0
6. I find it difficult to concentrate on what I'm doing because of worrying about other things.	2	1	0
7. I take tranquilizers (or other drugs) to relax.	2	1	0
8. I have difficulty finding enough time to relax.	2	1	0
9. Once I find the time, it is hard for me to relax.	2	1	0
10. My workday is made up of many deadlines.	2	1	0

Maximum total score = 20.   My total score: _____
[a]Circle the appropriate number for each item.

Source: Originally published in The American Way of Life Need Not Be Hazardous to Your Health *by John W. Farquhar, as a volume in* The Portable Stanford *series published by the Stanford Alumni Association. © 1978 by John W. Farquhar. Reprinted by permission of The Stanford Alumni Association.*

Farquhar identifies and discusses a stress management program consisting of the following six stages: (1) identifying the problem, (2) building confidence and commitment to change, (3) developing an awareness of stress sources and responses, (4) developing and implementing a stress management action plan, (5) evaluating the plan, and (6) maintaining the gains in effective stress management.[15] This stress management plan is similar to the self-modification-of-behavior plan presented in Chapter 8. (For further details, consult the reference by Farquhar.) Since both deal with the identification of the level of stress and related problem areas in stress management, the Simplified Self-scoring Test for Gauging Stress and Tension Levels and the Observer Behavior Rating Inventory are included here (see Tables 6.3 and 6.4).

The rating scale in Table 6.3 ranges from a score of 0–2 (considerably below average) to 14–18 (considerably above average). Each tension level is classified as a "zone":

Zone	Score	Tension level
A	14–18	Considerably above average
B	10–13	Above average
C	6–9	Average
D	3–5	Below average
E	0–2	Considerably below average

TABLE 6.4   Observer Behavior Rating Inventory[a]

	Never	Seldom (once or twice a week)	Often (almost every day)	Very Often (at least once a day)
1. Hurriedness: Eats and/or moves fast.	0	1	2	3
2. Talking: Speaks fast, in an explosive manner, repeats self unnecessarily, and/or interrupts others.	0	1	2	3
3. Listening: Has to have things repeated apparently because of inattentiveness.	0	1	2	3
4. Worries: Expresses worries about trivia and/or things he/she can do nothing about.	0	1	2	3
5. Anger/hostility: Gets mad at self and/or others.	0	1	2	3
6. Impatience: Tries to hurry others and/or becomes frustrated with own pace.	0	1	2	3

Maximum total score = 18   Subject's total score: _____

[a]Circle the number under the category that most accurately describes how often subject engages in the identified behavior.

Source: Originally published in The American Way of Life Need Not Be Hazardous to Your Health *by John W. Farquhar, as a volume in The Portable Stanford series published by the Stanford Alumni Association. © 1978 by John W. Farquhar. Reprinted by permission of the Stanford Alumni Association.*

Individuals who score in any zone but E should be interested in learning more about stress management. Anyone who completes Table 6.3 should seek the opinion of another person, who will use the rating inventory in Table 6.4. Compare the score you obtained with that of your "observer." Use the higher of the two scores; this is often the score of the observer, which is probably more objective. On the basis of this score, use either the self-modification-of-behavior plan in Chapter 8 or the plan presented by Farquhar. The important point is to use some systematic plan to change undesirable behavior patterns that are associated with coronary heart disease.

Type A Personality

Some individuals are believed to exhibit a personality profile that is associated with stress-filled activity. These persons do not manage stress effectively. They exhibit such behaviors as extreme competitiveness, hostility, impatience, and mistrust of others. Further, they are extremely time-conscious, success-driven, and anxiety-prone. These individuals try to meet too many poorly defined goals, frequently beginning new projects before completing old ones. They will let nothing interfere with their quest for "success." Things are more important to them than people. Friedman and Rosenman describe these individuals as Type A persons.[16]

The abnormal sense of "time urgency" and the fierce hostility exhibited by persons with Type A personalities are the main behaviors associated with coronary heart disease. However, a combination of stress-filled behaviors has been found to be more highly associated with coronary patients than noncoronary persons of the same age.

If you exhibit some of the behaviors of the Type A person, you are urged to modify these behaviors. It is hoped that you will try the self-modification-of-behavior plan presented in Chapter 8.

For people who are not physically active but can't seem to relax, participation in physical activity is suggested as a possible means of dealing with stress. Aerobic activities such as jogging, swimming, bicycle riding, and walking show promise as modalities in dealing with tensions and depression.[17] William Glasser, for example, feels that the "positive addiction" to running experienced by some running enthusiasts results because of the relaxation one enjoys while running.[18] A more in-depth discussion of the benefits of regular, vigorous exercise is presented in Chapter 7.

Are You at High Risk?

What is your overall risk of having a heart attack or stroke? Completion of the self-scoring test (Table 6.5) will provide some insights into your risk of having a heart attack or stroke. Be advised, however, that this test is not a substitute for sound medical advice and the need for

TABLE 6.5   Self-scoring Test of Heart Attack and Stroke Risk

Risk Factor	Increasing Risk				
I. Smoking cigarettes	None	Up to 9 per day	10 to 24 per day	25 to 34 per day	35 or more per day
Score	0	1	2	3	4
II. Body weight	Ideal weight	Up to 9 lbs. excess	10 to 19 lbs. excess	20 to 29 lbs. excess	30 lbs. or more excess
Score	0	1	2	3	4
III. Salt intake	$^1/_5$ average hard to do; no added salt, no convenience foods	$^1/_3$ average no salt at table, spare use of high-salt foods	U.S. average salt in cooking, some salt at table	Above average frequent salt at table	Far above average frequent use of salty foods
or Blood pressure upper level (if known)	Less than 110	110 to 129	130 to 139	140 to 149	150 or over
Score	0	1	2	3	4
IV. Saturated fat and cholesterol intake	$^1/_5$ average: almost total vegetarian; rare egg yolk, butterfat, lean meat	$^1/_3$ average: 2 meatless days/week, no whole-milk products, lean meat only	$^1/_2$ average: meat (mostly lean), eggs, cheese 12 times/week, nonfat milk only	U.S. average: meat, cheese, eggs, whole milk 24 times/week	Above average: meat, cheese, eggs, whole milk over 24 times/week
or Blood cholesterol level (if known)	Less than 150	150 to 169	170 to 199	200 to 219	220 or over
Score	0	1	2	3	4

a thorough medical examination at regular intervals. The test can be used as a general indicator to determine whether medical advice is needed.

The interpretation of the test scores is straightforward. The maximum number of points is 24.

TABLE 6.5 (*Continued*)

Risk Factor		Increasing Risk			
V. Self-rating of physical activity	Vigorous exercise 4 or more times/week 20 min each	Vigorous exercise 3 times/week 20 min each	Vigorous exercise 1 to 2 times/week	U.S. average: occasional exercise	Below average: exercises rarely
or Walking rating	Brisk walking 5 times/week 45 min each	Brisk walking 3 times/week 30 min each	Brisk walking 2 times/week 30 min each *or* Normal walking 4½ to 6 miles/day	Normal walking 2½ to 4½ miles/day	Normal walking less than 2½ miles/day
Score	0	1	2	3	4
VI. Self-rating of stress and tension	Rarely tense or anxious	Calmer than average	U.S. average: Feel tense or anxious 2 to 3 times/day	Quite tense, usually rushed	Extremely tense
or	Yoga, meditation, or equivalent 20 min, 2 times/day	Feel tense about 3 times/week	Frequent anger or hurried feelings	Occasionally take tranquilizer	Take tranquilizer 5 times/week or more
Score	0	1	2	3	4

Enter your total score here: _____

Notes:

a. Subtract 1 point if dietary fiber intake is high (almost all cereals whole grain, almost no sugar, and considerable fruit and vegetable intake).

b. Add 1 point if all exercise is competitive.

c. If you are a female taking estrogen or birth control pills, add 1 point if risk score is 12 or below, 2 points if score is 13 or above (especially if you smoke, are overweight, have high blood pressure or high blood cholesterol).

Source: Originally published in The American Way of Life Need Not Be Hazardous to Your Health *by John W. Farquhar, as a volume in The Portable Stanford series published by the Stanford Alumni Association. © 1978 by John W. Farquhar. Reprinted by permission of the Stanford Alumni Association.*

Zone A: 21–24 points. The probability of having a premature heart attack or stroke is about four to five times the U.S. average. Action is urgent. Try to drop four points within a month and three more points within six months.

Zone B: 17–20 points. Incidence of heart attack or stroke is about twice the U.S. average. Action is urgent. Try to drop four points within six months and continue reduction.

Zone C: 13–16 points. The U.S. average is 14. This is an uncomfortable and readily avoidable zone. Careful planning can result in a five- to six-point reduction within a year.

Zone D: 9–12 points. The likelihood of having a heart attack or stroke is about one-half the U.S. average. This is a zone rather easily achieved by most people within a year if they are now in zone B or C. Careful planning can result in a four- to six-point reduction within a year.

Zone E: 5–8 points. Incidence of heart attack or stroke is about one-fourth the U.S. average. This goal is achievable by many but often takes one or two years to reach.

Zone F: 0–4 points. Incidence of heart attack or stroke rates low, averaging less than one-tenth the rate in the U.S. 35–65 age group. This goal requires diligent effort and considerable family support and often takes three to four years to reach. Individuals in this range should be proud and gratified (and be committed to maintaining this low risk level).

If the test results indicate that you should change one or more health behaviors, check with a physician before embarking on a program of radical change. This book can provide physical activities that are useful in your behavior-change process. You are challenged to develop an active lifestyle and eating habits that reduce your risk of heart attacks or strokes.

Preventive measures such as diet, exercise, and sometimes drug therapy have been effective in reducing the premature development of coronary heart disease in many people with high-risk profiles. Unfortunately, however, some individuals have progressed to a point where conventional preventive measures are ineffective. They experience a heart attack. All is not lost for such persons. Modern methods of rehabilitation have been developed to provide help for patients with CHD who are beyond preventive measures of relief.

Cardiac Rehabilitation

Many methods are in use today for the restoration of the CHD patient to a complete and productive life. Rehabilitation includes restoring the physiological, psychological, social, vocational, and recreational aspects of human functions for the postcardiac patient. According to the American College of Sports Medicine (ACSM), many cardiac rehabilitation programs include the following intervention strategies: exercise therapy, psychological counseling, vocational counseling, and patient education and behavior modification regimens to encourage positive health lifestyles in the patients.[19]

Since the ability to function with greater independence and vigor is likely to foster positive attitudes regarding psychological and social aspects of life, an individually prescribed exercise program can be an especially useful and safe adjunct to any successful rehabilitation program for many kinds of postcardiac patients. Also, with the escalating cost of medical and health care, less costly means of rehabilitation must be sought and tried. The problem of costly medical care is especially acute in the black community, where unemployment is higher than the national average (almost double) and the income level is much lower than that of the average white American. Besides the therapeutic value of exercise as a rehabilitative modality, then, is its worth as an alternative to expensive medical procedures.[20]

Many medical centers provide cardiac rehabilitation services. For information on specific cardiac rehabilitation services, check with your local medical center. Also, use of a guide such as that developed by the ACSM or the American Heart Association's Committee on Exercise is recommended for persons developing exercise programs for individuals with cardiac problems.[21] It is imperative that each person, regardless of physical limitation, be helped to develop to an optimal level.

Notes

1. Elliot Rapaport, "Coronary Artery Disease," in American Heart Association, *Heartbook* (New York: Dutton, 1980), p. 180.
2. Henry Blackburn, "Risk Factors and Cardiovascular Disease," in ibid., p. 8.
3. Lipid Research Clinics Program, "The Lipid Research Clinics Coronary Primary Prevention Trial Results: I. Reduction in Incidence of Coronary Heart Disease" and "II. The Relationship of Reduction in Incidence of Coronary Heart Disease to Cholesterol Lowering," *Journal of the American Medical Association* 251 (1984):360, 373.
4. Jeremiah Stamler, "Population Studies," in B. Rifkind Levy et al., eds., *Nutrition, Lipids, and Coronary Heart Disease,* vol. I (New York: Raven Press, 1979), p. 78.
5. Richard J. Evans, J. Keith Thwaites, and John J. Witte, "Hazards of Smoking," in AHA, *Heartbook,* p 23.
6. A. W. Sloan, "Estimation of Body Fat in Young Men," *Journal of Applied Physiology,* 23 (1967):311–315; A. W. Sloan, J. J. Burt, and C. S. Blyth, "Estimation of Body Fat in Young Women," *Journal of Applied Physiology,* 17 (1962):967–970.
7. Arthur S. Leon and Henry Blackburn, "Physical Inactivity," in Norman M. Kaplan and Jeremiah Stamler, eds., *Prevention of Coronary Heart Disease* (Philadelphia: Saunders, 1974), p. 162.
8. Kenneth E. Powell and Ralph S. Paffenbarger, Jr., "Workshop on Epidemiologic and Public Health Aspects of Physical Activity and Exercise: A Summary," *Public Health Reports,* 100 (March–April 1985): 118.
9. David S. Siscovick, Ronald E. LaPorte, and Jeffrey M. Newman, "The Disease-specific Benefits and Risks of Physical Activity and Exercise," ibid., 187.
10. Ralph S. Paffenbarger, Jr., et al., "A Natural History of Athleticism and Cardiovascular Health," *Journal of the American Medical Association,* 252 (1984): 491.
11. Ibid., 495.
12. Hans Selye, *Stress Without Distress* (New York: Lippincott, 1974), p. 27.

13. Hans Selye, *The Stress of Life,* rev. ed. (New York: McGraw-Hill, 1976), pp. 36–38.

14. David C. Glass, *Behavior Patterns, Stress, and Coronary Disease* (New York: Wiley, 1977), pp. 10–22.

15. John W. Farquhar, *The American Way of Life Need Not Be Hazardous to Your Health* (New York: Norton, 1979), p. 59.

16. Meyer Friedman and Ray W. Rosenman, *Type A Behavior and Your Heart* (Greenwich, Conn.: Fawcett, 1974).

17. William P. Morgan, "Psychological Benefits of Physical Activity," in F. Nagle and H. Montoye, eds., *Exercise, Health, and Disease* (Springfield, Ill.: Thomas, 1981); William P. Morgan et al., "Psychological Effects of Chronic Physical Activity," *Medicine and Science in Sports* 2 (1970):213–217.

18. William Glasser, *Positive Addiction* (New York: Harper & Row, 1976).

19. American College of Sports Medicine, *Guidelines for Exercise Testing and Prescription,* 3d ed. (Philadelphia: Lea & Febiger, 1986), p. 53.

20. "Good Health," *Black Enterprise,* May 1983, pp. 36–43.

21. ACSM *Guidelines for Exercise Testing and Prescription;* American Heart Association Committee on Exercise, *Exercise Testing and Training of Individuals with Heart Disease or at High Risk for Its Development: A Handbook for Physicians* (Dallas, 1975).

CHAPTER 7

Values of Physical Activity

effects of exercise	values of exercise
older adult	work capacity

After reading this chapter, you should be able to:
1. Define and/or explain the key words listed above.
2. List and discuss the effects of physical activity on the systems of the body.
3. List and discuss the effects of physical inactivity on the systems of the body.
4. List the reasons people become engaged in programs of physical activity.
5. Compare and contrast the effects of physical activity on "normal" individuals and those with varying types of cardiovascular disease.
6. Compare and contrast the effects of physical activity on "normal" individuals up through adulthood.
7. Enumerate the three conditions and/or considerations said to be necessary to ensure the beneficial effects of physical activity.
8. Indicate the length of time the benefits of physical activity remain (the length of time before detraining occurs).
9. Develop a rationale for participating in regular, aerobic physical activity.

Myths and misconceptions abound regarding the benefits and dangers of engaging in strenuous physical activity. Some people refuse to engage in programs of physical activity because they feel either that it will be of no value or that it will damage their health. Conversely, many individuals have begun to participate in vigorous physical activity programs because they believe that such participation will prolong their life.

Media coverage given to isolated and unusual events associated with both famous and ordinary people as they participate in physical activity or avoid it helps to perpetuate extreme beliefs about physical activity. Some examples include the following: When former President Carter dropped out of a footrace in 1979, the headline on the front page of the *New York Times* was "Carter, Exhausted and Pale, Drops Out of 6-Mile Race."[1] The jogging death of a U.S. congressman in 1978 also received national attention.[2]

The most recent and highly publicized account of an exercise advocate who died while exercising was media coverage of the death of James Fixx, author of the best-selling text *The Complete Book of Running*. Fixx, the jogging advocate, died of a heart attack in July 1984 at the age of 52 while jogging in Vermont.

Fixx's heart attack while jogging points up the fact that although exercise does improve cardiovascular health, among other benefits, it does not guarantee immunity from coronary heart disease. In Fixx's case, according to news reports following his death, he failed to have medical examinations on a regular basis. An important principle of training, especially for individuals over 35 years old, is to undergo a medical examination (including an exercise stress test) before engaging in strenuous physical activity.

Since Fixx was aware of his family's history of coronary heart disease (his father died of a heart attack at the age of 43), he should have been even more diligent about getting regular checkups, including exercise stress tests with ECG monitoring.

The irony for Fixx, however, is that he showed no overt signs of coronary heart disease. In fact, during the ten years or so before his death, Fixx completed several marathons. He also quit smoking and reduced his weight from well over 200 pounds to approximately 160 pounds. These positive lifestyle changes notwithstanding, medical examination on a regular basis was advisable. Such examination might have revealed some latent coronary heart problem that could have been rectified, thus preventing a premature death.

Fixx's death certainly created a negative attitude toward physical activity in the minds of some people. Some who eschew physical activity will also echo the statement made by Dr. Robert M. Hutchins that when he got the urge to exercise, he would lie down until the sensation passed. Dr. Hutchins lived to be 78. In contrast, a person such as James Fixx, who changed from a sedentary to an active lifestyle, died of a heart attack at the age of 52 while jogging.

Although it is recognized that sudden death is a major cardiovascular complication of exercise, such deaths are rare. It has been estimated that the frequency of death among middle-aged joggers is only one death per 7620 joggers per year.[3]

This chapter summarizes the valuable contributions that a regular program of physical activity can provide, both for the healthy individual and for the person with cardiovascular disease. It cannot be stressed too strongly that the physical activity program must be designed and implemented in accordance with the principles of training discussed in Chapter 9 if the results are to be beneficial.

Reasons People Engage in Exercise Programs

Before discussing the values that can be derived from participating in a regular program of physical activity, it seems worthwhile to indicate the reasons people engage in exercise programs. Based on a survey of several of my physical fitness classes, the following reasons were consistently mentioned:

> To improve health
> For enjoyment
> To improve physical fitness
> To prevent disease
> To relieve tension and stress
> For weight control
> To keep from getting a heart attack
> To socialize and meet friends

The reasons cited by members of my fitness classes are consistent with those mentioned in other sources.[4] Does participation in physical activity programs enable individuals to achieve their objectives? Research evidence suggests that often the answer is yes.

Effects of Regular Physical Activity

A summary of the effects of regular physical activity on various components of physical fitness is presented in Table 7.1. The data that support the effects in the table come mainly from studies comparing well-conditioned and sedentary subjects. The data also indicate that the degree of change in physiological functioning as a result of participation in physical activity is variable. The type of activity; the frequency, intensity, and duration of the activity; and the age, sex, and physical condition of the people engaged in the program determine the degree of change in physiological variables.

S. J. Upton and colleagues examined the physiological profiles of 73 middle-aged women distance runners and sedentary women. The trained group consisted of 38 women who had run in at least one marathon who were currently training for another. The sedentary controls were 35 women who had not participated in an aerobic program within the past five years. The results of the testing revealed that the sedentary women possessed a significantly greater amount of total body weight

---

TABLE 7.1   **Possible Beneficial Effects of Regular Physical Activity**

IMPROVED CARDIORESPIRATORY ENDURANCE
Increased maximum cardiac output
Increased stroke volume
Decreased resting heart rate and smaller increase in heart rate during
   moderate work (in comparison with sedentary person)
Increased oxygen utilization during exhausting work
Increased blood volume
Decreased systolic and diastolic blood pressure
Increased coronary circulation
Increased mechanical efficiency of the heart muscle (myocardium)
More rapid return of heart rate and blood pressure to normal following
   physical activity
IMPROVED STRENGTH, MUSCULAR ENDURANCE, AND FLEXIBILITY
Increased muscle size
Increased capillarization and blood supply
More efficient internal respiration (O_2—CO_2 exchange)
Increased ability to move through full range of movement in various body
   parts
IMPROVED BODY COMPOSITION
Reduced overall body weight[a]
Reduced fat weight
Increased lean body mass
MISCELLANEOUS
Decreased serum cholesterol and triglycerides
Decreased low-density lipoprotein
Increased high-density lipoprotein
Reduction in anxiety and depression levels
More positive self-concept
Increased overall feeling of well-being

---

[a]In some cases there might be a slight increase in weight due to a large increase in lean body weight (muscle mass).

and fat weight (their percentage of fat weight was 27.8 percent, versus 15.5 percent for the trained subjects). The trained subjects had a 77 percent greater mean difference in maximum oxygen uptake and a significantly lower resting heart rate (55 versus 78 beats per minute).[5]

Jack Wilmore analyzed 55 studies dealing with the effects of physical activity on alterations of body composition in males and females. He concluded that alterations of body composition as a result of exercise training are minimal. An average of only 1.6 percent of relative body fat was reported to have resulted from training programs across all 55 studies. The training periods ranged from 6 to 104 weeks.[6] Although the average weight loss was only 1.6 percent, a high of 10.1 percent was reported (see Table 7.2).* Walk, jog, run was the mode of exercise that resulted in the largest weight loss (in the study of 19-year-old females).

* With one exception, only studies in which all the information sought was reported by Wilmore are included in Table 7.2. The study that was conducted for six weeks is not shown, since it did not contain all the information.

TABLE 7.2   **Alterations in Body Composition with Physical Training in Adults**[a]

		Training Program				Body Composition Alterations					
		Program Duration (wk)	Session Duration (min)	Frequency (days/wk)	Mode[b]	Weight (kg)		Lean Weight (kg)		Fat (%)	
Age	Sex					Before	After	Before	After	Before	After
39–59	M	104	60	2–3	a	80.3	77.0	64.4	62.7	19.8	18.6
55	M	20	30	3	a	79.1	77.9	62.2	62.5	21.4	19.8
49	M	20	40	4	a	77.6	76.3	60.5	60.4	22.0	20.9
35–46	M	16	30	3	a	88.1	83.6	64.5	63.3	26.8	23.9
42	M	26	40	6	a,d	79.6	79.7	63.7	65.7	20.0	17.5
40	M	22	35	3	a,d	84.4	81.9	66.3	64.9	21.4	20.7
39	M	20	45	2	a	81.3	80.4	62.4	62.0	23.3	22.9
39	M	20	45	2	a	79.4	78.7	61.2	61.3	22.9	22.1
28–39	M	20	30	2	a	80.2	80.3	65.8	65.1	18.0	18.9
28–39	M	20	30	4	a	79.7	76.8	64.1	62.5	19.6	18.6
38	M	20	30	3	a	84.7	83.4	66.3	64.4	21.7	20.4
38	M	20	30	3	a	85.2	83.9	66.1	67.6	22.4	19.4
38	M	20	30	3	c	84.1	82.9	66.4	66.5	21.0	19.8
38	M	8	30	3	a	84.7	83.9	60.8	62.1	27.9	25.4
38	M	8	30	3	e	86.2	87.2	63.7	66.8	25.9	23.1
37	M	20	30	3	c	85.7	85.3	66.4	67.4	21.2	19.6
37	M	16	30	3	a	79.5	77.1	60.9	60.8	23.3	21.1
37	M	16	30	4	a	79.4	78.5	62.8	64.7	20.7	17.4
37	M	16	30	2	a	80.6	79.8	62.0	61.5	22.8	23.2
36	M	20	30	3	a	79.8	77.9	63.6	63.5	19.8	17.8
21–35	M	20	45	3	e	85.4	85.9	64.6	66.4	24.4	22.7
21–35	M	20	45	3	a	82.1	81.6	64.3	66.0	21.7	19.1
33	M	10	20	3	a	79.6	78.6	64.2	64.4	18.9	17.8
25	M	16	90	5	a	99.1	93.4	75.8	76.0	23.5	18.6
44	F	17	60	2	a	76.2	72.0	45.2	46.3	40.4	35.4
19–39	F	15	30	5	a	48.7	49.5	41.6	42.7	14.1	13.2
16–23	F	26	60–90	3	e	79.0	78.6	58.0	58.4	24.4	23.9
18–22	F	16	60	5	f	58.6	59.0	45.2	44.7	22.8	24.2
18–22	F	16	120	5	b	60.1	60.3	48.0	46.3	20.1	23.2
22	F	12	15–33	3	e	57.9	56.2	43.4	42.7	25.0	24.0
21	F	7	16	3	c	57.9	59.3	45.5	46.6	21.4	21.1
21	F	9	40	3	e	58.1	58.5	40.1	41.6	30.8	28.7
20	F	15	60	3–5	a	83.4	77.7	56.9	54.2	31.8	30.2
19	F	8	—	6	a	67.1	64.7	49.0	51.9	38.6	28.5

[a]Wilmore provides individual references for the studies on pages 422–425.

[b]a = walk, jog, run; b = swim; c = bicycle, bicycle ergometer; d = calisthenics; e = circuit training, circuit weight training; f = tennis.

Source: Data derived from Jack H. Wilmore, "Appetite and Body Composition Consequent to Physical Activity," Research Quarterly *54 (1983):421. Reprinted by permission of the American Alliance for Health Physical Education, Recreation and Dance, 1900 Association Drive, Reston, Virginia 22091.*

In fact, the larger weight losses resulted from programs in which either walking, jogging, or running was the exercise modality.

One study was cited by Wilmore to answer the question: Does exercise therapy minimize the loss of lean weight that normally accompanies strict dietary regulation and decreased caloric intake, and are resulting alterations in body composition more likely to be permanent? In the study, body composition changes were evaluated in normal and obese middle-aged women following 12 weeks of training. The conclusion was that the obese individuals lost body weight and fat weight during the training program, but they returned to their pretraining weights when reevaluated 18 months after cessation of the training program. This conclusion is similar to the results of other studies.

Some authors indicate that detraining occurs much more rapidly. McArdle, Katch, and Katch, for example, report that significant reductions in working capacity can be measured after only two weeks of detraining, and almost all training improvements are lost within several months.[7] This information suggests that physical fitness programs must be engaged in on a regular, ongoing basis. A person cannot engage in an exercise program for 12 or 15 weeks and expect the benefits to continue indefinitely.

Effects of Physical Activity on Older Adults

Are the effects of participation in regular physical activity the same for older adults as they are for younger people? Although there are exceptions, the average older adult should not expect to improve on the various physiological parameters as much as younger people. Smith and Gilligan report that there is a 30 percent decline in work capacity (which is considered an overall indicator of physiological functioning) of the average sedentary person between the ages of 30 and 70.[8] These authors measured the maximum work capacity in a group of older adults, which they divided into the young-old (55 to 75) and the old-old (older than 75). The data are presented in Table 7.3. It can be seen that people in the young-old group have a maximum work capacity of between 5 and 7 METs (there is no appreciable difference between men and women). The maximum work capacity for the old-old group is much lower—an average of about 2.5 METs. Since one MET is the en-

TABLE 7.3   **Maximum Volitional Treadmill Exercise Tolerance Test in the Older Adult**

	Number in Group	Mean Age	MET Level	Heart Rate[a]
Young-old				
Men	13	72	4.9–6.6	122–139
Women	42	70	4.3–6.5	123–148
Old-old	24	85	2.0–3.4	102–128

[a]Ranges represent mean $\pm$ 1 SD (standard deviation).

Source: Everett L. Smith and Catherine Gilligan, "Physical Activity Prescription for the Older Adult, Physician and Sportsmedicine 11 (August 1983):92. Reprinted by permission of The Physician and Sportsmedicine, a McGraw-Hill publication.

ergy expended at rest, the old-old group has a work capacity that is low.

One would expect the older group to decline in physiological functioning, especially if individuals in the group do not participate in physical activity on a regular basis; however, as Herbert deVries notes, "to the extent that the functional capacity of the organism . . . declines as a result of aging per se, then to that extent the capacity for improvement should show an inverse correlation with age, if no real agewise change in training activity occurs during the middle and later years."[9] In other words, the older one gets, the capacity to improve one's physiological functioning decreases, assuming there is no significant change in physical activity during middle-age and after.

That there is a decline in physiological functioning during the aging process is well documented.[10] (The approximate magnitudes of change in various physiological functions between the ages of 30 and 70 appear in Table 7.4). However, as R. J. Shephard has noted, "it is far from clear whether the functional loss is an inevitable consequence of ageing, or whether it reflects merely a diminution of habitial physical activity."[11] To support a true aging process he cites research that indicates that the rate of loss of aerobic power is about the same for "master" athletes and for sedentary older individuals. This decline was indicated to be about 5

Effect of Exercise on the Aging Process

TABLE 7.4   **Biological Functional Changes Between the Ages of 30 and 70**

Biological Function	Change
Work capacity (%)	↓ 25–30
Cardiac output (%)	↓ 30
Maximum heart rate (beats/min)	↓ 24
Blood pressure (mm Hg)	
Systolic	↑ 10–40
Diastolic	↑ 5–10
Respiration (%)	
Vital capacity	↓ 40–50
Residual volume	↑ 30–50
Basal metabolic rate (%)	↓ 8–12
Musculature (%)	
Muscle mass	↓ 25–30
Hand grip strength	↓ 25–30
Nerve conduction velocity (%)	↓ 10–15
Flexibility (%)	↓ 20–30
Bone (%)	
Women	↓ 25–30
Men	↓ 15–20
Renal function (%)	↓ 30–50

Source: Everett L. Smith and Catherine Gilligan, "Physical Activity Prescription for the Older Adult," Physician and Sportsmedicine *11 (August 1983):92. Reprinted by permission of* The Physician and Sportsmedicine, *a McGraw-Hill publication.*

percent per decade from the age of 25 to 65 years. On the other hand, using the maximum oxygen intake as a criterion, Shephard indicates that the physically active athlete has a higher level of aerobic capacity (about 10 milliliters per kilogram per minute of oxygen transport at all ages) than his or her sedentary counterpart.[12]

Other research has also demonstrated the importance of exercise in curtailing the effects of aging. For example, regular participation in endurance-type exercise has been shown to improve endurance for dynamic work and maximum work capacity.[13] Also, physiological processes known to decline with age, including cardiac efficiency, arterial distensibility, pulmonary function, and bone calcium, have been reported to be modifiable by exercise.[14]

Based on the available evidence, it seems prudent to advocate increased physical activity during adult and later years not only as a means of slowing the aging process and improving physiological functioning but also to lessen the risks of serious medical problems associated with aging, such as arthritis and osteoporosis.

Effects of Physical Activity on Persons with Cardiovascular Disease

Dr. Nathan Pritikin, celebrity diet and fitness authority, writes that a high-complex-carbohydrate diet and exercise program enabled Eula Weaver at age 85 to train for and win gold medals in the 800 and 1500 meters at the Senior Olympics. Consider this account of Weaver's life before becoming involved in the diet and exercise program advocated by Dr. Pritikin:

> Eula Weaver developed heart disease with angina at 67, and at 75 was hospitalized with a severe heart attack. By age 81, she had developed congestive heart failure, hypertension, severe arthritis and claudication (insufficient blood flow to the legs). She could walk no more than 100 feet. Circulation to her hands was so bad that she had to wear gloves in the summer.[15]

After adopting the high-carbohydrate diet and the exercise program, Eula began to improve. She was off all medication in a year, had lost her symptoms, and was able to walk a mile. By the time she was 85, Eula accomplished the incredible feats at the Senior Olympics.

This is a highly unusual case of a person with cardiovascular problems responding favorably to a diet and exercise program. The question must also be raised as to the number of individuals with heart problems who would have the desire or need to become involved in competitive athletic events. In contrast to the story of Eula Weaver are stories of the many elderly persons—with cardiac problems or with other physical ailments—who receive little or no physical exercise. These are the extreme cases. Physical activity programs have beneficial effects for the vast majority of persons who have suffered some type of cardiovascular disease.

In the past decade or two, more and more health professionals are recommending increased physical activity for patients with cardiovascular problems. Yet the evidence to date regarding the effects of vigorous physical activity on physiological and psychological parameters in postcardiac patients is still equivocal and contradictory. Some authors even suggest that negative effects of intensive exercise therapy for these persons are possible. In 1974 Henry Blackburn, for example, questioned the widespread use of high-level intensive exercise therapy for coronary patients because "such therapy is not yet based on evidence of long-term benefit, it is potentially dangerous and costly, and it is unnecessary for good therapeutic results."[16]

Writing on physical inactivity with Arthur S. Leon in 1983, Blackburn indicates that there is indirect evidence of a protective effect of aerobic exercise through reduction of other CHD risk factors. Some of the possible protective effects of exercise for CHD patients listed by these authors are as follows:

1. Reduction of other coronary risk factors
2. Improved cardiovascular function and efficiency
3. Increased myocardial vascularity and coronary artery size
4. Increased resistance to ventricular fibrillation
5. Decreased tendency to thrombosis
6. Improved tolerance to stress[17]

Regarding the effects of exercise on patients with various types of cardiovascular disease, other researchers have made the following statements: They can achieve performance levels of sedentary normal subjects; properly executed training programs effectively improve the exercise tolerance of the majority of these patients with only small risks; they showed an improvement pattern similar to exercising normal subjects after a six-week training program, even though subjects with mild myocardial ischemia or arrythmias exercised at a lower level of intensity; and exercise training produced substantial improvements in the fitness level of these persons as determined by increased maximal oxygen uptake, oxygen pulse, ventilation, and physical work capacity.[18]

On the basis of the results of available research findings to date, it seems prudent to conclude that rhythmic, aerobic-type exercises, designed and conducted according to certain principles and under specific conditions (to be enumerated in the next section), will provide beneficial results for any participant. The alternative of inactivity or substantially reduced physical activity with resultant decreases in cardiovascular-respiratory functioning; reduced joint flexibility, muscle strength, and the support of ligaments and tendons (which are implicated in problems of low-back pain); and increases in total body weight and fat weight seems much less attractive or advisable.

Requisites for the Beneficial Effects of Physical Activity

Leaders in the professions of health, physical education, and recreation have long extolled the values of physical activity to the improvement of the quality of life for humans. Some have been accused of making claims regarding the benefits of physical activity that are not founded on scientific fact or empirical evidence. During the past two decades, many health professionals, including physical educators, have been especially careful in attempting to document the effects of physical activity on the human organism. An example of the combined efforts of health professionals from several disciplines to document the present state of knowledge regarding the effects of physical activity on the human organism is the papers contained in a special issue of *Public Health Reports.*[19] These articles present documented evidence of the beneficial effects of physical activity for cardiovascular health, weight control, and reduction of symptoms of depression, depressed mood, and anxiety.

In this chapter discussion of the effects of physical activity on various physiological variables and associated mechanisms has been designed to demonstrate the value of such activity to individuals. This approach is justified when one can show the relationship of the beneficial effects of physical activity to increased physical, emotional, and social well-being of normal persons as well as those who have restricted functioning because of age or some cardiovascular problem. At this point it is appropriate to indicate some of the conditions and considerations that are necessary to help ensure that physical activity will be of value to the individual participant.

Conditions and Considerations

Certain conditions must be met and practices adhered to if the effects of physical activity are to be beneficial. First, the principles of training that are outlined and discussed in Chapter 9 should guide program development. Care must be taken to adapt the exercise prescription to the special conditions of older adults and persons with cardiovascular problems or a high-risk profile for coronary heart disease. Second, the philosophy that "more is better" should not be practiced, especially for individuals with cardiovascular problems. For example, a 2- or 3-mile walk at a slow pace, rather than a 3-mile run in 30 minutes, might be advisable for certain patients who have suffered a myocardial infarction. Finally, the exercise program should be undertaken with other lifestyle changes or modifications, if necessary. The practice of sound nutritional habits, weight control, the ability to handle stress, control of blood pressure, and so forth, should all be stressed in addition to a regular exercise program in producing beneficial effects for individual participants.

Notes

1. Drummond Ayers, Jr., "Carter, Exhausted and Pale, Drops Out of 6-Mile Race," *New York Times,* September 16, 1979, p. 1.
2. B. Holt, "Ignoring Doctor's Orders, Byron Ran for His Life, Family Says," *Washington Star,* November 16, 1978, p. 1.
3. Paul D. Thompson, "Cardiovascular Hazards of Physical Activity," in Ronald L. Terjung, ed., *Exercise and Sport Science Reviews,* vol. 10 (Philadelphia: Franklin Institute Press, 1982), p. 230.
4. *Health Maintenance* (Newport Beach, Calif.: Pacific Mutual Life Insurance

Co., 1978); Wayne D. Van Huss et al., *Physical Activity in Modern Living,* 2d ed. (Englewood Cliffs, N.J.: Prentice-Hall, 1969).

5. S. J. Upton et al., "Comparison of the Physiological Profiles of Middle-aged Women Distance Runners and Sedentary Women," *Research Quarterly* 54 (1983):83–87.

6. Jack H. Wilmore, "Appetite and Body Composition Consequent to Physical Activity," *Research Quarterly* 54 (1983):415–425.

7. William D. McArdle, Frank I. Katch, and Victor L. Katch, *Exercise Physiology: Energy, Nutrition, and Human Performance* (Philadelphia: Lea & Febiger, 1981), p. 269.

8. Everett L. Smith and Catherine Gilligan, "Physical Activity Prescription for the Older Adult," *Physician and Sportsmedicine* 11 (August 1983):91.

9. Herbert A. deVries, "Physiological Effects of an Exercise Training Regimen upon Men Aged 52 to 88," *Journal of Gerontology* 25 (1970):334.

10. J. L. Hodgson and E. R. Buskirk, "Physical Fitness and Age, with Emphasis on Cardiovascular Function in the Elderly," *Journal of the American Geriatrics Society* 25 (1977):385–392.

11. R. J. Shephard, "Physical Fitness: Exercise and Ageing," in M. S. J. Pathy, ed., *Principles and Practice of Geriatric Medicine* (London: Wiley, 1985), p. 164.

12. Ibid.

13. Hodgson and Buskirk, 385.

14. N. W. Bolduan and S. M. Horvath, "Survey of Exercise and Aging," in Edward J. Masoro, ed., *CRC Handbook of Physiology in Aging* (Boca Raton, Fla.: CRC Press, 1981), p. 443.

15. Nathan Pritikin, "Given the Right Diet, a Champion Can Be Made at Any Age," *Runner's World,* March 1984, p. 120.

16. Henry Blackburn, "Disadvantages of Intensive Exercise Therapy After Myocardial Infarction," in F. Ingelfinger, ed., *Controversy in Internal Medicine* (Philadelphia: Saunders, 1974), p. 162.

17. Arthur S. Leon and Henry Blackburn, "Physical Inactivity," in Norman M. Kaplan and Jeremiah Stamler, eds., *Prevention of Coronary Heart Disease* (Philadelphia: Saunders, 1974), p. 162.

18. William C. Adams, Malcolm M. McHenry, and Edmund M. Bernauer, "Long-Term Physiologic Adaptations to Exercise with Special Reference to Performance and Cardiorespiratory Function in Health and Disease," *American Journal of Cardiology* 33 (1974):765. Jan Praetorius Clausen, "Circulatory Adjustments to Dynamic Exercise and Effect of Physical Training in Normal Subjects and in Patients with Coronary Artery Disease," *Progress in Cardiovascular Disease* 18 (1976):459; deVries, 335; Joseph A. Bonanno and James E. Lies, "Effects of Physical Training on Coronary Risk Factors," *American Journal of Cardiology* 33 (1974):720.

19. "Public Health Aspects of Physical Activity and Exercise," *Public Health Reports* 100 (1985):113–202.

Behavior Change Through Behavior Modification

Key Words

behavior modification
contingency contracting
contingency intervention plan
motivation

positive reinforcement
reinforcement
self-modification of behavior
social reinforcement

Key Words

After reading this chapter, you should be able to:
1. Define and/or explain the key words listed above.
2. Use the Health and Exercise Behavior Report Form to determine whether you should use the self-modification-of-behavior plan.
3. Use the self-modification-of-behavior plan to modify or eliminate undesirable behavior and reinforce desirable behavior.
4. Identify eight reasons some people give for not exercising and eating nutritious meals and indicate the counterpoint for each reason.
5. Develop appropriate contingency reinforcement strategies.
6. Identify three negative mental images that are deterrents to desirable behavior change and indicate three positive mental images to replace them.

Chapter Highlights

Information presented in Chapters 6 and 7 might prove sufficient to get some individuals started on a fitness program that they will continue. Others might need more direct intervention by a fitness instructor or some other exercise or health care professional. However, the primary responsibility for controlling behavior rests with each individual. The major thrust of this chapter is based on this premise. The overall objective is to present information to help people develop and maintain desirable behaviors and eliminate or at least alter undesirable behaviors related to selected risk factors associated with cardiovascular disease.

The centerpiece of this chapter is a self-modification-of-behavior plan and suggestions for motivating individuals to begin and adhere to a physical fitness program. The self-modification-of-behavior plan may be used to modify behaviors related to other risk factors as well as inactivity. In essence, the skills and techniques of behavior modification will be used to help you achieve self-directed change.

Your Health and Exercise Behavior

Some individuals may not need to change their behavior related to health and fitness. They are the fortunate ones who maintain a healthy and physically active lifestyle. How is your health and fitness behavior? You will be able to answer this by completing the checklist that follows. Furthermore, you will be able to modify undesirable behavior by using the self-modification-of-behavior plan presented thereafter.

Health and Exercise Behavior Report

The following statements to which you are to respond will provide an overview of your behaviors relevant to selected aspects of health and fitness (specifically, those identified as risk factors in cardiovascular disease). If you check "yes" for all statements, you are exhibiting exemplary behavior. Maintain these positive behavior patterns.

If you check "no" for any item, you should either complete the more precise self-scoring test for heart attack and stroke presented in Chapter 6 or begin the self-modification plan. The item for which you check "no" and the number of items checked should determine the next course of action you take. For example, if you check "no" for item 2, dealing with the intensity, frequency, and duration of exercise, you might begin using the self-modification-of-behavior plan. You are advised, however, to get a medical checkup before beginning a vigorous exercise program. This is especially relevant if you have not engaged in physical activity on a regular basis for the past year. If you are over 35, the physician will probably suggest an exercise stress test as part of the examination. Once you get medical clearance from the doctor, you can proceed with the self-modification-of-behavior plan.

If you check "no" for item 6, dealing with blood pressure, or item 8, dealing with diet, you should complete the self-scoring test for heart attack and stroke risk to get more precise information regarding these risk factors. The higher your risk profile (determined by the number of risk factors and the extent of each risk factor), the more concerned you should be with seeking medical advice before proceeding with the self-modification-of-behavior plan.

Self-scoring checklist for heart attack and stroke risk
Check "Yes" or "No" opposite each statement.*

	Yes	No
1. I get a complete medical examination at least once each year.	_____	_____
2. I exercise and get my heart rate to between 70 and 85 percent of my age-adjusted maximum heart rate for 15 to 30 minutes as least three times a week.	_____	_____
3. I am within the normal weight range for my age, sex, height, and body frame.	_____	_____
4. I do not smoke cigarettes.	_____	_____
5. My resting pulse rate is within an acceptable range.	_____	_____
6. My blood pressure is within a normal range.	_____	_____
7. I am able to handle stress adequately.	_____	_____
8. I eat a balanced diet and do not consume an excessive amount of foods high in saturated fats and cholesterol.	_____	_____

Self-Modification-of-Behavior Plan

The self-modification-of-behavior plan focuses on human behavior, applies the principles of the laws of learning, and emphasizes relevant reinforcement strategies (positive reinforcement, social reinforcement, contingency contracting, self-reward, and so on). Moreover, this plan includes techniques for accurate observation of behavior, and all who desire to modify their behavior are able to design and execute their own program.

The self-modification-of-behavior plan consists of the following six steps:[1]

1. Identify the problem and select the goal.
2. State the problem behavior(s) you need to change to achieve the goal.
3. Make observations of how often the problem behavior occurs, the antecedents that precede it, and the consequences that follow it.
4. Develop a plan to intervene by contingently reinforcing some desirable behavior and by arranging situations to increase your chances of performing desirable behaviors.

Steps in the Self-Modification-of-Behavior Plan

---

* If you are unable to reply to a statement because of a lack of knowledge of the specific information required, refer to the appropriate chapter in this book. (Consult the index, if necessary.)

5. Monitor the results.
6. Maintain, adjust, and finally terminate the intervention program.

You should be systematic in your use of the self-modification-of-behavior plan, regardless of the goal of your program—the elimination of some undesirable behavior or the increase of occurrence of some desirable behavior. Each of the steps of the plan should be addressed in the sequential manner in which it is presented.

Using the Plan

The general approach to the use of the self-modification-of-behavior plan is illustrated by presenting abridged case studies of two individuals who used the plan and making clarifying comments as needed for the various steps of the plan. Both subjects had a weight problem. They are remarkably similar in physical stature—5 feet 3 inches tall, of medium body build, and weighing 170 pounds at the start of the program. They differ in age and occupation. Ann, an elementary school physical education teacher, is 46 years old. Iola is a 38-year-old dance instructor.

Identification of the Problem and Selection of the Goal.   Both subjects used the Health and Exercise Behavior Report to identify the general problem or problems as a prelude to selecting the goal of the program. Among other problem areas, both checked that they were overweight. Each selected slightly different goals to achieve. Ann, the 46-year-old physical education teacher, established a goal of losing 30 to 35 pounds in six months. Her final weight goal was 135 to 140 pounds. Iola, the 38-year-old dance instructor, set a goal of reducing her weight from 170 to 130 pounds in eight months (a total of 40 pounds to be lost).

It is very important to establish realistic goals. Many times people with good intentions and great commitment fail to adhere to a program of behavior change simply because they set unrealistically high goals. In fact, Iola initially wanted to lose 40 pounds in three months but on reflection decided to give herself more time. If she loses the weight in three or four months instead of the projected eight months, that would be fine. However, if Iola had kept the goal of three months to lose 40 pounds and did not achieve it, she might have become discouraged and quit the program. She should be encouraged to continue the program even if her present goal is not achieved in the established time period. If undesirable behavior patterns are changed, the weight will eventually be reduced.

Statement of Problem Behavior.   The problem behavior, often called the "target behavior," is the behavior that you wish to change. When stating the behavioral problem or problems, you should include a precise description of the behavior, the conditions under which the behavior should or should not occur, and the acceptable level of change for the identified problem behavior.

Both Ann and Iola realized that being overweight was a problem; however, they also recognized that the overweight condition was a result of several undesirable behaviors rather than the target behavior itself. After giving some thought to their daily activity pattern, each individual indicated that the problem behavior related to eating and activity habits.

Two Week Weight Information Form

NAME _*Iola*_
BODY FRAME____(S)_____(M)__✓__(L)_____
BEGINNING WEIGHT ___*170*___ Date_*11.28.86*_
DESIRED WEIGHT ___*130*___ Date_*7.31.87*_

Day	Date	Beg. Wt.	Current Wt.	Difference
1 M	11/28/86	170	170	0
2 Tu	11/29/86	170	168	-2
3 W	11/30/86	170	$167\frac{1}{2}$	$-2\frac{1}{2}$
4 Th	12/1/86	170	$167\frac{1}{2}$	$-2\frac{1}{2}$
5 F	12/2/86	170	167	-3
6 S	12/3/86	170	166	-4
7 Su	12/4/86	170	167	-3
8 M	12/5/86	170	$166\frac{1}{2}$	$-3\frac{1}{2}$
9 Tu	12/6/86	170	167	-3
10 W	12/7/86	170	$167\frac{1}{2}$	$-2\frac{1}{2}$
11 Th	12/8/86	170	167	-3
12 F	12/9/86	170	166	-4
13 S	12/10/86	170	166	-4
14 Su	12/11/86	170	166	-4

Figure 8.1
Completed Two-Week
Weight Information
Form.

After reviewing the nutrition, exercise and weight control information in Chapter 4, each individual was able to state her behavioral problems in measurable terms. Ann stated that she sometimes did not eat at least three nutritious meals a day, and she also failed to engage herself in aerobic activities a minimum of three times a week for 30 or more minutes at each workout. Iola, while teaching aerobic dance two days a week, also indicated that she failed to become involved in aerobic activities at least three times a week.

Observations Regarding Problem Behavior.   The next step is to make careful observations of how often the problem behavior occurs, the conditions and/or events that precede it, and the consequences that follow the problem behavior. The idea is to obtain an accurate account of the frequency of the problem behavior and the probable reinforcing events and/or conditions surrounding the behavior in question. Both Ann and Iola made careful observations of their target behaviors (that is, food consumption and activity habits) for two weeks.

Forms were provided for them to record target behaviors. Figure 8.1 shows the recording of Iola's weight and Figure 8.2 the transfer of this information to a graph. It is important to record the weight about the same time each day and to use a heavy-duty medical scale. It should also be noted that baseline measures should be recorded for at least two weeks to get an accurate indication of the target behavior. Record the target behavior as soon after it occurs as possible.

Ann's recordings of daily activities (Figure 8.3) and eating behaviors (Figure 8.4) demonstrate suggested means of recording these behaviors.

Daily Weight Graph Form

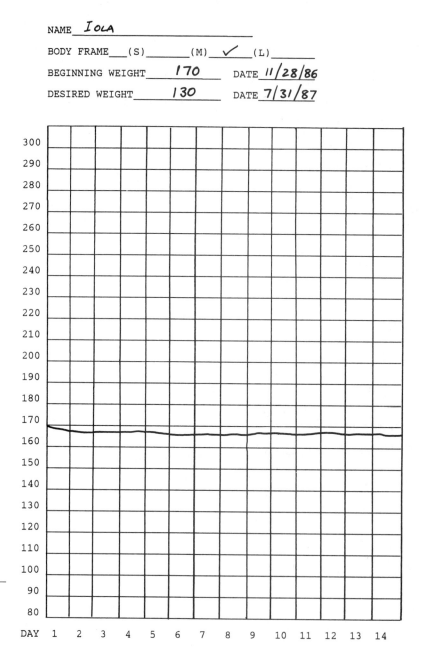

NAME *Iola*

BODY FRAME___(S)_____(M) ✓ (L)_____

BEGINNING WEIGHT____170____ DATE 11/28/86

DESIRED WEIGHT____130____ DATE 7/31/87

Figure 8.2
Completed Daily
Weight Graph Form.

The Daily Activity Record Form (Figure 8.3) enables a person to record all activities engaged in during a 24-hour period. The objective is to determine the types of activities one engages in as well as to determine the amount of Calories one burns up during a day. This information, when compared with the amount of Calories consumed, will enable a person to compare caloric consumption with energy expenditure and thus determine weight gain or loss. Moreover, specific activity and eating patterns may be noted by examining these forms.

Using Ann's completed charts for one day, for example, it can be seen that she consumed 1094 Calories and burned up 2335 Calories. Further,

Activity Record Chart

Name ANN			Wt. 171 1/2-hr MET 39.28 Date		11/30/86
		1/2 MET		1/2 MET	Total METS per hr
A.M. 6:00 GET UP/BRUSH TEETH	1.5		6:30 SHOWER & DRESS	1.5	3
7:00 DRESS / EAT B'FAST	1.5		7:30 DRIVE TO SCHOOL /STAND	1.5	3
8:00 PREPARE FOR CLASS	1.5		8:30 TEACH (STANDING)	2	3.5
9:00 STAND & TALK	1.5		9:30 SIT & WRITE	1.5	3
10:00 LIGHT MOVING / SIT	2		10:30 TEACH	2	4
11:00 TEACH/PREPARE FOR LUNCH	2		11:30 WASH HANDS / EAT	1.5	3.5
1200 SIT & EAT	1.5		12:30 CLEAN UP / TALK	1.5	3
P.M. 1:00 TEACH (STANDING)	2		1:30 TEACH	2	4
2:00 TEACH	2		2:30 PUT AWAY EQUIPMENT	2	4
3:00 DRIVE HOME / WASH HANDS & FACE	1.5		3:30 SIT, WATCH T.V.	1	2.5
4:00 WASH DISHES / LIGHT HOUSE WORK	2		4:30 LIGHT HOUSEWORK	2	4
5:00 PREPARE DINNER	1		5:30 PREPARE DINNER/WATCH T.V.	1.5	2.5
6:00 WATCH T.V.	1		6:30 WATCH T.V.	1	2
7:00 SIT, NODDING	1		7:30 SIT / DRIVE TO TRAIN STATION	1.5	2.5
8:00 EAT DINNER	1.5		8:30 SIT, WATCH T.V.	1	2.5
9:00 SIT, WATCH T.V.	1		9:30 SIT, WATCH T.V.	1	2
10:00 WASH CLOTHES	1.5		10:30 WASH CLOTHES	1.5	3
11:00 WASH CLOTHES & DISHES	1.5		11:30 WASH DISHES	1.5	3
12:00 FLOSS TEETH	1.5		12:30 BATHE	1.5	3
A.M. 1:00 PREPARE FOR BED	1		1:30 IN BED	.85	1.9
2:00 SLEEP	.85		2:30 SLEEP	.85	1.7
3:00 SLEEP	.85		3:30 SLEEP	.85	1.7
4:00 SLEEP	.85		4:30 SLEEP	.85	1.7
5:00 SLEEP	.85		5:30 SLEEP	.85	1.7
			Total METS per day (add down)		66.7
			Multiply by your 1/2-hr MET value		35
			Total calories burned this day		2,335

Figure 8.3
Completed Daily
Activity Record Form.

it can be seen that she spent most of her day in sedentary activities (those requiring the use of less than 3 METs).*

If you are considering using the activity form presented here, the computation of total Calories burned may be a concern. The procedure is simple. Each of the activities has a MET value. Place the appropriate MET value opposite each activity you engage in during the day in ques-

---

* Remember that a MET is the amount of energy expended at rest. The higher the MET value, the greater the energy expenditure.

Eating Behavior Record Form

NAME __ANN__   DAY & DATE __MON 11/17/86__

ANTECEDENT EVENTS (When, where, time and mood before & during eating)	Food	Amount	Calories	CONSEQUENT EVENTS (Activities & mood following eating)
BREAKFAST — 7.15 A.M. KITCHEN RELAXED & HAPPY	EGG (OVER LIGHT) / SAUSAGE PATTY / ORANGE JUICE	1 / 1 / 4 OZS.	85 / 60 / 110	RINSED MOUTH, WASHED HANDS, DROVE TO SCHOOL. RELAXED.
IN-BETWEEN —	NONE	—	—	—
LUNCH — 11.15 A.M NURSES OFFICE AT SCHOOL. HUNGRY.	EGG SALAD SANDWICH / POPCORN / APPLE JUICE	1 / 1 CUP / 1 CUP	225 / 50 / 120	FLOSSED TEETH, RINSED MOUTH, WASHED HANDS, & SAT AND TALKED WITH COLLEAGUES
IN-BETWEEN — 3.15 P.M. IN KITCHEN. HUNGRY	ORANGE / GRAPEFRUIT	1 SMALL / 1 MEDIUM	65 / 90	SAT, RELAXED. WATCHED T.V.
DINNER — 10.30 P.M IN KITCHEN. TIRED & HUNGRY	SMOKED SAUSAGE SANDWICH / WATER	1 / 8 OZS.	254 / 35	SAT, RELAXED. WATCHED T.V. FLOSSED TEETH
AFTER DINNER —	NONE	—	—	—

Figure 8.4
Completed Eating Behavior Record Form.

Total Calories= __1,094__

tion. Add these values up and multiply this number by the half-hour MET (or caloric expenditure) value for your weight (all this information is contained in Chapter 4). Using Ann's figures as an example, her total of METs for the day was 66.7 and her half-hour MET value (caloric expenditure) was 35 (that's the value for a woman weighing 170 pounds). A total Calorie count (of 2335) was obtained by multiplying the total METs for the day (66.7) by the half-hour MET value (caloric expenditure) of 35. The half-hour MET value will vary according to your weight as indicated in Table 4.3 in Chapter 4.

An examination of information in Ann's eating chart revealed that she had a good breakfast and lunch with no snacks between the two meals. The dinner meal, though low in Calories, is not nutritious and is high in fat content. The snack eaten between lunch and dinner is nutritious.

By carefully recording both eating and activity behaviors for two weeks, Ann and Iola were able to get accurate baseline measures regarding time and conditions surrounding these events. (That Ann's eating behavior on the day used for this text is not typical of her normal eating habits is justification for recording baseline measures for at least two weeks.) An analysis of the information generated by Ann and Iola enabled them to determine the contingencies responsible for controlling their problem behaviors. They were thus able to develop contingency intervention plans to change the problem behaviors.

It should be mentioned that the forms shown in this text are not the only ones that might be used. For example, some people prefer to use small notebooks in which to keep diary accounts of their activities, instead of separate forms for recording eating and activity behaviors. Use whatever form will be practical and convenient. However, make sure that the form enables you to record the target behaviors accurately. *Do not substitute convenience or brevity for accuracy.*

One final suggestion concerning the observation and recording of baseline data is to presevere in your record-keeping efforts. At first glance, for example, you might be thinking that the activity form is too detailed to complete for two weeks. Initially, both Ann and Iola had the same reaction. As they began to complete the forms, however, they found that it was easy to use. You too can become adept at observing your behavior and recording it on the forms provided in this text.

Develop a Contingency Intervention Plan.   Once the target behaviors have been observed and recorded for at least two weeks, a plan to reinforce desirable behaviors can be developed. Undesirable behaviors you wish to change should not be reinforced.

After carefully analyzing their eating and exercise behaviors, Ann and Iola concluded that the pleasure derived from eating and the enjoyment gained from sitting and watching television were the major positive reinforcers for their eating and activity behaviors, respectively. Accordingly, the following strategies for contingency management were devised:

1. I acknowledge that my eating habits and lack of adequate aerobic exercise have caused me to reach a weight I am unhappy with.
2. I will establish a positive attitude that I am willing to change my eating and exercise behaviors to reach my weight goal and maintain that weight.
3. I will establish the following environmental controls:[2]
    a. Eat in one place. Make it a habit not to eat all over the home, especially not in my work area.
    b. Prepare only enough food for one meal at a time. (I will not eat leftovers at a meal.)
    c. Always sit down to a carefully set place at the table and eat only one helping of the food prepared for that meal.
    d. Make a conscious effort to eat four or five small meals each day rather than three large meals and several snacks in between each meal. Limit my food consumption to no more than 1200 Calories a day (based on a weekly average).
4. I will establish the following self-controls:
    a. Eat slowly. Put down the utensils after every mouthful.
    b. Partway through the meal, stop and sit relaxed, without eating for two or three minutes.

    c. Avoid becoming really deprived of food. Plan to lose an average of one to two pounds each week.

    d. Eat a nutritiously balanced diet so that no food group is completely eliminated.

    e. Reward myself for actually changing my eating and exercise behaviors. If I reach my weekly goals, I will go to a movie I've been wanting to see or buy myself a new dress. When I reach my monthly goal, I will get a ticket to see a dance performance (Iola) or a play (Ann).

5. I will use these specific techniques to increase my activity level:

    a. Perform the aerobic activity before I allow myself to engage in activities I enjoy (watching television, attending a dance concert, eating out, and so on). I will not cheat!

    b. Work with another person who is also trying to lose weight. I will seek support from that person and give whatever support I can. I will seek also the help and support of family members to aid me in my attempt to reach my goal.

This is a comprehensive contingency program established by Ann and Iola. They are using a variety of behavior modification strategies, including positive reinforcement (watching television only after exercising), self-reward (going to a dance performance or play when the monthly goal is reached), social reinforcement (the use of family members and the companionship and support of another person with a similar goal), and stimulus control (eating in one room). The overall plan is a form of self-contract.

Even though the contingency plan used by these two individuals is extensive, it is not all-inclusive. Other intervention strategies can be used. Token reinforcement (using money as a reinforcer) and response-cost punishment (giving money to charity, for instance, if the desired behavior is not exhibited) are reinforcement contingencies that have been used successfully.[3] Use the behavior modification techniques you feel will work for you. You might wish to consult some of the sources on behavior modification in the notes for this chapter for more information and examples of self-modification-of-behavior strategies that have proved successful for others.

It is good practice to display your intervention plan in a prominent place and refer to it frequently. Ann keeps her self-contract on a small table in the kitchen. Iola has her self-contract in a handbag that she carries with her every day.

Monitor the Results.   It would be rewarding to hear that all who have used this book to help change some undesirable behavior have succeeded. Realistically, however, some of you may have trouble achieving your goals. If you are experiencing difficulty in achieving the behavior change you seek, examine the intervention plan you developed. You might discover that the original goal is too difficult, that you need to plan more short-term goals, or that environmental stimuli need to be altered (for instance, associate with individuals who are active rather than sedentary). Sometimes it just might be that you have lost the desire to adhere to the intervention plan and need to make a renewed commitment to succeed.

What kind of progress are Ann and Iola making toward their goals? To refresh your memory, Ann's goal was to reduce her weight from 170 pounds to between 135 and 140 pounds (a total loss of 30 to 35 pounds) in six months. The goal for Iola was to lose a total of 40 pounds in eight months. Both subjects developed self-contracts with a variety of intervention strategies to help them change undesirable behaviors and facilitate goal attainment. Each sought to increase her aerobic activity participation level and decrease her caloric intake, especially of foods high in fats and cholesterol.

An evaluation of the results of the intervention plans of both individuals to date has produced some interesting revelations. While the weight of both persons has fluctuated between 160 and 170 pounds, their overt exercise and eating behaviors have changed.

Let's monitor Ann's results first. For the past three weeks, Ann has made a conscientious effort to eat three small nutritious meals each day. She eats her last meal by 6:00 P.M. For the past two weeks, Ann also has been engaged in aerobic exercises at home for 20 to 30 minutes, four to six days a week. She exercises at a target heart rate of between 130 and 140 beats per minute. Since she has been following this new routine of eating and exercising, Ann has indicated that she feels better and has more energy.

Although Iola has attempted to change her eating and exercise habits, she has not completely succeeded. She has reduced the amount of junk food she used to eat, for example. But she has not been able to eat three or four small nutritious meals due to her work schedule. She eats a light breakfast at home and lunch in the college cafeteria. Many times during the week she eats dinner after eight o'clock at night because she works late those days. Iola also finds it difficult to engage in aerobic activities more than two days a week on a regular basis. She teaches aerobic dance at a college, and the class meets only two days a week. She works with the dance group and gets some physical exercise but not much of the aerobic type.

Maintain, Adjust, and Finally Terminate the Program. Based on a careful analysis of the results of the contingency intervention program, you are now ready to proceed to the next step. Keep all aspects of the plan that produce positive results. Adjust the reinforcement strategies that are not working. By all means terminate the intervention program if you are now able to maintain your goal without the aid of reinforcement contingencies.

Ann has decided to maintain her intervention program in its present form. She feels that a continuation of increased physical activity and lowered caloric intake will eventually produce a reduction in her weight. Ann has indicated that she can detect a reduction in the fat tissue in certain trouble spots. An assessment of her percentage of body fat using skinfold calipers indicated that she had indeed reduced her fat weight. Ann is determined to reach her overall weight goal and maintain it.

After carefully monitoring the results of her plan, Iola indicated that she was going to make some changes. One proposed change is to engage in racquetball or handball and enroll in a dance class as a means of increasing her cardiorespiratory fitness. She is also going to ask a co-worker, who is also attempting to lose weight, to join her. Iola plans to continue monitoring her eating habits and substitute fruits for sweets, eat less of the nuts she likes, and generally eat fewer Calories but more nutritious food.

Where Do We Go from Here?

Those of you who have been able to develop lifestyles that avoid the risk factors associated with cardiovascular disease should continue your present behaviors. You are to be commended. For those of you who started the self-modification-of-behavior plan but did not continue for whatever reason, start at the first step of the plan and try again. Here are a few suggestions.

1. Carefully and accurately identify the problem behavior(s) and select the goal to be achieved. Establish realistic goals! It is better to exceed a modest goal than to fail to achieve an unrealistically grandiose goal.
2. Once you have identified the target behavior and set realistic goals, you must make a commitment to change the undesirable behavior with unshakable confidence. Remove all negative thoughts (such as "I'm destined to be fat"; "I gain weight no matter what I eat"; "I don't have time to exercise, and if I did I would be too tired to exercise") and substitute positive mental images ("If I exercise more and eat less, I will lose weight"; "Others tell me that they have more energy after they exercise, so I'm going to fit some exercise into my schedule").
3. Keep complete and accurate records when you are monitoring your behavior and recording the results. You need to get a true picture of your behavior pattern for at least two weeks. Use recording devices that are practical and convenient so that they are available when you need them. Record the behavior as soon after it occurs as possible.
4. Select a variety of activities to participate in. Alternate the activities in which you participate to add variety and help eliminate boredom. Schedule the activity on a regular basis (remember to engage in continuous aerobic activities). Review the target heart rate information in Chapter 9 if you are not sure of the intensity level at which to exercise.
5. In your selection of activities, make sure to choose ones you enjoy and have the skill to participate in successfully. Consider the availability and location of the facility that is required for you to engage in a particular activity. Is it close enough to your home or your job? Can you afford the cost? These and other practical questions should be considered before finally choosing activities for your program; otherwise you might not proceed beyond the point of selecting the activities.[4]

6. Consider activities that can be incorporated into your regular daily schedule. For example, take the stairs instead of the elevator; get off the subway or bus one or two stops earlier than usual and walk the remaining distance to your destination. Take a walk during lunch and eat a light snack (a fruit and soup, maybe) instead of sitting and eating a heavy meal every day at lunch time. Think of other ways to live a more active, stress-reduced life. You can do it!

7. Do not overstrain. For instance, you don't have to work out for two hours every day to stay in shape. Try exercising on alternate days, thus giving the body a chance to rest between two strenuous workouts. For those of you who choose jogging or running as your means of physical activity, remember that a 2-mile jog or run (in 15 to 20 minutes) is enough to develop adequate cardiorespiratory fitness. You should also remember the principle of progression. If you are beginning a jogging program, for example, you would not begin by jogging 2 miles. In fact, those of you who have not been active in the past year or two and those who are obese should probably begin with a brisk walk for the first few weeks. (This book should provide you with the necessary information to begin to adhere to a safe and rewarding physical activity program.)

8. Reward yourself when you make a desirable change in your behavior. The reward need not always be expensive or even materialistic. For example, it might be a mental self-reward such as "I feel proud that I did not eat any candy today," or it might be a little more tangible reward like "After that exhilarating workout, I'm going to watch a movie on television this evening." Try to progress to the point where external rewards become unnecessary. Once you are working out on a regular basis for three or four months, the physiological and psychological benefits you receive from the activity should be ample reward.

If several people were to complete the Self-scoring Test for Heart Attack and Stroke, three groups would probably be identified. One would consist of people whose score indicated that they had a low-risk profile and did not need to modify their behavior. A second group would include those who began the self-modification-of-behavior plan but did not complete it or failed to benefit from it. People in the first group were encouraged to maintain their positive behaviors, and those in the second group were urged to try the plan again.

Those Who Doubt

A third group exists, however, made up of the "doubting Thomases." Individuals in this group are often pessimists who question the effectiveness of plans such as the one presented in this chapter. Often persons in this group have experienced failure in using diets and have begun several exercise programs only to drop out before realizing any positive results. Frequently, individuals who have tried several different diets have lost weight on some of them but have regained the lost weight and have often added additional pounds. Many of these individuals have thus become weary of trying new plans for losing weight and adopting a more active lifestyle.

Individuals in this third group will not only resist the new plans for changing their undesirable behavior, but they also will give what they consider to be legitimate reasons for maintaining their present behavior patterns. Upon close examination, however, these reasons are not sound. In fact, many of the so-called reasons are simply alibis or excuses to avoid situations that might lead to another failure.

What kind of reasons do people usually give for not exercising and eating nutritiously well-balanced meals? Students in several of my fitness classes, as well as other persons with weight problems, have provided the answer to this question. I will cite reasons given by large numbers of people and provide a rebuttal for each.

REASON: "I don't have the time. My schedule is too hectic to allow me to prepare special diet meals and exercise regularly."

REBUTTAL: If you examine your schedule carefully, you will discover that you have more than enough time to exercise on a regular basis. Remember that it takes only three hours per week to accomplish this exercise goal. The food you prepare for the family should be nutritious. You should not have to prepare any special diet for yourself. Eat less of the food that you prepare, and make sure that it is nutritiously sound. Consider the benefits that will be gained from eating properly and exercising regularly.

If you do not have a family, you will have to prepare food for yourself only. Planning a special diet for one should be easier than planning for several people. If you do not cook, many restaurants prepare low-calorie meals that are nutritiously sound. When planning to eat out, call the restaurant in advance to determine whether special meals are prepared for diners on a diet.

REASON: "Participation in physical activity will not be of any benefit to me. Besides, I get enough physical activity on my job."

REBUTTAL: Exercise stimulates you and gives you more energy. You might wish to exercise in the morning before going to work. Or maybe exercising during the lunch hour will be perfect for you. Arrange some time in your schedule for exercise on a regular basis and you will probably increase your energy level.

REASON: "No diet works for me; I've tried them all. I guess I was just born to be fat."

REBUTTAL: A special diet is not required. If you eat fewer Calories of nutritiously prepared food and exercise regularly, you will reduce your weight. Try eating some of the food combinations suggested in this text; choose those foods that you like.

REASON: "Even when I lose weight on a diet, I put it back on in one or two weeks. So why bother with diets?"

REBUTTAL: As was indicated in Chapter 4, when you go on a diet that restricts or drastically lowers one food group (such as high-carbohydrate and low-protein diet), you do not lose weight permanently. A combination of eating fewer Calories of food that is nutritiously well balanced and engaging in an exercise program on a regular basis will reduce your weight and your "risk for heart attack" profile.

REASON: "I'm too heavy to exercise."

REBUTTAL: Absolutely not. Some types of exercise might be difficult for you, but get started with those that you can perform. Begin to walk more. Get a bicycle and ride it on nice days. If you can swim, go to a pool and swim off those pounds. There are many activities you can become engaged in to lose those extra pounds, no matter how many of them you've got!

REASON: "I don't need to exercise because I'm too thin now."

REBUTTAL: Weight loss is not the only reason to exercise. A regular program of aerobic exercise will help to reduce several of the risk factors associated with cardiovascular disease and make you feel better. You might want to review Chapters 6 and 7 to recognize the benefits that a program of physical activity can offer you.

REASON: "When I get my life together, I'm going to go on a diet and get some exercise. Right now I'm too depressed to do anything."

REBUTTAL: Exercise might just be the thing to help you relieve your depression. Research has demonstrated that vigorous exercise reduces depression and anxiety in some people. Think positive and begin an exercise program today. Begin to eat a more nutritious diet at the same time you start your exercise program (today) to develop a "new" you.

If these or other conditions or situations are preventing you from practicing positive behavior patterns, you are urged to think positively and change those undesirable behaviors. The self-modification-of-behavior plan presented in this text is designed to aid you in this endeavor. Give it a try.

Notes

1. Robert A. Sherman, *Behavior Modification: Theory and Practice* (Belmont, Calif.: Wadsworth, 1973), pp. 36–37; David L. Watson and Roland G. Tharp, *Self-directed Behavior: Self-modification for Personal Adjustment,* 2d ed. (Monterey, Calif.: Brooks/Cole, 1977), p. 2.

2. Based on information in Alvin N. Deibert and Alice J. Harmon, *New Tools for Changing Behavior* (Champaign, Ill.: Research Press, 1973), p. 111.

3. John E. Martin and Patricia M. Dubbert, "Exercise Application and Promotion in Behavioral Medicine: Current Status and Directions," *Journal of Consulting and Clinical Psychology,* 50 (1982):1004–1017; Robert J. Presbie and Paul Brown, *Physical Education: The Behavioral Modification Approach* (Washington, D.C.: National Education Association, 1977), pp. 96–103; Albert J. Stunkard and Michael J. Mahoney, "Behavioral Treatment of Eating Disorders," in Harold Leitenberg, ed., *Handbook of Behavioral Modification and Behavior Therapy* (Englewood Cliffs, N.J.: Prentice-Hall, 1976), pp. 53–61.

4. John Dietrich and Susan Waggoner, *The Complete Health Club Handbook* (New York: Simon & Schuster, 1983).

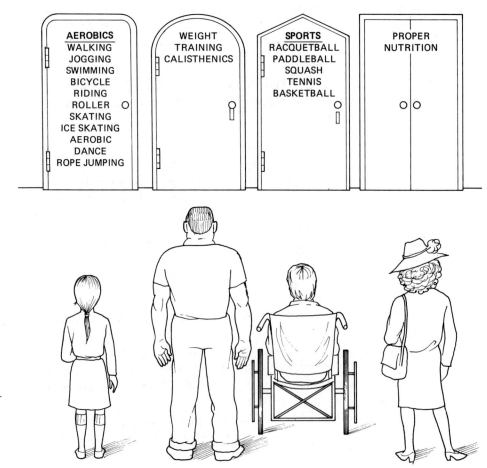

AEROBICS
WALKING
JOGGING
SWIMMING
BICYCLE
RIDING
ROLLER
SKATING
ICE SKATING
AEROBIC
DANCE
ROPE JUMPING

WEIGHT
TRAINING
CALISTHENICS

SPORTS
RACQUETBALL
PADDLEBALL
SQUASH
TENNIS
BASKETBALL

PROPER
NUTRITION

There are many
pathways to fitness for
both the able-bodied
and the handicapped.

APPLICATIONS FOR FITNESS

This section indicates how to develop a fitness program and recommends suitable activities for health-related fitness. Also included is information of special concern, such as fitness for the handicapped, for children and youth, for the elderly, and for women who are pregnant, and considerations for exercising under extreme environmental conditions (at high altitude, in extreme heat or cold, and others).

CHAPTER 9

Principles and Procedures for Developing a Physical Fitness Program

duration
exercise prescription
frequency
intensity
principles of training

overload
progression
specificity
threshold level
training effect

After reading this chapter, you should be able to:
1. Define and/or explain the key words listed above.
2. Identify and discuss the five principles of training identified in the chapter.
3. Identify and discuss the factors that should be considered in choosing activities for a fitness program.
4. Develop your own individualized fitness program.
5. Determine your resting heart rate.
6. Determine your age-adjusted maximum heart rate, your target heart rate, and your target heart rate range.
7. Discuss the rationale for spacing training sessions on alternate days.
8. Identify and discuss the three phases of an exercise workout.
9. Differentiate between maximum oxygen uptake and maximum heart rate as methods of determining the intensity level of participation in an activity.

Having assimilated the foundation information in Section One and the motivation arguments in Section Two, you should be ready to begin a physical fitness program. To aid you in developing a suitable individualized fitness program, this chapter presents several principles of training; important considerations in program planning, such as the types of exercise programs to consider; and a discussion of the three phases of an exercise program.

Recognize that physical fitness improvement will occur only if the principles and program planning considerations are adhered to. Further, you must realize that your choice of activities for fitness development is critical. You should choose an activity that you can perform and are interested in as well as one that will produce fitness benefits. You must know that you can gain access to the facility for participation in such activity. For example, swimming is an ideal exercise for cardiorespiratory development. However, you must be able to swim and have access to a swimming pool before you can decide to use swimming as an activity for cardiorespiratory development.

Principles of Training

Physiologists and physical fitness specialists have identified several principles of training that should guide the development and implementation of a physical fitness program. Principles of training or conditioning refer to general statements based on scientific evidence or logical reasoning that are applied as systematic guidelines to aid in the development of a safe and effective fitness program. The principles of training included in this text are the principles of a sound foundation, progression, overload, specificity, and fitness balance and maintenance. Each of these principles will be discussed briefly.

A Sound Foundation

It is important to know your state of health before engaging in a strenuous fitness program. This is the principle of a sound foundation. A complete medical examination will help to determine your present state of health and the types of activities to choose as well as the intensity level at which you can begin to exercise. For example, a medical examination may reveal that you have a physical impairment such as scoliosis (a lateral curvature of the spine). Such a condition might cause the doctor to advise against running or jogging as an aerobic activity for the development of cardiorespiratory endurance. Swimming or some such activity that would not aggravate the existing physical condition might be advised instead.

As was indicated in Chapter 5, it is important for each person to be examined by a medical doctor before engaging in a strenuous exercise program. It is obligatory, however, for persons over 35 years of age, those who have any overt symptoms of cardiac impairment, and those who have led sedentary lives to get a thorough medical examination, including an exercise stress test.

The design and implementation of your fitness program should be based on the results of the medical examination, your present level of fitness, and your overall fitness goal. Even though the principles are general, they should guide the development of a sound individualized physical fitness program.

These two principles are interrelated. Progression refers to a systematic increase in the intensity level or duration of the activity (or both). For improvement to occur, it is important for each person to begin at a level of intensity that he or she can tolerate and progressively to increase the amount of work performed. For example, a person who has not been engaged in any aerobic activities for the past two years should not attempt to run two miles in 15 minutes. It would be more reasonable for such a person to begin a walking program and build up to a program of jogging or running or to engage in some other aerobic activity more strenuous than walking.

Overload refers to the increase in workload of the body or body parts above the present level. The procedures for accomplishing an overload would be determined by the type of activity. In general, an overload can be achieved by manipulating the frequency, intensity, and duration of the activity. For cardiorespiratory endurance activities, the overload would be accomplished by increasing the intensity level or duration of the activity, or both. For instance, a person might engage in an aerobic dance routine for 15 minutes at a working heart rate of 75 percent of that person's age-adjusted heart rate maximum. The overload principle would be in effect if the person were to increase the intensity level to 80 percent of the age-adjusted heart rate maximum for the aerobic dance routine or perform the activity for 20 or 30 minutes instead of 15.

One may overload for strength and muscular endurance by (1) increasing the resistance on the muscle or muscle group (Example: work with a weight of 110 pounds after you have lifted 90 pounds for a few workouts); (2) increasing the number of repetitions to be performed (Example: execute 15 repetitions of a particular exercise rather than 10); and (3) increasing the speed of the repetitions (Example: Perform 50 sit-ups in one minute instead of 30 sit-ups).

Progression and Overload

The principle of specificity dictates that improvement in physical fitness will depend on the degree to which one chooses activities and methods of training that are specific to the outcome desired. To develop strength in the biceps muscle, for example, one would engage in an activity such as arm curls to overload the biceps muscle. On the other hand, one would not perform arm curls to develop cardiorespiratory endurance. Rather, one would engage in activities such as jogging, swimming, or aerobic dance. The activity must be specifically related to the goals and objectives of the fitness program.

The specificity principle might be viewed on two levels. First, the activity chosen must be specific to the development of the general fitness goal. The list of activities indicated for the development of cardiorespiratory endurance illustrates the specificity principle on the first level. Second, activities must be chosen to produce a training effect for the specific body part or parts in need of fitness development or maintenance. There-

Specificity

fore, to develop the triceps muscles, one would use push-ups and bench press exercises rather than arm curls.

Balance and Maintenance

While the principle of specificity stipulates that the activity chosen must be specific to the general goals and specific objectives of the fitness program, it should not preclude the development of the entire body. This means, for instance, that one should not develop cardiorespiratory endurance to the exclusion of minimal levels of strength, muscular endurance, and flexibility. Although the development of cardiorespiratory endurance is vitally important, the other components of fitness should also be developed to the extent that they will aid in the overall development of total body fitness. Think of the track sprinter who has great leg strength but suffers frequent hamstring pulls because of a lack of adequate flexibility.

Just as it is important to develop all components of fitness to ensure balanced development, it is equally important to engage in physical fitness activities with a degree of regularity and continuity for optimal fitness goals to be reached and maintained. Once your fitness goals are realized, it is no longer necessary to use the overload principle. At that point you should maintain participation in the activity or activities at the intensity, duration, and frequency that will enable you to maintain your desired level of fitness. Continual overloading beyond the body's capacity to handle such overloading usually leads to injury. Discontinuance of the exercise regimen or a sharp curtailment of the program will cause a loss in the training effect and thus reduced fitness benefits.

Besides the principles of training, other important aspects to consider in planning a fitness program are the types of activities to include and the intensity, duration, and frequency of participation. These factors or aspects of a fitness program are often called the *exercise prescription*.

Types of Activities to Consider

The types of activities one would include in a fitness program would depend on the goals and objectives of the program. A first step in determining the type of activity to engage in is to observe the principle of specificity: Choose activities that will aid in the development of the fitness component under consideration. For example, progressive resistance exercises (weight training) would be recommended to develop strength and muscular endurance.

Kuntzleman and the editors of *Consumer Guide*[1] have rated 14 popular sports and exercises according to their value in the development of the basic fitness components and important aspects of general well-being. A summary of the ratings appears in Table 9.1.

Table 9.1 reveals that some activities are good for the development of some fitness components but not so good for the development of other components. Therefore, their overall ranking might be lower. Jogging, for

TABLE 9.1   **The Fitness Value of Fourteen Sports and Exercises**[a]

Sport or Exercise	Cardio-respiratory Endurance	Muscular Endurance	Muscular Strength	Joint Flexibility	Total Points for All Components
Swimming	21	20	14	15	70
Handball or Squash	19	18	15	16	68
Jogging	21	20	17	9	67
Skiing (Nordic)	19	19	15	14	67
Basketball	19	17	15	13	64
Skating (Ice or Roller)	18	17	15	13	63
Skiing (Alpine)	16	18	15	14	63
Bicycling	19	18	16	9	62
Tennis	16	16	14	14	60
Calisthenics	10	13	16	19	58
Walking	13	14	11	7	45
Golf[b]	8	8	9	9	34
Softball	6	8	9	9	30
Bowling	5	5	5	7	22

[a]This is a summary of the rankings of 14 sports and exercises by seven experts on physical fitness and exercise. Ratings are on a scale of 0 to 3, with a rating of 21 indicating maximum benefit (a score of 3 by all seven judges). Ratings were made on the basis of regular (minimum of four times per week), vigorous (duration of 30 minutes to one hour per session) participation in each activity.

[b]Ratings for golf are based on the fact that many Americans use golf carts or caddies. Walking the links increases the physical fitness value appreciably.

Source: Adapted from Charles T. Kuntzleman et al., Rating the Exercises (New York: Morrow, 1978), p. 243.

example, is rated tops for developing cardiorespiratory endurance; however, it is rated poorly as an activity for the development of joint flexibility. Handball or squash is rated lower than jogging in cardiorespiratory endurance development, but these activities have a higher overall rating because of their consistently good ratings on all four fitness components. As mentioned previously, activities should be chosen with a view toward helping to meet fitness goals and objectives. It might be necessary to participate in several activities to achieve total fitness.

The value of the activity in developing selected physical fitness components should be an important criterion in deciding which activities to engage in. However, it should not be the only determining factor. Other important practical considerations include your interest and skill in the activity, the availability of equipment and facilities, and the need (or lack of need) for a partner or group to participate in the activity. For instance, swimming is rated number one as a developer of total fitness and is highly recommended on the basis of its value in helping to meet the overall goal of total fitness. However, in order for swimming to be used as fitness activity one must be able to swim continuously for 30 minutes or more and have access to a swimming pool.

One final comment about activity selection is that the fitness values of activities ultimately depend on the effort put into the activity (intensity), the length of time the activity is engaged in (duration), and the

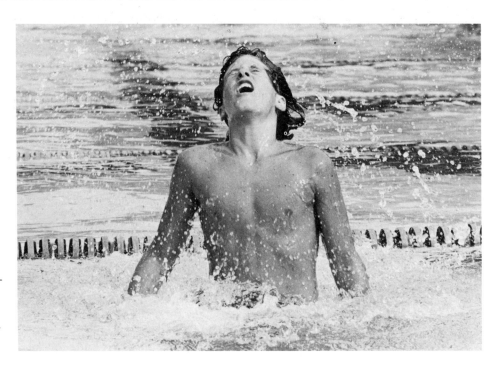

Swimming can be quite a refreshing activity during the heat of the summer.

number of times per week of such engagement (frequency). The fitness values of the activities are directly proportional to the degree of intensity, duration, and frequency—the higher the intensity level, the longer the time of participation, and the greater the frequency of engagement in the activity, the greater will be the fitness value in terms of training effect. In this text training effect refers to the improved physiological changes that take place due to participation in physical activity. Examples include an increased ability of the heart to pump blood to the working muscles and increased oxygen consumption and use due to participation in aerobic activities.

Intensity: How Hard Should You Exercise?

A certain amount of effort or exertion is necessary to develop and maintain a physically fit body. Contrary to some advertising slogans, there is no effortless way to achieve and maintain good physical fitness. Conversely, one does not have to exercise to the point of exhaustion to achieve an optimal level of fitness. How much effort should one put forth during a workout? While it is recognized that each individual is different in some respects and will require an individualized exercise prescription, there are some general guidelines for determining the intensity level at which activities should be engaged in.

A determination of the intensity of the overload needed to produce the training effect necessary to improve one's fitness level is related to the maximum oxygen uptake (vO_2 max) one can achieve. Results of thousands of tests in exercise physiology laboratories have shown that there is generally a linear relationship between vO_2 and heart rate (HR). This simply means that as O_2 consumption increases, maximum heart rate increases in a corresponding manner.

It should be realized that some accuracy is sacrificed when estimating the percent vO_2 max from percent HR max. The stated degree of inaccuracy varies among experts. For example, McArdle, Katch, and Katch indicate that there is an error of about $\pm$ 8 percent,[2] whereas Astrand and Rodahl state that there is an error variance as high as $\pm$ 15 percent in estimating oxygen uptake from heart rate.[3] Even with such inaccuracies, using heart rate to determine the relative intensity of the exercise bout needed to produce a training effect is viewed by these exercise physiologists as an acceptable procedure, since it is impracticable for most individuals to determine their vO_2 max directly because of the unavailability of sophisticated equipment that is needed.

The threshold or lower level at which aerobic capacity will improve is said to be at a heart rate of 70 percent of the maximum heart rate. This is equivalent to approximately 50 to 55 percent of the maximum aerobic capacity. The upper limit of training intensity is estimated to be about 90 percent of the maximum heart rate (which corresponds to about 85 percent of vO_2 max).

Instead of actually having people perform an activity at an intensity level to elicit their maximum heart rate, which would require the individuals to be extremely motivated and to have had medical clearance, age-adjusted maximum heart rates are used. It is recognized that maximum heart rates differ among individuals even in the same age group (by an estimated $\pm$ 10 beats per minute).[4] However, predicted age-adjusted maximum heart rates are acceptable and have been established. (See Table 9.2)

The age-adjusted target heart rate range chart in Table 9.2 provides some latitude for people of different levels of physical fitness to improve by overloading the fitness component being developed.

These ranges allow one to work at an intensity level of between 70 and 90 percent of one's maximum heart rate, adjusted for age. The age-adjusted maximum heart rate is 220 minus the person's age.

Table 9.2 contains both the age-adjusted maximum heart rates and the target heart rate ranges for individuals between the ages of 20 and 60. The fitness goal as well as the person's present fitness status will determine the intensity level necessary to produce increases in aerobic capacity. For example, a 33-year-old man who has been sedentary for the past few years might wish to engage in a walking program whereby he overloads at the threshold level (that is, 70 percent of HR max, or 131 beats per minute). A well-conditioned person of the same age might be able to exercise at the upper level of the target heart rate range, at 168 beats per minute (or 90 percent of HR max).

Many people might need to exercise at an intensity level somewhere between the lower and upper limits of the target heart rate range (70 and 90 percent of HR max). The intensity level at which one exercises is called the target heart rate (or training heart rate). The target heart rate is the percentage of the age-adjusted maximum heart rate at which one

TABLE 9.2   **Age-adjusted Maximum Heart Rates and Heart Rate Ranges**

Age	Age-adjusted Maximum Heart Rates	Target Heart Rate Ranges	
		Lower Level (70%)	Upper Level (90%)
20	200	140	180
21	199	139	179
22	198	139	178
23	197	138	177
24	196	137	176
25	195	137	176
26	194	136	175
27	193	135	174
28	192	134	173
29	191	134	172
30	190	133	171
31	189	132	170
32	188	132	169
33	187	131	168
34	186	130	167
35	185	130	167
36	184	129	166
37	183	128	165
38	182	127	164
39	181	127	163
40	180	126	162
41	179	125	161
42	178	125	160
43	177	124	159
44	176	123	158
45	175	123	158
46	174	122	157
47	173	121	156
48	172	120	155
49	171	120	154
50	170	119	153
51	169	118	152
52	168	118	151
53	167	117	150
54	166	116	149
55	165	116	149
56	164	115	148
57	163	114	147
58	162	113	146
59	161	113	145
60	160	112	144

exercises. Let's use the 33-year-old man as the example again. Suppose he wanted to jog at a pace that would cause his heart rate to increase to 80 percent of the maximum heart rate. To do so he would have to achieve a target heart rate of 150 beats per minute (80% $\times$ 187 max/hr = 150 bpm).

As a general rule, most people can improve their aerobic capacity if they train at an intensity level in the target heart rate range for their age (refer to Table 9.2). However, individuals at either end of the continuum (those so out of condition that they need to train at a level lower than 70 percent of HR max or those well-conditioned individuals who can train at a level above the 90 percent upper level) who need to calculate their target heart rate would simply multiply the desired percent of maximum heart rate times the age-adjusted maximum heart rate for their age. A formula is presented here to aid those who wish to exercise at a target heart rate other than those appearing in Table 9.2.

Formula for calculating your target heart rate

1. Calculate the age-adjusted maximum heart rate by subtracting your age from 220.

    $$220 - \text{your age} = \text{age-adjusted maximum heart rate}$$

2. Multiply the desired percent of the maximum heart rate by the age-adjusted maximum heart rate.

    $$\% \text{ of maximum heart rate desired} \times \begin{array}{c} \text{age-adjusted} \\ \text{maximum HR} \end{array} = \begin{array}{c} \text{target} \\ \text{heart rate} \end{array}$$

The Karvonen Formula

Another method for estimating target heart rate ranges, which takes into account the present fitness level of the individual, is the technique proposed by Karvonen, Kentala, and Mustala.[5] The minimal threshold level for cardiorespiratory improvement in the Karvonen et al. formula is 60 percent of the maximum heart rate reserve. The maximum heart rate reserve is the percent difference between the resting and maximal heart rates plus the resting heart rate. The upper level of the target heart range is 90 percent of the age-adjusted maximum heart rate reserve. The formulas for determining the lower level or threshold and the upper level of the age-adjusted heart rate range and examples for a hypothetical exerciser are shown in Table 9.3.

What is the difference between the two techniques for calculating the target heart rate range? Besides the fact that the resting rate is used in the Karvonen method, this method also results in higher lower and upper levels of the target heart rate range than the other method. It is estimated that the first method underestimates the target heart rate range by an average of about 15 percent.[6] Only at extremely high resting heart rates do the discrepancies in target heart rate ranges approximate 15 percent when using the two methods. For instance, by comparing the heart rate range of the hypothetical person used as an example in Table 9.3 with a 20-year-old in Table 9.2, it can be seen that the lower level of the target heart rate range using the Karvonen formula is only a little higher (144 versus 140) than the other method. Similarly, the Karvonen formula results in only a slightly higher upper limit of the target heart rate range (186 versus 180) than the other method. The figures for the Karvonen formula were based on a person with a resting heart rate of 60.

Continuing to use the 20-year-old for illustrative purposes, let us

TABLE 9.3   **Steps in Calculating the Target Heart Rate Range for a 20-Year-Old Person with a Resting Heart Rate of 60 Beats per Minute (bpm)**

1.	*Calculate the maximal heart rate*	
	220 − age (in years) = maximal heart rate	220 − 20 = 200
2.	*Calculate the maximal heart rate reserve*	
	Maximal heart rate − resting heart rate = maximal heart rate reserve	200 − 60 = 140
3.	*Calculate the lower level of the age-adjusted maximal heart rate range*	
	Maximal heart rate reserve × .60 + resting heart rate = lower level target heart rate range	140 × .60 = 84 + 60 = 144
4.	*Calculate the upper level of the age-adjusted maximal heart rate range*	
	Maximal heart rate reserve × .90 + resting heart rate = upper level of target heart rate range	140 × .90 = 126 + 60 = 186
5.	*Indicate the target heart rate range*	
	Lower level of target HR range and upper level of target HR range	144 to 186 bpm

assume that this person has a resting heart rate of 100. Using the Karvonen formula, this person would have a heart rate range of 160 to 190 beats per minute. The lower level (160) would be 20 beats per minute higher than in the other method, and the upper level (190) would be 10 beats per minute higher. (See Table 9.2 to check these comparisons.) You can see that a person with this high resting heart rate will experience a rather large divergence in heart rate range when using the two methods of computation.

It also should be noted that the percentage of the maximal working capacity in the two methods is different. The Karvonen formula requires the use of 60 to 90 percent of the *maximal heart rate reserve,* whereas the other formula requires the use of 70 to 90 percent of the *maximal heart rate.*

Each person should learn to calculate his or her target heart rate range. The formulas in Table 9.3 can be used to make such calculations. Remember to take the resting pulse rate upon awakening in the morning, and use this pulse rate in the Karvonen formula.

Rating of Perceived Exertion

A third measure of exercise intensity is the Rating of Perceived Exertion (RPE) model proposed by Gunnar Borg.[7] The gist of the theory is that a person can determine the level of exercised intensity by his or her subjective feeling of the strenuousness of an exercise task. The RPE response to graded exercise correlates highly with oxygen uptake and heart rate, among other cardiorespiratory and metabolic variables, and is a valid and reliable instrument to indicate the level of physical exertion in continuous, aerobic exercises. It is thus an appropriate tool to use for the establishment of exercise intensity levels for cardiorespiratory endurance development.[8]

Borg's perceived exertion scale provides a means to quantify subjective exercise intensity. The perceived exertion of an exercise task is arrived at by noting the strenuousness of the task and adding a zero to the appropriate rating in Table 9.4. The corresponding heart rate for a very hard task, number 17 according to the RPE scale, would be 170.

Borg has devised another RPE scale with a range of 0 (nothing at all) to 10 (very, very strong). This scale appears in Table 9.5. Borg recommends the old RPE scale (Table 9.4) for most simple applied studies of perceived exertion, for exercise testing, and for predictions and prescriptions for exercise intensities in sports and medical rehabilitation; the new scale is thought to be suitable for determining other subjective symptoms such as breathing difficulties and aches and pains.[9]

Regardless of the method used to calculate the target heart rate, the principles of progression and overload should be observed when undertaking a fitness program. As the body adapts to the increased demands

TABLE 9.4   **The Rating of Perceived Exertion (RPE) Scale**

6		14	
7	very, very light	15	hard
8		16	
9	very light	17	very hard
10		18	
11	fairly light	19	very, very hard
12		20	
13	somewhat hard		

Source: Gunnar Borg, "Perceived Exertion: A Note on History and Methods," Medicine and Science in Sports 5 (1973): 90. © by American College of Sports Medicine, 1973.

TABLE 9.5   **The New RPE Scale**

0	Nothing at all	
0.5	Very, very weak	(just noticable)
1	Very weak	
2	Weak	(light)
3	moderate	
4	Somewhat strong	
5	Strong	(heavy)
6		
7	Very strong	
8		
9		
10	Very, very strong	(almost maximal)
	Maximal	

Source: Gunnar Borg, "Psychophysical Bases of Perceived Exertion," Medicine and Science in Sports and Exercise 14 (1982): 380. © by American College of Sports Medicine, 1982.

of training intensities, one must periodically overload to continue to produce a training effect. Keep in mind that age and present level of fitness should help to determine the training intensity at which you will exercise. It can be seen from Table 9.2, for example, that a 20-year-old might work out at a target heart rate range of 140 to 180 heart beats per minute, while a 60-year-old person should exercise at an intensity level of between 112 and 144 heart beats per minute.

The pulse rate is a close approximation of the heart rate. The pulse rate should be taken *immediately* following the exercise activity (if the conditioning bout is long, the pulse rate may be taken at intervals during the exercise). The pulse count can be taken for six seconds or ten seconds. If you take the pulse for six seconds, add a zero; if you take the pulse for ten seconds, multiply by 6. Both procedures give the heart rate for one minute. Practice taking your pulse a few times to achieve accuracy in the procedure. (Instructions for determining the pulse rate are given in Chapter 5.)

A stopwatch or watch with a second hand is needed to keep time when counting the pulse rate.

Duration: How Long Should You Exercise?

The length of time that one exercises depends on a number of factors, an important one being the type of activity in which one engages. For instance, a person would need to walk for an hour at a normal pace to burn up approximately 423 Calories, whereas a person could run at a pace of seven minutes per mile for 30 minutes and burn up approximately 468 Calories. To account for the many variable factors that affect the optimal length of time of participation in an activity for improvement in fitness to occur, a duration of 15 to 60 minutes is recommended. (Keep in mind that an additional 45 minutes to an hour will be needed to warm up, cool down, shower, and so on).

The actual length of time devoted to an activity is related to the intensity level at which the person participates in the activity and is dependent on the type of activity, training frequency, and the fitness level of the participant. Although the 15- to 60-minute time period for exercise duration is recommended as a general rule, there are situations where shorter durations might be used. When participating in an activity at an intensity level of 70 percent of maximal heart rate, for instance, a poorly conditioned person would probably benefit from bouts of exercise lasting only 5 to 10 minutes, whereas a well-conditioned person would require about 30 minutes of exercise to produce a training effect at the same intensity level.

The use of high-intensity, short-duration activities to develop cardiorespiratory endurance is especially effective with interval training techniques. Interval training is a method in which high-intensity exercises of short duration are combined with intermittent periods or intervals of rest or light exercise.

Using the interval training technique, Edward Fox and colleagues studied the relative importance of intensity and distance on maximal aerobic power (vO_2) on untrained college students.[10] Three programs were used: (1) high-intensity, short-distance sprints (Group S); (2) low-intensity, long-distance runs (Group L); and (3) a combination of both (Group M).

Although all groups showed significant increases in vO_2 max (when measured in liters/min) following 7½ weeks of training 5 days per week, increases in vO_2 max (when measured in ml/kg/min) were significant only for Groups S and M. Further, a significant relationship ($p < .05$) was found between the change in vO_2 max and training intensity. The researchers thus concluded that intensity rather than distance of the interval training program is the more important factor in improving vO_2 max.

It is advisable to design exercise programs for beginners at a low level of intensity and longer duration to minimize injuries and discourage individuals from dropping out of the exercise program. The threshold level of 70 percent of the maximum heart rate or 60 percent of the heart rate reserve (if resting heart rate is known) may be used as a guide. However, individuals should experiment with many intensity levels and durations to determine the best combination.

Frequency: How Often Should You Exercise?

Must you work out on a daily basis to improve your fitness level? Or is it better to exercise every other day? A precise answer cannot be provided. However, after reviewing numerous studies dealing with the intensity, duration, and frequency of training, for example, the American College of Sports Medicine has recommended that exercise sessions be participated in three to five days per week.[11] In a 20-week study of the effects of various combinations of frequency and duration on attrition and incidence of injury, Michael Pollock and colleagues noted that the greatest increase in cardiorespiratory fitness occurred in groups that exercised 45 minutes a day, five days a week.[12] However, they did not recommend programs of that duration and frequency for beginning joggers at the training intensity of between 85 and 90 percent of maximum heart rate that was used in the study. The rationale was that participating at a lower intensity for fewer days per week would result in fewer injuries and fewer dropouts.

The duration and intensity of your training regimen as well as the goal of your fitness program should help to determine the ultimate choice of training frequency. For example, the American College of Sports Medicine has reported that training programs conducted for at least 20 minutes' duration and at an intensity level to expend about 300 kilocalories require only three days per week for weight reduction. (If the intensity level expends 200 kilocalories, four days a week is required.) So if weight control is the goal, participation must be at least three days per week, with each exercise session lasting a minimum of 20 minutes at a training intensity sufficient to burn at least 300 kilocalories per session. (A listing of the caloric expenditures of various household, recreational, and sports activities can be found in Tables 4.4 and 4.5 and in Appendix F.) If, on the other hand, the goal is cardiorespiratory fitness, high-intensity training sessions of short duration (15 to 20 minutes) may be recommended for well-conditioned individuals.

A training frequency of three days per week is recommended for beginners and for people in poor physical condition. As the level of fitness improves, a gradual increase to four- or five-day training sessions is recommended. (I favor a four-day schedule.) Although the practice has been questioned by one group of researchers,[13] it is recommended that training sessions be spaced—that is, conducted on alternate days. The main reason for such a recommendation is to allow the body time to rest between aerobic exercise sessions of moderately high intensity levels to minimize the incidence of injuries and to combat attrition due to boredom. This recommendation is supported by the American College of Sports Medicine and a joint group of the American Heart Association and the President's Council on Physical Fitness and Sports.[14]

Phases of an Exercise Workout

There should be at least three phases or parts of an exercise workout: (1) warm-up, (2) conditioning bout, and (3) cool-down. Each of these phases is important in designing the overall exercise prescription.

Warm-up

A five- to ten-minute warm-up is necessary to get the body ready for the main conditioning bout. Sometimes warming up has served as a precaution to muscle pulls and other injuries. The warm-up should consist of activities that will slowly activate the body systems that will be used in the conditioning bout. For example, if jogging is to be used in the conditioning bout, the warm-up might consist of stretching, bending, and twisting exercises to stimulate the heart and activate the leg muscles for the more strenuous activity to follow. Beginning the jog at a slow pace for the first few minutes will also act as a warm-up to the main conditioning bout. The idea is gradually to increase blood and muscle temperatures to increase blood flow and muscle elasticity and contractility. (Chapter 11 contains numerous exercises that can be used for warming up.)

The conditioning bout refers to the time spent engaging in the activities designed to achieve your fitness goals. In training to improve strength, for instance, progressive resistance (weight training) exercises such as the bench press, arm curls, and leg lifts would constitute the conditioning bout. The length of time for the conditioning bout will depend on the several factors discussed earlier in the chapter. The chapters that follow contain exercises and activities for the development of each of the fitness components.

Conditioning Bout

Some of the activities that are used in the main conditioning bout can also be used for the warm-up and cool-down. Examples include stretching exercises and calisthenics. The feature that distinguishes how the exercise is to be used is the intensity of the exercise. Whereas the intensity level of the exercise for warm-ups and cool-downs should be low, the level of intensity of activities during the conditioning bout should be within the target heart rate range of 70 to 90 percent of the age-adjusted maximum predicted heart rate. It should be emphasized again, however, that beginners and people with symptoms of cardiovascular disease should begin an exercise program at an intensity level that they can tolerate safely. For some, this may be only 40 to 50 percent of HR max. The intensity level should be gradually increased according to the principles of progression and overload.

I have emphasized repeatedly that cardiorespiratory fitness is of paramount importance and should be the main feature of any exercise program. However, activities to develop minimal levels of strength, muscular endurance, and flexibility should also be incorporated in a fitness program. This is especially critical when one uses an aerobic activity such as jogging or walking for the conditioning bout. These activities are good for cardiorespiratory development but poor for the development of strength, muscular endurance, and flexibility, especially of the upper body.

A recommended strategy for developing cardiorespiratory endurance and the other components is to include an activity such as jogging as the conditioning bout three days a week and strength-building activity such as weight training two days a week. The strength activities should be devoted to the upper body, and the front of the thighs (quadriceps muscles) for joggers. Flexibility and muscular endurance exercises can be a part of the warm-up and cool-down and can also be incorporated in the strength exercise workout days. The exercises for flexibility should focus on the total body, with special attention being paid to the muscles in the back of the thighs (hamstrings) for those who jog.

If you design an exercise program for five days a week, it does not mean that you do nothing on the other days. Although no formal exercise program should be conducted on these days, you should be as physically active as possible as you go about your normal activities. Take the stairs instead of the elevator; walk the several blocks to the office instead of taking public transportation; go window shopping instead of having a large lunch; mow the lawn with a manual lawn mower instead of a power mower. An active lifestyle is conducive to health and happiness.

Cool-down

The cool-down or gradual reduction of body systems to normal after a vigorous workout is of vital importance. The time needed to cool down will vary according to the type of activity engaged in and the intensity and duration of the activity. For instance, only two to three minutes might be needed to cool down after a brisk 15-minute walk. On the other hand, a much longer period of time (10 to 15 minutes) might be needed to recover from a 45-minute run at a seven-minutes-per-mile pace.

The cool-down might consist of a continuation of the activity of the main conditioning bout, but at a slower pace or intensity level. The runner might jog slowly and then walk for a few minutes to begin the cool-down period; the jogger might walk at a slow pace to cool down. Stretching exercises should be included as part of the cool-down regimen for joggers and runners.

Cool-down exercises permit the body to return gradually to its normal resting state. In continuous, rhythmic, aerobic activities such as running, swimming, cycling, and aerobic dance, a cool-down period in which the body continues to move at a reduced intensity level keeps the blood from pooling in the extremities. It also aids in the return of blood to the heart and helps to buffer out lactic acid and other metabolic waste materials from the tissues by providing adequate oxygen to the muscles.

A person should be considered recovered from an exercise bout if he or she has ceased breathing heavily and has recovered from any feelings of discomfort. The heart rate is also a good indicator of the time needed to cool down after a conditioning bout. The heart rate should approach the resting level during the cool-down period. If not at the resting level, it should certainly be below 100 before one should consider the recovery period to be adequate.

Developing an Individualized Exercise Prescription

Use the information in this chapter to develop your own exercise program. Personal interests, present fitness status, physical capabilities, and physical fitness goals as well as practical factors such as availability of facilities and time available to participate in the activity will undoubtedly influence the program design. For example, some people with busy schedules might wish to increase the intensity level of the activity and engage in it for shorter periods of time. Others might wish to participate at a lower intensity level for a longer duration and with less frequent exercise sessions to cut down on the number of times required to travel to the exercise facility and engage in the chores related to exercising, such as showering and changing clothes.

The type of activity one chooses might also be influenced by several factors. One such factor is age. Jogging has been mentioned as an excel-

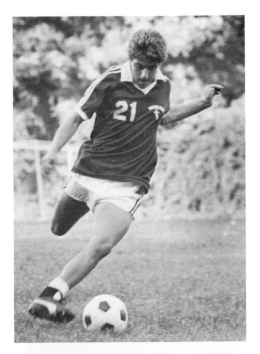

One should become fit before engaging in an activity such as soccer.

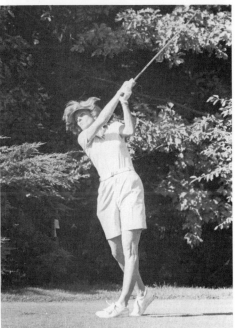

Golf requires flexibility and strength, among other fitness components.

lent activity for the development of cardiorespiratory endurance. But the stress to the joints would make such an activity less appealing to some older adults. These individuals might wish to engage in other activities such as walking, swimming, and cycling. One or a combination of these activities would be appropriate for the development of cardiorespiratory fitness in older adults.

Manipulation of the various stimulus variables (intensity, duration, frequency, and type of activity) is encouraged. However, the principles of training and the general guidelines presented in this chapter should

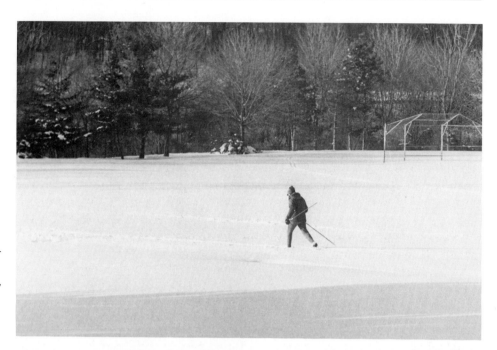

Cross-country (Nordic) skiing can be a solitary activity. However, some people might use the time to contemplate.

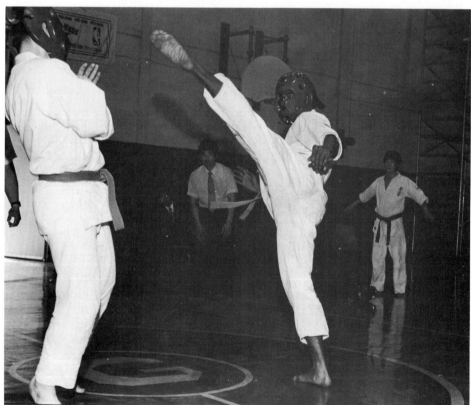

Adequate fitness development is a prerequisite to success in karate.

guide the development and conduct of fitness programs. It would not be prudent, for instance, for a person who has been extremely sedentary for the past few years to increase the intensity level of an activity to 80 or 90 percent of the maximum heart rate the first few weeks to reduce the time spent in the activity. The principle of progression dictates that one should start at a level of intensity that is safe for the individual and increase the intensity gradually by applying the overload principle—place increasingly more stress on the cardiorespiratory system until the desired training effect is realized.

Adherence to the principles and guidelines in this chapter, along with the exercise of good personal judgment, should enable each person to establish and maintain a safe and productive physical fitness program. Remember that although it takes some effort to develop and maintain an acceptable level of physical fitness, the training regimen does not have to cause pain or discomfort. The exercise program should be one that you plan to engage in for the remainder of your life. In this regard you should consider a program with a *variety* of activities, one where the intensity level is moderate and the duration and frequency are manageable in terms of time devoted to the fitness program.

Finally, your fitness program should be reevaluated at four- to six-month intervals to determine whether program goals and objectives are being met. During the periodic reevaluation, changes can be made in aspects of the program as needed. You might wish to substitute different activities, for example, or change the intensity or duration of an activity. The reevaluation should allow you to determine the present state of the fitness program and to change those aspects that will make the program better for you.

Notes

1. Charles T. Kuntzleman et al., *Rating the Exercises* (New York: Morrow, 1978), p. 243.
2. William D. McArdle, Frank I. Katch, and Victor L. Katch, *Exercise Physiology: Energy, Nutrition, and Human Performance,* 2d ed. (Philadelphia, Lea & Febiger, 1986), p. 365.
3. Per-Olof Astrand and Kaare Rodahl, *Textbook of Work Physiology,* 2d ed. (New York: McGraw-Hill, 1977), p. 456.
4. Ibid., p. 189.
5. M. Karvonen, K. Kentala, and O. Mustala, "The Effects of Training on Heart Rate: A Longitudinal Study," *Annals of Medicine and Experimental Biology* 35 (1957): 307–315.
6. American College of Sports Medicine, *Guidelines for Exercise Testing and Prescription,* 3d ed. (Philadelphia: Lea & Febiger), 1986, p. 35.
7. Gunnar Borg, "Perceived Exertion: A Note on History and Methods," *Medicine and Science In Sports* (1973): 90–93.
8. ACSM, p. 36.
9. Gunnar Borg, "Psychophysical Bases of Perceived Exertion," *Medicine and Science in Sports and Exercise* 14 (1982): 380.
10. Edward L. Fox et al., "Intensity and Distance of Interval Training Programs and Changes in Aerobic Power," *Medicine and Science in Sports* 5 (1973): 18–22.
11. ACSM, "The Recommended Quantity and Quality of Exercise for Developing and Maintaining Fitness in Healthy Adults," *Medicine and Science in Sports* 10 (1978): vii–x.
12. Michael L. Pollock et al., "Effects of Frequency and Duration of Training on Attrition and Incidence of Injury," *Medicine and Science in Sports* 9 (1977): 31–36.

13.   Robert J. Moffatt, Bryant A. Stamford, and Robert D. Neill, "Placement of Tri-weekly Training Sessions: Importance Regarding Enhancement of Aerobic Capacity," *Research Quarterly* 48 (1977): 581–591.

14.   ACSM, *Guidelines for Graded Exercise Testing and Exercise Prescription,* 3d ed. (Philadelphia: Lea & Febiger, 1986); Lenore L. Zohman, *Exercise Your Way to Fitness and Heart Health* (American Heart Association and the President's Council on Physical Fitness and Sports: CPC International, 1974).

Pathways to Cardiorespiratory Endurance

aerobic dance
cardiorespiratory
endurance
continuous training

interval training
jogging
running

Key Words

Chapter Highlights

After reading this chapter, you should be able to:
1. Define and/or explain the key words listed above.
2. Identify and discuss the advantages and disadvantages of six pathways to cardiorespiratory endurance.
3. Compare and contrast walking and running as pathways to cardiorespiratory endurance.
4. Explain the proper mechanics of jogging and running.
5. Compare and contrast the philosophy and techniques of interval and continuous training as modalities for the development of cardiorespiratory fitness.

This chapter is designed to present specific activities and exercises to aid in the development and maintenance of cardiorespiratory endurance. I have tried to include from the vast number of activities that can be used to develop cardiorespiratory endurance enough so that each user of this book might choose one or more that are suitable. All activities in this chapter meet the criteria outlined in Chapter 9.

To enjoy the full benefits of the activities contained in this chapter, you must follow the guidelines for program development presented in Chapter 9. For example, you should choose an activity that you can enjoy and can perform; you must start slowly and work up to an intensity level that will produce a training effect (improve the condition of the heart, blood vessels, and lungs) and that you can sustain continuously for 15 to 30 minutes. Also remember to warm up before and cool down after the aerobic conditioning bout. (Review Chapter 9 before beginning your exercise program, if necessary.)

Activities That Develop Cardiorespiratory Endurance

Basic activities recommended for the development of cardiorespiratory endurance include walking, jogging or running, bicycling, swimming, aerobic dance, rope jumping, ice and roller skating, and the sports activities of raquetball, paddleball, squash, tennis, and basketball. (See Table 9.1 for the fitness values of other activities not included here.)

Some of the program progressions presented in this chapter are adapted from Dr. Kenneth Cooper's Aerobics Chart Pack, the data for which are based on the extensive research conducted at the Aerobics Center in Dallas, Texas. Since only five of the activities from Dr. Cooper's work are used here, Dr. Cooper's book, *The Aerobics Way,* is recommended for persons interested in developing cardiorespiratory endurance on an individual basis.

All the program progressions are age-adjusted and require you to begin exercising at a level that you can safely perform and to increase gradually the level of intensity (overload) to produce a training effect. Following the weekly progressions that are suggested for the programs

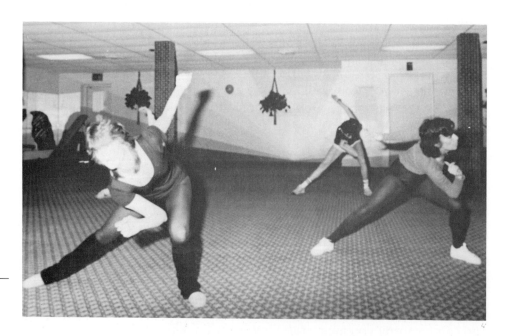

An aerobic dance
workout

will enable you to attain this objective. However, be sure to monitor your pulse rate about 10 to 15 minutes into the activity and again immediately after the activity to determine the intensity level at which you are exercising. Make adjustments in the intensity level as needed to achieve a training effect.

1. Select one activity and follow as closely as possible the recommended progression for that activity during the program.
2. Aim to achieve the time goals by the end of the week. However, if you can start the week within the recommended time limits, do so.
3. Once you have completed the number of weeks suggested for a particular activity progression, continue with that activity at the intensity level that will enable you to maintain your desired level of cardiorespiratory fitness. A suggested level at which you should attempt to continue exercising is indicated by an "M" (for maintenance) opposite the appropriate week with the distance and time goal recommended. (Remember that you are not bound to complete a particular program simply because you started it. You may change the activity initially selected and choose another activity. For instance, you may start a running program and find that it is too damaging to your joints. You might find walking to be more appropriate. (Begin the walking program even if you have been running for three or four weeks.)
4. Select activities from Chapter 11 to aid you in the development of minimal levels of strength and joint flexibility necessary to complete your total fitness program.
5. Warm up before the aerobic activity and cool down after it.

Walking

Although walking is not rated as highly as some of the other activities that can be used for the development of cardiorespiratory endurance, it is included for its overall value for physical fitness. It is especially recommended for persons with heart problems, those who are obese, and those who are beginning an exercise program after a long period of sedentary living.

The appeal of walking is that it can be performed alone or in a group situation, it requires no special athletic skill, no special facilities are needed, and it is much easier on the joints than jogging or running and sports activities. Walking may also be used as a starter activity for those interested in a more strenuous activity such as jogging or running.

A suggested walking program progression is presented in Table 10.1. You will note that this program is age-adjusted and has time goals. Although you should ultimately strive to reach the time goals, do not feel that you must reach them immediately. Above all, do not become obsessive about reaching time goals. Walk at a pace that is comfortable for you, and increase the intensity level (pace) as your fitness improves. After a few weeks you should be able to reach the time goals and thereby produce a training effect. You might even wish to begin the jogging/running program.

TABLE 10.1   **Walking Program Progression**[a]

Age	Week	Distance (miles)	Time Goal (minutes)	Times per Week
Under 30	1	1.0	18:00	4
	2	1.0	17:00	4
	3	1.0	16:00	4
	4	2.0	32:00	5
	5	2.0	31:00	5
	6	2.0	30:00	5
	7	2.0	29:00	5
	8	2.0	28:00	5
	9	2.5	34:00	5
	10 (M)	2.5	33:00	5
	11	3.0	42:00	5
	12	3.0	41:00	5
30–39	1	1.0	18:30	4
	2	1.0	18:00	4
	3	1.0	17:00	4
	4	2.0	32:00	5
	5	2.0	31:00	5
	6	2.0	30:00	5
	7	2.0	29:00	5
	8	2.0	28:00	5
	9	2.5	35:30	5
	10 (M)	2.5	34:30	5
	11	3.0	43:30	5
	12	3.0	42:30	5
40–49	1	1.0	19:00	4
	2	1.0	18:00	4
	3	1.0	17:30	4
	4	2.0	34:00	5
	5	2.0	33:00	5
	6	2.0	32:00	5
	7	2.0	31:00	5
	8	2.0	29:00	5
	9	2.5	36:00	5
	10 (M)	2.5	35:30	5
	11	3.0	43:00	5
	12	3.0	42:30	5
50–59	1	1.0	20:00	4
	2	1.0	19:00	4
	3	1.0	17:00	4
	4	1.5	30:00	4
	5	1.5	28:00	4
	6	1.5	26:00	4
	7	2.0	32:00	4
	8	2.0	31:00	4
	9	2.5	38:00	4
	10	2.5	37.30	4
	11	2.5	37:00	4

TABLE 10.1 (*Continued*)

Age	Week	Distance (miles)	Time Goal (minutes)	Times per Week
	12 (M)	2.5	37:00	5
	13	3.0	44:00	4
	14	3.0	43:00	4
60 and over	1	1.0	20:00	4
	2	1.0	19:00	4
	3	1.0	18:00	4
	4	1.5	29:00	4
	5	1.5	28:00	4
	6	1.5	27:00	4
	7	2.0	38:00	4
	8	2.0	36:00	4
	9	2.0	43:00	4
	10	2.5	42:30	4
	11	2.5	41:30	4
	12	2.5	40:00	4
	13	3.0	55:00	4
	14 (M)	3.0	53:00	5
	15	3.0	51:00	4
	16	3.0	49:00	4

[a]You may use walking to warm up before the conditioning bout and to cool down after the main exercise. Walk at a slower pace than recommended for that week for about three minutes to warm up, and for three to five minutes at a slower pace after the conditioning bout to cool down.

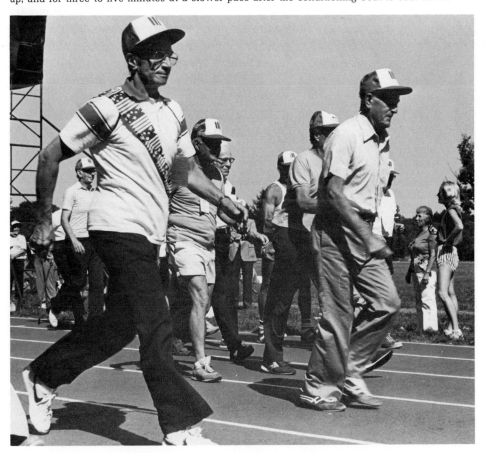

Walking

Jogging/ Running

A jogging/running program is an excellent activity for the development of cardiorespiratory endurance. Like walking, jogging or running requires neither special facilities nor expensive equipment. Only a good pair of running shoes and comfortable clothing are needed. The importance of quality footwear cannot be overemphasized. (See Chapter 14 for information on this topic.)

Running is the act of moving continuously at an 8- to 10-minute-mile pace. Jogging is at a slightly slower pace (11 to 12 minutes per mile). Some experts might give slightly different definitions of jogging and running, but the idea is to move continuously at a pace fast enough to produce a training effect. Remember the overload principle: work at progressively higher intensity levels to increase cardiorespiratory endurance.

At a jogging or running pace, one can get a good workout in 15 to 30 minutes. It is advisable to begin by jogging slowly and gradually increase the tempo after the first few weeks. Monitor your heart rate to ensure that you are exercising within your target heart rate range. If you are 40 years old, for instance, you should get your working heart rate to between 126 and 162 beats per minute. Refer to Table 9.2 for the age-adjusted target heart rate ranges. Remember that the American College of Sports Medicine estimates that the formula used to calculate these heart rate ranges underestimates the heart rate range by an average of 15 percent.[1] So individuals who feel that these heart rates are too low can either add 15 percent to the heart rate ranges for their age in Table 9.2 or calculate their heart rate range using the Karvonen formula (Table 9.3).

Mechanics of Running.   Incorrect running form can cause unnecessary injuries. The body should be erect, with the back straight and the shoulders parallel to the running surface. The running stride should be short, with a heel-to-ball-of-foot landing. The feet should land on the ground directly under the knees with the legs slightly bent. The arms should be held at approximately right angles and should be allowed to swing parallel to the body. There should be a natural rhythm between arm action and leg movement; that is, the left arm should be moved forward at the same time as the right leg, and the right arm should likewise move with the left leg. The hands should be closed with the fingers slightly cupped (the exact hand position should be one that feels naturally comfortable). Breathe through both mouth and nose when running.

Do not forget that adequate strength and flexibility workouts should supplement aerobic training programs. Chapter 11 contains activities for the development of strength, muscular endurance, and flexibility. These activities are recommended to serve as a part of your overall fitness training program. The suggested running programs are presented in Table 10.2.

Limit your running program to no more than four days per week. More injuries are likely to occur if you run long distances more often. Engage in a weight training program, either on alternate days or after the running workout. You should stretch for flexibility before and after the conditioning bout of running. Remember that you might start the running program by alternating walking and jogging with running until you are

TABLE 10.2   **Jogging/Running Program Progression**[a]

Age	Week	Distance (miles)	Time Goal (minutes)	Times per Week
Under 30	1	1.0	16:00	4
	2	1.0	15:00	4
	3	1.0	13:30	4
	4	1.5	20:00	4
	5	1.5	19:00	4
	6	1.5	18:30	4
	7	1.5	18:00	4
	8	2.0	22:00	4
	9	2.0	21:00	4
	10 (M)	2.0	19:00	4
	11	2.0	18:00	5
	12	2.0	17:00	5
30–39	1	1.0	16:00	4
	2	1.0	15:00	4
	3	1.0	14:00	4
	4	1.5	21:00	4
	5	1.5	20:00	4
	6	1.5	19:00	4
	7	2.0	24:00	4
	8	2.0	23:00	4
	9	2.0	22:00	4
	10 (M)	2.0	21:00	4
	11	2.0	20:00	5
	12	2.0	19:00	5

(continued)

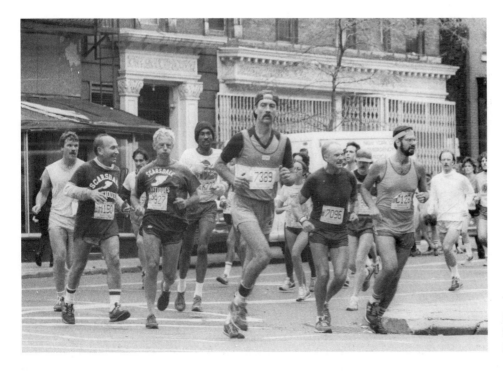

Some joggers progress to competitive road racing.

TABLE 10.2 (*Continued*)

Age	Week	Distance (miles)	Time Goal (minutes)	Times per Week
40–49	1	1.0	17:00	4
	2	1.0	16:00	4
	3	1.0	15:00	4
	4	1.5	22:00	4
	5	1.5	21:00	4
	6	1.5	20:00	4
	7	2.0	25:00	4
	8	2.0	24:00	4
	9	2.0	23:00	4
	10 (M)	2.0	22:00	4
	11	2.0	20:00	5
	12	2.0	19:00	5
50–59	1	1.0	18:00	4
	2	1.0	17:00	4
	3	1.0	16:00	4
	4	1.5	23:00	4
	5	1.5	22:00	4
	6	1.5	21:00	4
	7	1.5	20:00	4
	8	2.0	26:00	4
	9	2.0	25:00	4
	10 (M)	2.0	24:00	4
	11	2.0	23:00	5
	12	2.0	22:00	5

[a]If necessary, start the program by walking, then walk and jog, or run, to achieve the time goals. You may also start the program by covering less than one mile and gradually build up to the distance and time goals.

able to run continuously for 15 to 30 minutes. The maximum length of time you run will depend on your fitness goal and the intensity at which you run.

Safety Considerations. Besides the careful preparation needed to avoid injuries, persons who run should also be concerned with problems caused by running in traffic and running under extreme weather conditions. Chapter 14 contains information for exercising during hot or cold weather conditions; it should be read carefully.

Those who jog or run in areas where there is traffic should be aware of the traffic laws and obey them. Although pedestrians have the right-of-way, runners should always be ready to yield such a right to drivers who lose control of their vehicle or who may simply ignore the rules of the road. Avoid running in traffic-congested areas where the concentration of carbon monoxide is high. When jogging at night, wear clothing with bright reflective coloring.

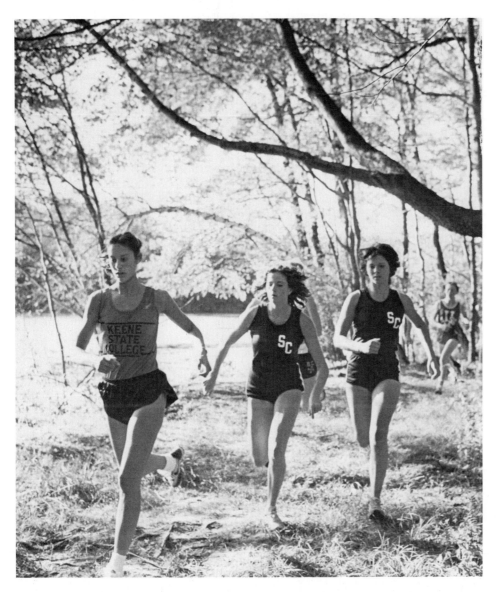

Cross-country running

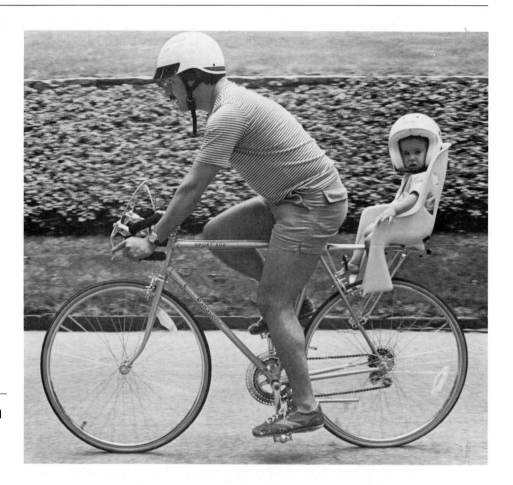

Bicycling can be used as a means of transportation as well as a fitness activity.

Bicycling

Although it requires more time for each workout in comparison with running, bicycling can provide equally effective improvement in the cardiorespiratory system. And bicycling can be fun.

There are three types of cyclists. The cross-country cyclist rides a bicycle 100 to 200 miles at a time. The "ordinary" cyclist rides to and from school or work or rides with friends for enjoyment. A third type of bicyclist rides a stationary cycle for physical fitness only.

For the more adventuresome, there is also cycle touring and cycle racing. The tour cyclist might take the bike for an overnight trip or spend the summer touring abroad. (One famous tour cyclist, Lloyd Summer, took a 28,478-mile four-year bicycle tour of the world!) Cycle racing is the competitive form of cycling. It can be performed on a track, on a road, or through fields and woods. Bicycle racing is one of three events in the triathlon (swimming and running are the other two). Probably the most spectacular of the bicycle racing events is long-distance road racing, which reaches its apotheosis in the Tour de France, the month-long race staged primarily in France during the month of July each year.

If you plan to use bicycling as an activity to develop cardiorespiratory endurance, be aware that the price ranges from about $100 to $800 for a ten-speed bike. A lightweight racing bike can cost $1000 or more. Some stationary bicycles cost more than $2000.

Those who can afford the cost of a bicycle and can ride it will discover that cycling is an excellent means of developing cardiorespira-

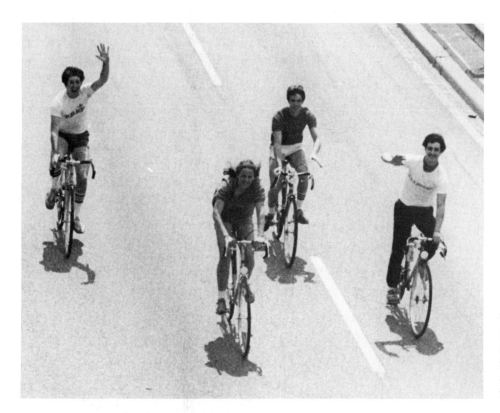

Long distances on the bicycle are necessary for the development of cardiorespiratory fitness.

tory fitness. They will also join the 72 million individuals who were reported to have engaged in cycling during 1982 by an A. C. Nielsen sports participation survey.

Persons who would like to use cycling as an activity for the development of cardiorespiratory endurance but do not possess the riding skills are urged to enroll in a cycling course. Check with the continuing-education department of your local high school or higher-education institution. The local recreation department might also offer a cycling course. Bicycling (other than stationary cycling) is not recommended for persons with conditions that affect their balance or for persons 60 years of age and older who have not ridden a bicycle in years.

Bicyclists using public roads should be aware of traffic regulations in their state. A significant number of traffic accidents involving bicyclists occur each year. If possible, use the bike trails that are provided in many communities. These trails are free of traffic and are much safer than public roads and highways. Besides reflective apparatus that is required on bicycles, cyclists who ride on public roads at night should also wear light-colored reflective clothing.

Age-adjusted cycling program progressions are presented in Tables 10.3 and 10.4. Review the information in Chapter 9, if necessary, before beginning the cycling program.

TABLE 10.3   **Bicycling Program Progression**

Age	Week	Distance (miles)	Time Goal (minutes)	Times per Week
Under 30	1	1.0	5:00	4
	2	1.0	4:00	4
	3	2.0	8:00	4
	4	2.0	7:00	4
	5	3.0	10:00	4
	6	3.0	9:00	4
	7	4.0	14:00	4
	8	4.0	13:00	4
	9	5.0	17:00	4
	10 (M)	5.0	16:00	4
	11	6.0	22:00	4
	12	6.0	21:00	4
30–39	1	1.0	6:00	4
	2	1.0	5:00	4
	3	2.0	9:00	4
	4	2.0	8:00	4
	5	3.0	11:00	4
	6	3.0	10:00	4
	7	4.0	15:00	4
	8	4.0	14:00	4
	9	5.0	18:00	4
	10 (M)	5.0	17:00	4
	11	6.0	22:00	4
	12	6.0	21:00	4
40–49	1	1.0	7:00	4
	2	1.0	6:00	4
	3	2.0	10:00	4
	4	2.0	9:00	4
	5	3.0	12:00	4
	6	3.0	11:00	4
	7	4.0	16:00	4
	8	4.0	15:00	4
	9	5.0	19:00	4
	10 (M)	5.0	18:00	4
	11	6.0	23:00	4
	12	6.0	22:00	4
50–59	1	1.0	8:00	4
	2	1.0	7:00	4
	3	2.0	11:00	4
	4	2.0	10:00	4
	5	3.0	13:00	4
	6	3.0	12:00	4
	7	4.0	17:00	4
	8	4.0	16:00	4
	9	4.0	15:00	4
	10 (M)	5.0	20:00	4
	11	5.0	19:00	4
	12	5.0	19:30	5

TABLE 10.4   Stationary Bicycling Program Progression

Age	Week	Speed (mph/ rpm)	Time Goal (minutes)	Pulse Rate After Exercise	Times per Week
Under 30	1	15/55	8:00	134–140	4
	2	15/55	10:00	134–140	4
	3	15/55	12:00	134–150	4
	4	17/65	12:00	141–150	4
	5	17/65	14:00	141–150	4
	6	17/65	16:00	141–150	4
	7	17/65	16:00	151–160	5
	8	17/65	16:00	151–160	5
	9	20/75	18:00	161–170	5
	10 (M)	25/75	18:00	161–170	5
	11	25/90	20:00	161–170	5
	12	25/90	25:00	161–170	4
30–39	1	15/55	7:00	127–140	4
	2	15/55	9:00	127–140	4
	3	15/55	11:00	127–140	4
	4	15/55	13:00	140–150	4
	5	15/55	15:00	140–150	4
	6	15/55	17:00	140–150	4
	7	15/55	19:00	151–159	5
	8	17/65	18:00	151–159	5
	9	17/65	20:00	151–159	5
	10 (M)	20/75	18:00	151–159	5
	11	20/75	22:30	161–169	5
	12	25/90	25:00	161–169	4
40–49	1	15/55	6:00	125–139	4
	2	15/55	8:00	125–139	4
	3	15/55	10:00	125–139	4
	4	15/55	12:00	140–149	4
	5	15/55	14:00	140–149	4
	6	15/55	16:00	140–149	4
	7	15/55	18:00	140–149	5
	8	15/55	20:00	140–149	5
	9	17/65	18:00	150–159	5
	10 (M)	17/65	20:00	150–159	5
	11	20/75	18:00	150–160	5
	12	20/90	23:00	150–160	4

(continued)

TABLE 10.4 (*Continued*)

Age	Week	Speed (mph/rpm)	Time Goal (minutes)	Pulse Rate After Exercise	Times per Week
50–59	1	15/55	4:00	119–134	4
	2	15/55	6:00	119–134	4
	3	15/55	8:00	119–134	4
	4	15/55	10:00	135–139	4
	5	15/55	10:00	135–139	4
	6	15/55	12:00	135–139	4
	7	15/55	14:00	135–139	5
	8	15/55	16:00	135–139	5
	9	15/55	18:00	135–139	5
	10	15/55	20:00	135–139	5
	11	17/65	18:00	140–149	5
	12 (M)	17/65	20:00	140–149	5
	13	20/75	20:00	140–149	5
	14	20/75	25:00	150–159	4
60 and over	1	15/55	4:00	90–100	3
	2	15/55	4:00	90–100	3
	3	15/55	6:00	90–100	3
	4	15/55	6:00	101–109	4
	5	15/55	8:00	101–109	4
	6	15/55	10:00	101–109	4
	7	15/55	12:00	101–109	4
	8	15/55	14:00	101–109	4
	9	15/55	16:00	101–109	4
	10	15/55	16:00	110–119	5
	11	15/55	18:00	110–119	5
	12	15/55	20:00	110–119	5
	13	17/65	18:00	110–119	5
	14 (M)	17/65	20:00	110–119	5
	15	20/75	20:00	120–129	5
	16	20/75	23:00	120–129	4

Swimming

Swimming is widely recognized as the best activity for the development of total fitness. In rating activities for their physical fitness value, swimming was ranked number one by both Kuntzleman and Pipes and Vodak.[2] What's more, swimming is an appropriate activity for a wide spectrum of age groups and persons with varying handicaps. The President's Council on Physical Fitness and Sports states: "Swimming is one of the best physical activities for people of all ages and for many of the handicapped."[3]

Besides being an excellent activity for cardiorespiratory development as well as other fitness components, swimming results in fewer injuries than jogging or running and sports activities. Persons who swim don't have the stress placed on the joints that is common to joggers and runners or others who participate in sports activities. They therefore avoid the shin splints, muscle pulls, and stress fractures that are sometimes experienced by persons involved in these activities.

The two main disadvantages of using swimming as an activity for the development of cardiorespiratory fitness are the difficulty of finding a place to swim and the need to be able to swim well enough to move continuously for 10 to 15 minutes.

People who can swim but do not have access to a swimming facility are urged to check with the local municipal recreation department, school district administration, college, and YMCA about the use of their facility. Usually for a nominal fee these facilities can be used. Also, many of these agencies and institutions offer swim classes for both beginners and intermediate swimmers. Enroll in a class or become involved in a swim club and develop your swimming skills to the point where you will be able to swim for cardiorespiratory fitness.*

When swimming for cardiorespiratory endurance, use the crawl stroke as the basic stroke. The swimming program progression is presented in Table 10.5.

*Research has revealed that exercises performed in water at certain temperatures produce a lower heart rate than exercises requiring the same type of muscle action and intensity performed on land. For example, in their study of a group of swimmers, Magel and Faulkner noted that the heart rate during maximal work in water averaged ten beats per minute slower than during land exercise.[4] The water temperature in their study was 25° to 27°C.

TABLE 10.5   **Swimming Program Progression (Overhand Crawl)**[a]

Age	Week	Distance (yards)	Time Goal (minutes)	Times per Week
Under 30	1	300	12:00	4
	2	300	10:30	4
	3	300	10:15	4
	4	500	20:00	5
	5	500	18:00	5
	6	500	17:00	5
	7	200	4:00	5
	8	300	6:00	5
	9	400	8:00	5
	10 (M)	500	10:00	5
	11	600	12:00	5
	12	800	15:00	4
30–39	1	200	8:00	4
	2	300	12:00	4
	3	300	10:00	4
	4	500	20:00	5
	5	500	18:00	5
	6	500	17:00	5
	7	200	4:00	5
	8	300	6:00	5
	9	400	8:00	5
	10 (M)	500	10:00	5
	11	600	12:00	5
	12	800	16:00	4
40–49	1	200	8:00	4
	2	200	7:00	4
	3	300	12:00	4
	4	300	10:00	5
	5	400	16:00	5
	6	400	14:00	5
	7	200	6:30	5
	8	200	5:30	5
	9	300	6:15	5
	10	400	9:00	5
	11	500	11:00	5
	12 (M)	600	13:00	5
	13	700	15:00	4
	14	800	16:30	4

TABLE 10.5 (*Continued*)

Age	Week	Distance (yards)	Time Goal (minutes)	Times per Week
50–59	1	150	6:00	4
	2	200	8:00	4
	3	200	7:00	4
	4	300	12:00	5
	5	300	10:30	5
	6	400	16:00	5
	7	100	2:30	5
	8	150	3:45	5
	9	200	4:45	5
	10	250	5:30	5
	11	300	6:45	5
	12	400	9:15	5
	13	500	11:30	5
	14 (M)	600	13:45	5
	15	700	16:00	4
	16	800	18:00	4
60 and over	1	100	5:00	4
	2	150	7:30	4
	3	200	10:00	4
	4	200	9:00	5
	5	300	15:00	5
	6	300	12:00	5
	7	100	4:00	5
	8	100	3:30	5
	9	150	5:30	5
	10	200	6:30	5
	11	250	7:00	5
	12	300	8:30	5
	13	350	9:00	5
	14	400	10:30	5
	15	450	11:00	5
	16 (M)	500	12:25	5
	17	550	13:30	5
	18	600	Under 15:00	5

Note: Before each workout, warm up by walking back and forth across the shallow end of the pool for a minimum of five minutes. Cool down by walking slowly for three minutes at the end of the exercise.

During the first six weeks, the objective is to swim the distance, but not continuously. Swim a distance that is comfortable to you, rest, and then continue the swimming-resting cycle until the required distance is covered. Beginning with the seventh week, attempt to cover the distance without stopping.

[a]The breaststroke, backstroke, and sidestroke are less demanding. The butterfly is considerably more demanding.

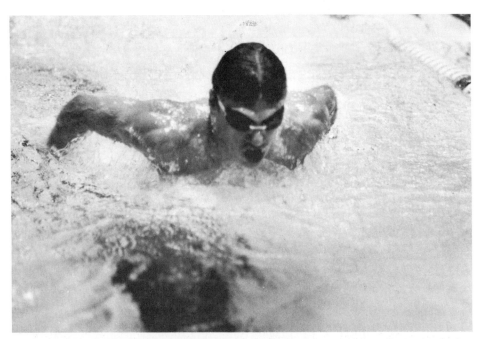

Lap swimming

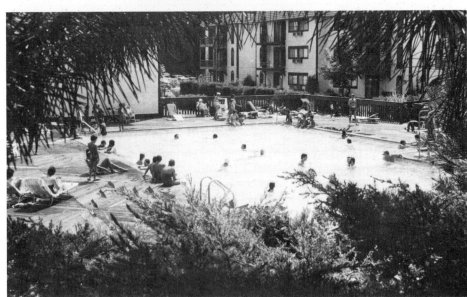

Many planned housing
communities include
swimming pools for
recreational use.

Rope Jumping

For people who possess the necessary coordination, agility, balance, and muscular endurance, rope jumping can be an inexpensive, quick, and convenient activity for the development of cardiorespiratory endurance. It should be pointed out, however, that rope jumping is strenuous and places great stress on the ankle, knee, and hip joints. It also often causes considerable pain and discomfort in the muscles of the lower legs. To minimize injuries, persons who jump rope should do so on a soft surface (a thick carpet, for example) and should wear a good pair of shoes with adequate support.

There are many types of ropes from which to choose: leather, cord, nylon, and plastic. Many types of ropes have handles with ball bearings. A recommendation is to go to the local hardware store and buy a No. 10 sash-cord rope and tie a knot at both ends for the handles. Whatever type of rope you decide to use, it should be long enough to reach under both armpits when you stand on it.

The type of rope described above is for single jumping. Jumping with others in pairs or groups has been practiced by children for years. In many communities there are "double Dutch" rope jumping contests. This activity is especially popular in large urban inner-city neighborhoods. In New York City a double Dutch rope jumping club has been established for adult women 21 years old and over.

The American Alliance for Health, Physical Education, Recreation and Dance has been using famous personalities to stress cardiovascular fitness through rope jumping with its "Jump Rope for the Heart" program. School districts throughout the United States are urged to sponsor a rope jumping team as a part of this effort. Besides the cardiorespiratory endurance it develops, rope jumping with groups fosters socialization. It is also fun.

A rope jumping progression is presented in Table 10.6. This progression requires between 70 and 80 jumps per minute. It also requires the jumper to gradually increase the time of the jumping (people under 30, for instance, should begin by jumping two to three minutes and increase to 17 minutes over ten weeks).

Because of the great stress that is placed on the joints by jumping rope and the strenuousness of the activity, it is recommended that rope jumping be used as a supplement to some other aerobic activity. Rope jumping is not recommended for people 60 years of age and older.

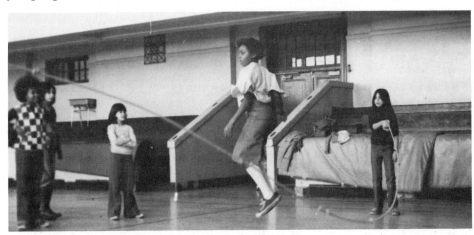

Rope jumping requires coordination and timing.

TABLE 10.6   **Rope Jumping Program Progression**

Age	Week	Steps per Minute	Time Goal (minutes)	Times per Week
Under 30	1	70–75	2:00–3:00	5
	2	70–75	4:00–5:00	5
	3	70–75	6:00–7:00	5
	4	70–75	7:00–8:00	5
	5	75–80	10:00	4
	6	75–80	12:00	4
	7	75–80	13:00	4
	8 (M)	75–80	15:00	5
	9	75–80	16:00	5
	10	75–80	17:00	4
30–39	1	70–75	2:00–3:00	5
	2	70–75	3:00–4:00	5
	3	70–75	4:00–5:00	5
	4	70–75	5:00–6:00	5
	5	70–75	7:00–8:00	5
	6	75–80	10:00	4
	7	75–80	12:00	4
	8	75–80	13:00	5
	9	75–80	14:00	5
	10	75–80	15:00	5
	11 (M)	75–80	16:00	5
	12	75–80	17:00	5
40–49	1	70–75	2:00–3:00	5
	2	70–75	3:00–4:00	5
	3	70–75	4:00–5:00	5
	4	70–75	5:00–6:00	5
	5	70–75	6:00–7:00	5
	6	70–75	7:00–8:00	5
	7	70–75	10:00	5
	8	75–80	11:00	4

TABLE 10.6 (*Continued*)

Age	Week	Steps per Minute	Time Goal (minutes)	Times per Week
	9	75–80	12:00	4
	10	75–80	13:00	5
	11 (M)	75–80	14:00	5
	12	75–80	15:00	5
	13	75–80	16:00	5
	14	75–80	17:00	5
50–59	1	70–75	1:00–2:00	5
	2	70–75	2:00–3:00	5
	3	70–75	3:00–4:00	5
	4	70–75	4:00–5:00	5
	5	70–75	5:00–6:00	5
	6	70–75	5:00–7:00	5
	7	70–75	6:00–8:00	5
	8	70–75	7:00–9:00	5
	9	75–75	10:00	5
	10	75–80	11:00	4
	11 (M)	75–80	12:00	4
	12	75–80	13:00	4
	13	75–80	14:00	4
	14	75–80	15:00	5
	15	75–80	16:00	5
	16	75–80	17:00	5

Note: You might not be able to exercise continuously for the first four or five weeks. Rest frequently, and as long as necessary, but continue either to skip very slowly or to walk while resting. Progress at your own pace. It might take you longer to reach the time goals than someone else. Warm up before beginning to jump for time and cool down after the timed jumps.

Remember to exercise on a soft surface and to wear athletic shoes with good arch support. Skip with both feet together, or step over the rope, alternating feet. If this jumping style is too strenuous, try the "rhythm hop": a leap (take off on one foot and land on the other) followed by a small hop (take off on one foot and land on the same foot) for each turn of the rope; then leap on the other foot to repeat the sequence (leap, rhythm hop, leap, rhythm hop, leap, rhythm hop).

Source: From Jump Rope! © *1974 by Peter L. Skolnik. Workman Publishing, New York. Reprinted with permission of the publisher.*

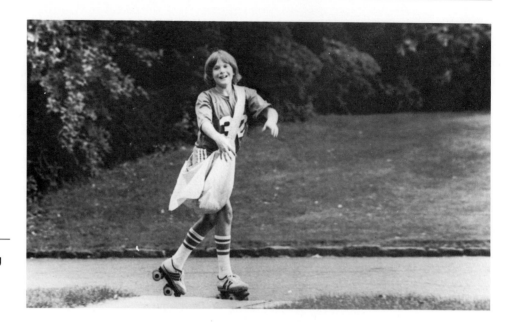

This youngster is using roller skates as a means of transportation.

Skating

Both ice and roller skating are rated good to excellent activities for the development of cardiorespiratory endurance by several sources.[5] Despite the lack of adequate facilities, skating is enjoying increased popularity and participation in the United States. The 1982 A. C. Nielsen Sports Participation Survey revealed that 30 million people participated in roller skating and 18 million in ice skating.

It is surmised that many more individuals would participate in skating activities if it were not for the scarcity of facilities and the cost of equipment. Another disadvantage in using skating as an activity for the development of cardiorespiratory endurance is that one must possess the skills necessary to skate. Although it is much easier to learn to skate while you are young, adults have been able to learn to skate. Check with your local recreation department, school system, or YMCA to inquire about classes in roller skating and ice skating.

The extent of cardiorespiratory fitness development one gets will depend on the intensity, duration, and frequency of skating, just as with other aerobic activities. Since skating is such a social activity, many people have a tendency to skate for a few minutes and then sit and talk with friends. To develop cardiorespiratory endurance, one must skate at an appropriate intensity level for 20 to 30 minutes or more. Those interested in recreational skating would need to skate for an hour or more. A suggested skating progression for speed skating is presented in Table 10.7.

TABLE 10.7   **Skating Program Progression**[a]

Week	Laps[b]	Distance (miles)	Time Goals[c] (minutes)	Times per Week
1	16	1	9:00	3
2	16	1	7:00	3
3	32	2	14:00	3
4	32	2	13:00	3
5	32	2	12:00	4
6	48	3	15:00	3
7	48	3	14:00	4
8	64	4	20:00	4
9	64	4	18:00	4
10	64	4	17:00	4
11 (M)	64	4	16:00	3
12	80	5	25:00	4
13	80	5	24:00	4

[a]This is a skating progression geared for individuals under 30 years of age who engage in speed skating. (The intensity level and thus the energy expenditure will vary according to the skill level of the skater.) Older individuals should skate at a slower pace, using the age-adjusted target heart rate as a guide. Take the pulse rate immediately after the activity to determine the intensity level at which you are exercising. Make adjustments in the intensity or duration of the activity as needed.

[b]Based on a facility with a track that measures 16 laps to the mile.

[c]These are time goals for speed skaters. Those interested in recreational skating should skate for an hour or more at a slower pace to improve cardiorespiratory endurance. Monitor your pulse rate to determine the intensity level of the workout.

Aerobic Dance

Aerobic dance is a series of specially choreographed movement routines that incorporate a combination of dance step patterns and other whole-body movements including walking, jogging, hopping, skipping, jumping, and kicking. Aerobic dance is performed to the rhythmic beat of popular music and might draw from various dance forms, such as jazz, folk, modern, ballet, and rock.

The use of aerobic dance as a means of developing and maintaining cardiorespiratory endurance has become popular during the past few years. The many aerobic dance classes being offered in schools, colleges, and universities, health spas, and elsewhere attest to its widespread popularity. That it is an enjoyable activity for many persons and can be performed at varying intensity levels makes aerobic dance suitable for individuals of various fitness levels and of all ages.

Careful attention should be paid to the type of floor surface on which aerobic dance workouts are performed. Wooden spring floors are best. Do not perform aerobic dance routines on hard surfaces such as concrete-based floors. It would be wise for individuals intersted in taking aerobic dance classes to check the flooring of the facility offering the classes. Performing aerobic dance exercises on the proper floor surfaces can help to avoid unnecessary injuries.

Aerobic dance workouts, like other exercise programs, should consist of three phases: warm-up, the conditioning bout, and cool-down. To realize some fitness benefits, aerobic dance workouts should be of sufficient intensity and duration to produce a training effect. The workouts

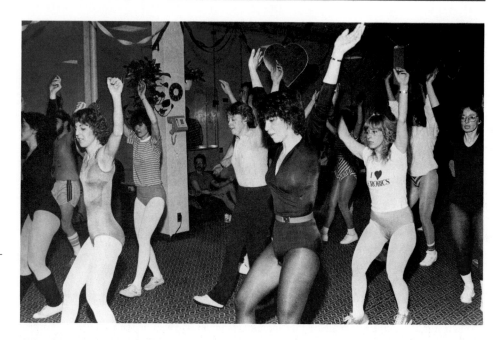

Some exercise enthusiasts prefer group activities such as aerobic dance.

should also be engaged in on a regular basis to maintain fitness gains. General guidelines for determining the intensity, duration, and frequency of exercising are presented in Chapter 9.

Research studies have indicated that aerobic dance workouts can be performed at intensity levels that will result in energy expenditures near those produced by participating in squash, rugby, football, swimming, skating, and skiing and higher than the energy expenditure needed for participation in tennis, archery, and hockey.[6] Aerobic dance routines will result in improvements in cardiorespiratory fitness if the conditioning bout is at an intensity level of between 70 and 90 percent of maximal heart rate and the workouts are performed at least three times per week with a conditioning bout of 15 to 30 minutes at each session.[7] Following an adequate warm-up, the conditioning bout should be performed at an intensity level that is geared to the present fitness level of the participants and gradually increased to achieve the desired training effect.

The options for dance routines are many and varied. Jacki Sorensen, a pioneer in the aerobic dance movement, and many others have produced records containing dance routines and instructions for their use. Some individuals might wish to compose their own aerobic dance routines. Appendix K contains an aerobic dance routine developed by Iola Thompson, dance instructor at Medgar Evers College of the City University of New York. It features a warm-up, a conditioning bout, and a cool-down.

Sports Activities

In general, sports activities such as racquetball, paddleball, squash, tennis, and basketball should be used with some other aerobic activity to meet the objective of cardiorespiratory fitness. Although squash, racquetball, and basketball are rated high as developers of cardiorespiratory endurance,[8] it must be remembered that variables such as skill level, interaction with other players, and the stop-and-go nature of these activities greatly influence the possible fitness benefits. Therefore, the

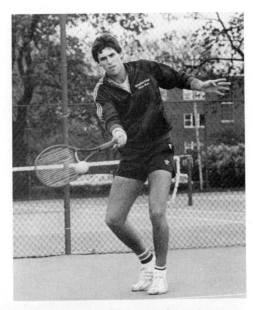

Tennis

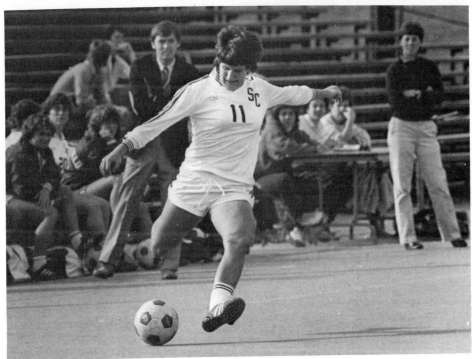

A sport like soccer
requires one to be fit
to engage in it.

value of these sports activities might vary widely, depending on the
interaction of the variables.

Beyond these considerations, participation in sports activities requires other measures of fitness and motor skill: muscular endurance,
strength, power, flexibility, and agility. Add to these prerequisites for
participation in sports activities the fact that special facilities are needed
to participate in the activities. Many of these facilities are inaccessible
to some people because of their cost. For these reasons, sports activities
become less attractive to many as a means of developing cardiorespiratory endurance.

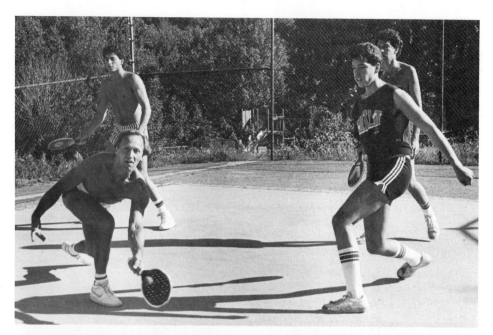

Paddleball is an ideal group activity.

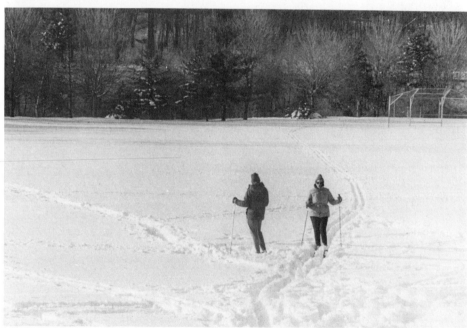

Cross-country skiing is an excellent activity for the development of cardiorespiratory endurance.

However, some people like to participate in sports activities. They will do whatever is necessary to engage in a favorite sport. For such individuals it is suggested that they use some other aerobic activity to get in shape before engaging in sports activities. It is recommended that sports activities be used to maintain an acceptable level of cardiorespiratory fitness.

When engaging in sports activities to develop cardiorespiratory endurance, follow the basic principles of training—a sound foundation, progression and overload, specificity, and balance and maintenance. For example, start at a low intensity level and increase the amount of effort gradually. Check the pulse rate immediately after the activity (and sometimes at a rest break during an activity) to determine the intensity level at which you are exercising. The main conditioning bout, which should be preceded by an adequate warm-up and followed by a cool-down, should range from 30 to 60 minutes. Most sports activities will require participation for close to 60 minutes for physiological benefits to accrue.

Interval Training

To this point the emphasis has been on continuous training in discussing pathways to cardiorespiratory fitness. An alternate method of achieving optimal fitness is interval training. In fact, Fox and Mathews,[8] among others, feel that interval training—alternating work bouts with rest periods (intervals) or intervals with activity of light intensity such as walking—is superior to programs using continuous exercise protocols.

The basic rationale they cite in support of interval training is the promise that more work and less fatigue will result. Other purported advantages are the possibility of working at higher levels of intensity and for longer periods of time because of the introduction of rest intervals and a reduction in boredom because of the increased variety that can be added to the workouts.

Opponents of the interval training system feel that some of the advantages cited are actually disadvantages for some individuals. For example, they contend that business people and others who operate on a busy schedule do not wish to take a great deal of time to spend on exercise programs. It is asserted that many of these people are looking for some activity that can be performed in as short a period of time as possible. The contention about intensity is that many people would prefer to exercise at a moderate intensity level for slightly longer periods of time than exercise at a high intensity levels for short time periods.

Anyone who is interested in exploring interval training to improve fitness levels should consult a book on the subject for more detailed information. The book by Fox and Mathews contains a good introduction on interval training as well as many examples of fitness programs using interval training techniques.

Notes

1. American College of Sports Medicine, *Guidelines for Exercise Testing and Prescription,* 3d ed. (Philadelphia: Lea & Febiger, 1986), p. 35.
2. Charles T. Kuntzleman et al., *Rating the Exercises* (New York: Morrow, 1978); Thomas V. Pipes and Paul A. Vodak, *The Pipes Fitness Test and Prescription* (Los Angeles: Tarcher, 1978).
3. Quoted in Pipes and Vodak, p. 157.
4. J. R. Magel and J. A. Faulkner, "Maximum Oxygen Uptake of College Swimmers," *Journal of Applied Physiology* 22 (1967):929–933.
5. Works cited in Note 2; C. C. Conrad, "How Different Sports Rate in Promoting Physical Fitness," *Medicine Times,* May 1976, pp. 4–5.

6. Carl Foster, "Physiological Requirements of Aerobic Dancing," *Research Quarterly* 46 (1975): 120–122; Veronica Igbangu and Bernard Gutin, "The Energy Cost of Aerobic Dancing," *Research Quarterly* 49 (1978): 308–316.

7. Monica L. Clearly et al., "The Effects of Two- and Three-Day-per-Week Aerobic Dance Programs on Maximal Oxygen Uptake," *Research Quarterly* 55 (1984): 172–174.

8. Edward L. Fox and Donald K. Mathews, *Interval Training* (Philadelphia: Saunders, 1974), p.v.

CHAPTER 11

Pathways to Flexibility, Strength, and Muscular Endurance

ballistic stretching
calisthenics
circuit training
concentric contraction
eccentric contraction

isokinetic training
repetition
repetitions maximum
set
static stretching

After reading this chapter, you should be able to:
1. Define and/or explain the key words listed above.
2. Design a training program to develop and maintain flexibility for the total body.
3. Discuss the advantages and shortcomings, if any, of isometric, isotonic, and isokinetic training.
4. Explain how the overload principle can be applied to a strength training program and to a program for muscular endurance.
5. Compare and contrast the essential features of a fitness program for the development of muscular endurance and strength.
6. Design a training program to develop and maintain muscular endurance and strength.
7. Describe the procedure for determining a proper starting weight.
8. Indicate when an overload (more weight) should be applied during a weight training program.

In addition to the development of cardiorespiratory endurance, which was discussed in Chapter 10, it is important to develop adequate levels of flexibility, strength, and muscular endurance if optimal fitness is to be achieved. Flexibility exercises are needed to prevent body stiffness and muscle-boundness, to prevent injuries, and to improve circulation within internal organs. Exercises for strength and muscular endurance help to maintain good body posture, among other important benefits. Weak lower back muscles, for example, often result in low-back problems.

This chapter presents a series of exercises and programs for developing flexibility, strength, and muscular endurance for the entire body. Unlike cardiorespiratory endurance, which can be developed by an activity such as swimming, the fitness components of flexibility, strength, and muscular endurance are "area-specific"; that is, each body part must be developed with specific programs and exercises. A person might be strong in the legs, for instance, because he or she uses weight training exercises that deal with the leg muscles. However, the leg exercises would not develop arm strength. Specific exercises for the arms would have to be used to develop strength in the arms. Therefore, not only must exercises be included to develop all fitness components, but different exercise regimens must also be included for different body parts. In this chapter are exercises intended to develop flexibility, strength, and muscular endurance in all major muscle groups and body segments. (This is an application of the principle of specificity discussed in Chapter 9.)

Flexibility

Flexibility has been defined as the ability of the body parts to move through a full range of motion. The natural aging process causes a decrease in flexibility as one gets older. However, people who engage in a systematic program of physical activity that includes flexibility exercises will maintain remarkable flexibility throughout their life span. Besides the flexibility exercises presented in this section, individuals should concentrate on improving their flexibility during everyday activities. For instance, use the complete range of arm movement when showering, washing the car, hanging curtains, and the like.

Flexibility exercises include movements that require bending, twisting, reaching, and stretching. Flexibility exercises presented in this section, especially the stretching movements, can be used as the general warm-up and cool-down for all-body aerobic-type activities such as jogging and cycling. Use the flexibility exercise (or exercises) for a specific body part (or body parts) to get the body ready for a particular activity. For example, after a general warm-up before a game of racquetball, stretching exercises for the arm and shoulder girdle and the legs and hip area should be performed.

When engaging in stretching exercises, always make slow, rhythmic, sustained movements. Do not bounce or jerk; such actions might result in an injury to the muscle fiber or tendon because of the stretch reaction that accompanies ballistic stretching (quick, high-force movements). The best way to improve flexibility is to stretch the muscle to the point of slight discomfort and hold the position for a period of time (start with three to five seconds and work up to 20 seconds). If you feel pain in the muscle area, you know you are overstretching. This type of slow, deliberate, continuous stretching is called static stretching. As you continue to engage in this type of stretching regimen, the muscle fibers and connecting tendons will become more elongated and the joints more flexible. At that point you will be able to stretch fully and without discomfort.

A sequence of 14 flexibility exercises is presented after the following general recommendations:

1. Precede the exercises with a slow walk and then a brisk walk or jog in place.
2. Perform the exercises the first time in the order in which they appear. Next, pick out exercises that focus on the specific body parts that will be used in the subsequent activity. (Where two exercises are presented for the same body part or muscle, use the one that you prefer.)
3. In the stretch-and-hold exercises, the hold time is a recommendation only. You might wish to hold the position for a longer period of time. If you hold the stretching position for long periods (20 to 30 seconds), fewer repetitions will be necessary.
4. When performing the exercises, breathe in and out—do not hold your breath. Exhale as you execute the exercise.
5. Perform the stretching exercises before vigorous physical activity and at one or two other times during the day. Include some stretching exercises in your daily activities.

Flexibility Exercises

1.   Head Rotation (Figure 11.1)

Target Area(s):   Neck muscles

Instructions: From a standing position, slowly move head forward to the front, then slowly to the right, then slowly to the rear, and finally to the left. Hold each position for 4 counts, and return to the starting position.

Repetitions: 2 or 3

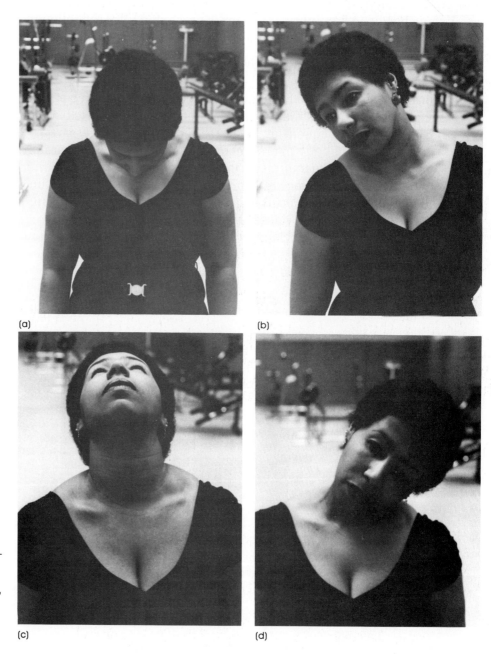

Figure 11.1
Head rotation: (a) front, (b) right, (c) back, (d) left.

2. Double-Shoulder Shrug (Figure 11.2)

Target Area(s):   Neck and shoulders

Instructions: From a standing position, with arms at the sides, slowly raise and lower the shoulders. Hold each position for 4 counts.

Repetitions: 5

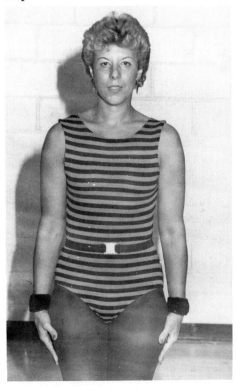
(a)

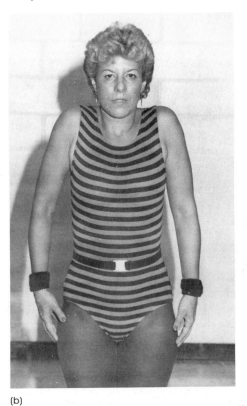
(b)

Figure 11.2
Double-shoulder shrug:
(a) start, (b) finish.

3. Double-Arm Circle (Figure 11.3)

Target Area(s):   Shoulder girdle

Instructions: From a standing position, with arms at the sides, make slow, wide circles with the arms. Keep the elbows straight and swing from the shoulders. Make circles forward and backward.

Repetitions: 10 forward and 10 backward

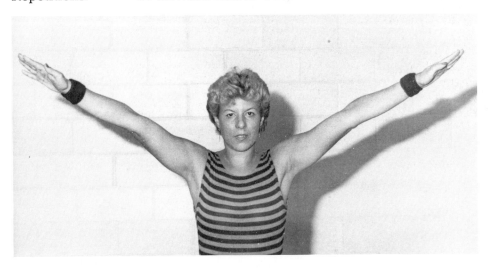

Figure 11.3
Double-arm circle.

4. Side Stretch (Figure 11.4)

Target Area(s):   Hips and lower back

Instructions: Standing with arms at the sides, reach up over the head with one arm. Stretch the other hand as far down the side of the leg as possible. Hold this position for 5 to 10 seconds. Repeat to the other side.

Repetitions: 5 to each side

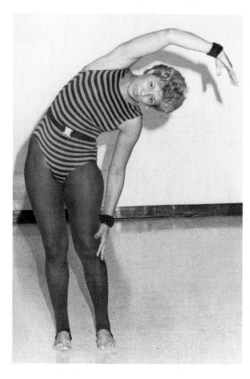 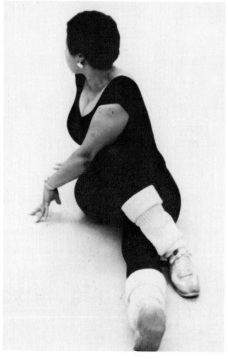

Figure 11.4 (right)
Side stretch.

Figure 11.5 (far right)
Trunk twist.

5. Trunk Twist (Figure 11.5)

Target Area(s):   Trunk, groin, and shoulder

Instructions: Sitting with legs crossed, slowly twist your trunk to the right and place both hands on the floor outside the right leg. Hold for 5 seconds, and repeat to the other side.

Repetitions: 5 to each side

6. Leg-over (Figure 11.6

Target Area(s):	Hips and lower back
Instructions:	Lying prone with arms extended to the side at shoulder level, raise the right leg to a vertical position, with the leg straight and the toes pointed. Lower the leg slowly until the right leg touches the floor near the left hand. Keep the shoulders, arms, and back on the floor as you lower your leg to the floor. Hold for 3 to 5 seconds and then return to the starting position. Repeat with the other leg.
Repetitions:	5 to each side

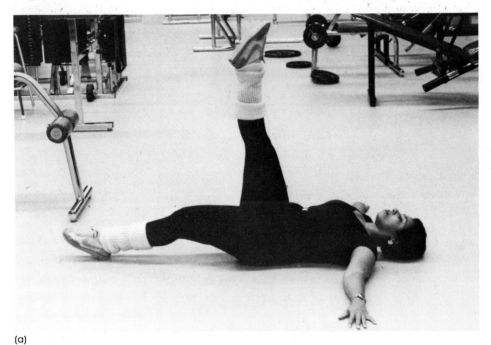

(a)

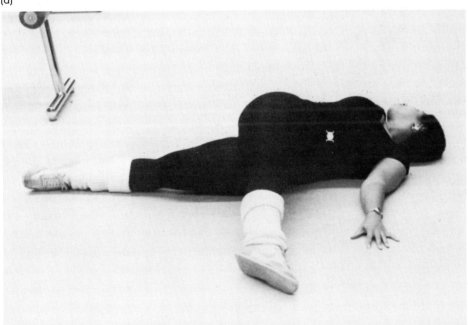

(b)

Figure 11.6
Leg-over: (a) start,
(b) finish.

7. Side Leg Raise (Figure 11.7)

Target Area(s):   Hips

Instructions: Lie on your left side, with the body straight and your head resting on your left hand and forearm. Raise your right leg as far off the floor as possible (keeping the knee locked and the toes pointed). Hold for 3 seconds and then return to starting position. Repeat to the opposite side.

Repetitions: 5 to each side

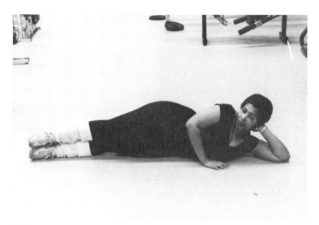

(a)

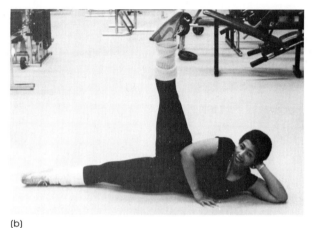

(b)

Figure 11.7
Side leg raise: (a) start, (b) finish.

8. Lying Knee-Pull (Figure 11.8)

Target Area(s):   Lower back and hips

Instructions: Lie on back with legs fully extended. Slowly pull the right knee to the chest, holding the leg just below the knee with both hands. Hold for 5 seconds and then return to the starting position. Repeat with the opposite leg.

Repetitions: 5 with each leg

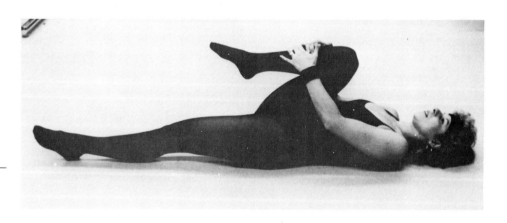

Figure 11.8
Lying knee pull.

9. Quadriceps Stretch (Figure 11.9)

Target Area(s):	Anterior leg and thigh muscles
Instructions:	Sit with the left leg extended and the right leg bent, with the heel of the foot touching the buttocks (modified hurdler's position) and hands on the floor opposite the hips. Keeping the right leg and knee in contact with the floor, lean backward until the back is flat on the floor (or as far back as you can go without raising the leg off the floor). Hold this position for 5 seconds and then return to the starting position. Repeat alternately with the other leg.
Repetitions:	5 with each leg

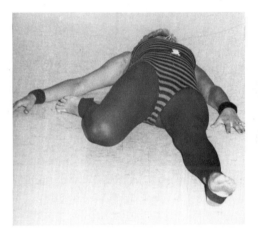

Figure 11.9
Quadriceps stretch.

10. Hamstring Stretch & Sit and Reach (Figure 11.10)

Target Area(s):   Lower back and posterior leg and thigh muscles

Instructions: *Standing Hamstring Stretch.* Stand with one leg crossed over the other, with the heel of the crossed leg off the floor and the other foot flat on the floor. Bend over and reach for the floor where the front leg is located. Hold this position for 5 seconds and then return to the starting position. Repeat alternately with the other leg.

Sit and Reach. Sit with your legs straight out in front of the body. Reach for your toes (or beyond them) with your hands in a palms-down position. Hold this position for 5 seconds and then return to the starting position. Repeat alternately with the other leg.

Repetitions: 5 with each leg

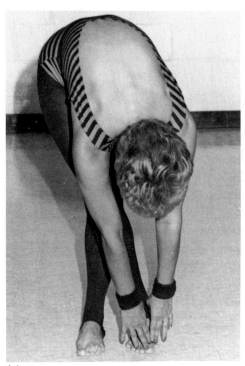

(a)

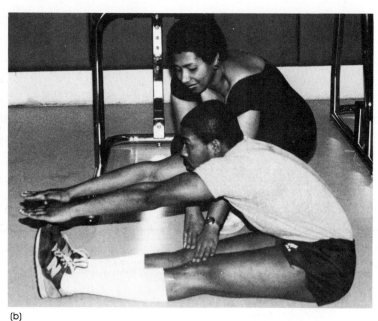

(b)

Figure 11.10
(a) Hamstring stretch,
(b) sit and reach.

11. Groin Stretch (Figure 11.11)

Target Area(s):   Groin and medial leg muscles (inner sides of legs)

Instructions: Stand with the feet spread more than shoulder-width apart. Turning the toes of the right foot to the right and keeping the toes of the left foot straight ahead, shift the weight of the body to the left leg. Hold this position for 5 seconds and then return to the starting position. Repeat alternately with the right leg.

Repetitions: 5 with each leg

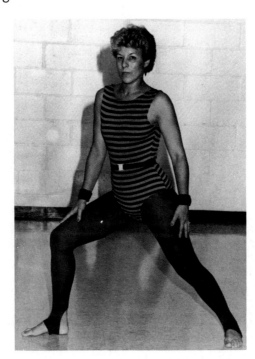

Figure 11.11
Groin stretch.

12.   Calf and Achilles Stretch (Figure 11.12)

Target Area(s):   Calf muscle (gastrocnemius) and heel cord (Achilles tendon)

Instructions: Stand facing a wall at arm distance away, with heels flat on the floor. Place your hands on the wall and lean forward, bending your elbows slowly so that your calf and Achilles tendon are stretched. Keep the knees locked and the heels flat on the floor. Hold for 5 seconds and then return to the starting position.

Repetitions: 5

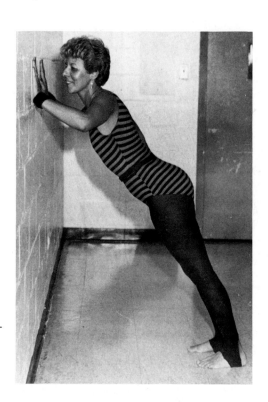

Figure 11.12
Calf and Achilles
stretch.

13. Curl and Stretch (Figure 11.13)

Target Area(s):   Lower back, hips, and knees

Instructions: Kneel on hands and knees. Curl one leg up so that the knee moves toward the nose as the head is lowered, and then slowly extend the leg behind and parallel to the floor (bring the head back up so as to form a straight line from head to toes). Repeat alternately with the other leg.

Repetitions: 5 with each leg

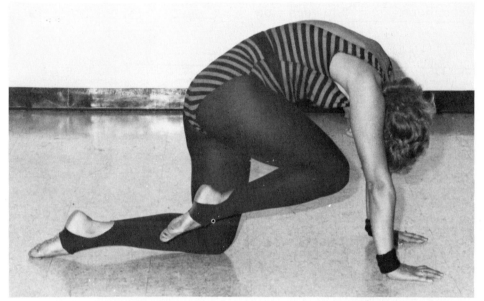

(a)

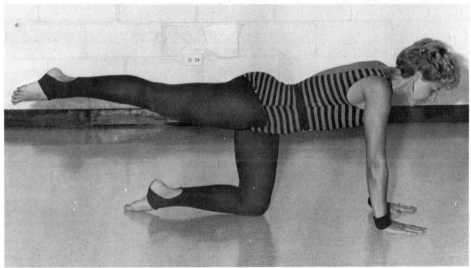

(b)

Figure 11.13
Curl and stretch:
(a) curl, (b) stretch.

14.   Side Bend (Figure 11.14)

Target Area(s):   Pelvic girdle (hip abductor muscles)

Instructions: Stand with feet together (flat on the floor) and right side to wall, about 24 inches from the wall. Place the right hand and forearm against the wall at shoulder level. Supporting the body's weight with the hand and arm, move the hips toward the wall (try to touch the right hip to the wall). Hold for 3 seconds and then return to the starting position. Repeat alternately to the other side.

Repetitions: 2 to each side

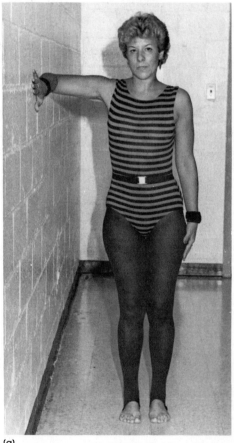 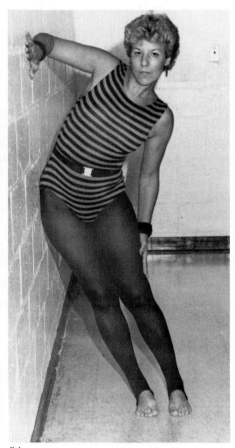

(a)   (b)

Figure 11.14
Side bend: (a) start, (b) finish.

Strength and Muscular Endurance

Strength is the maximal force that a muscle or muscle group can generate in a single contraction. *Muscular endurance* refers to the ability of a muscle or muscle group to exert several contractions against a resistance for a period of time or to maintain an isometric contraction for an extended period of time. Three general types of training for strength and muscular endurance are isometric, isotonic, and isokinetic training.

Isometric Training.   Isometric training involves muscle contractions against a resistance that is immovable. In this type of training the joints are placed at a certain angle and the muscles contract without changing in length at the angle where the movement stops. Isometric contractions do not permit the joints to move through a full range of motion. An example of an isometric training exercise is a person performing a bent-arm hang (Figure 11.15). Pushing the hands against each other with equal force so that no movement occurs is another example of an isometric exercise (Figure 11.16).

Types of Training for Strength and Muscular Endurance

The main attraction of isometric training techniques is the claim that they can produce gains in strength similar to those using isotonic training methods but in a much shorter time period. Gains in strength were noted in persons who performed as little as six-second isometric contractions per day.[1] The initial enthusiasm for isometrics is based largely on the work of two German physiologists, Hettinger and Muller, in the 1950s. Subsequent research studies have failed to support the claims of these researchers. Moreover, isometric training is potentially dangerous for older persons and those with symptoms of cardiovascular disease. Isometrics, which is usually accompanied by breath holding for a period of time, restricts the flow of blood to the heart and brain and elevates the blood pressure. The resulting effects of these physiological changes include dizziness, fainting, and sometimes heart attack. Because of these observations, isometrics should be used with great caution.

Isotonic Training.   Isotonic training methods result in contractions in which the muscle either shortens (concentric contractions) or lengthens (eccentric contractions). Weight training is a classic example of isotonic training. An obvious advantage of isotonic training over isometric training is that body parts can be made to move through their entire range of motion in isotonic training. However, the resistance is constant throughout the movement in isotonic training. Therefore, the force that must be exerted by the muscle varies at different points during the movement, usually requiring greater force at the beginning.

The uneven generation of force during isotonic training with weights occurs because the resistance is normally set at the greatest load that permits one to complete the movement. Consequently, the resistance can

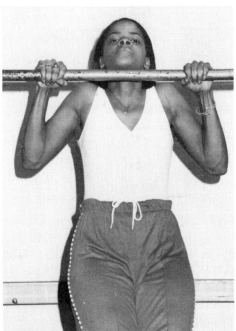

Figure 11.15
Bent-arm hang, an
isometric exercise.

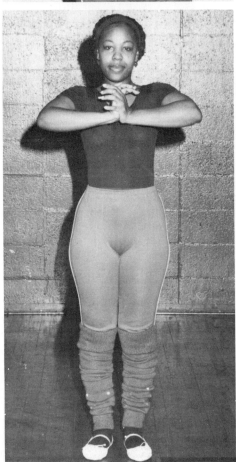

Figure 11.16
Hand press, an
isometric exercise.

be no greater than the maximum strength of the weakest muscle or muscle group responsible for the movement. The resulting uneven generation of force during an isotonic movement with weights is undesirable because the muscle is not exercised fully throughout the movement. This is especially evident at the end of a biceps curl, for example.

Isokinetic Training.   Isokinetic training, the most recent of the three methods, is said to have an advantage over isotonic training programs because it provides a variable or accommodating resistance in which the level of resistance corresponds to the tension or force created by the muscle throughout the movement. *Isokinetic* means "same speed," so the speed of movement can also be controlled in an isokinetic contraction. In other words, isokinetic training allows a muscle group to contract at a set speed and against a resistance that is equal to the force of the contraction throughout the movement. Some individuals feel that a disadvantage of isokinetic training is the lack of feedback that results from the weights' being moved at a set speed. Also, isokinetic training requires the use of rather expensive machines that are beyond the means of the average person. Examples of isokinetic equipment include the Exergenie and Mini-Gym and the Orthotron and Cybex, which are well suited for training and rehabilitation.

Regardless of the type of training program used, the overload principle must be applied. The overload principle may be applied by using any one or a combination of the following methods:
1. Increasing the resistance or load (or the time force is applied)
2. Increasing the number of repetitions*
3. Increasing the number of sets†

Applying the Overload Principle

The training objective sought will help to determine the manner in which the variables are manipulated. For example, greater strength development will result when the resistance is progressively increased and the number of repetitions is held constant. On the other hand, development of muscular endurance will be facilitated when the number of repetitions is increased and the resistance is kept constant. The number of sets used in the overloading process will depend on the amount of gain desired and the experience of the person engaged in the weight training program. It is recommended that from one to three sets be used by beginners. Experienced bodybuilders‡ might design a program that contains three to five sets. For most persons interested in developing minimal strength and muscular endurance to complement a cardiorespiratory development program, one to three sets should be sufficient.

*A *repetition* ("rep") is a single complete execution of an exercise. An example is the performance of one sit-up.
†A *set* is the number of consecutive repetitions performed. A set is followed by either a rest or the performance of another exercise. For example, the execution of ten arm curls and then ten leg lifts would represent one set of ten repetitions of each exercise.
‡*Bodybuilding* is a competitive sport whose aim is to increase muscle size and definition; *weight training* is the primary mode of training to accomplish this goal.

Women and Muscular Strength

Women in many of my classes have questioned the propriety of their using weight training. They voiced their belief that women who engage in weight training will develop bulging muscles and a figure that is unfeminine.

Research does not support the assertions that weight training by females will result in unsightly muscles and masculine physiques. Since women have less muscle mass and lower levels of testosterone, the male sex hormone that stimulates muscular development, they will gain the benefits of weight training without significant enlargement (hypertrophy) of the muscle. In fact, more and more women are discovering that weight training can produce bodies that are firm and taut yet feminine in appearance.

A Program for the Development of Strength and Muscular Endurance

A program using both calisthenics and weight training has been selected for this text. The calisthenics—formal exercises performed without equipment or with a minimum of small equipment—can be performed by anyone almost anywhere. The weight training program can either be performed using free weights (barbells and dumbbells) or weight machines such as those made by Universal or Nautilus.

The specific training technique suggested for both calisthenics and weight training is circuit training. This system of training involves a series of exercises arranged in a logical sequence to develop different muscle groups. In circuit training, exercises should be performed in a sequential order so that no one muscle group is overworked and fatigue does not limit lifting ability. The sequence should be arranged so that the same muscle group is not used consecutively. For example, in designing a circuit of the calisthenic exercises in this chapter, the first exercise might be one for the arm muscles, the second for the abdominals, the third for the quadriceps, and so forth. One set of a specified number of repetitions of each exercise is performed before moving to the next exercise station. One to three complete circuits is the usual routine for developing strength and muscular endurance using the circuit training technique.

Calisthenic Exercises. A group of calisthenic exercises is included on the following pages, and a circuit using some of these exercises is presented in Table 11.1. More than one variation of most exercises is included to permit adaptation by people of varying fitness levels. The exercises in the sample circuit were chosen to develop the major muscle groups of the body. Other exercises can be used; a chart is included in Appendix I for you to develop your own calisthenic program.

TABLE 11.1 **Sample Calisthenics Exercise Circuit**

Station/ Exercise	Target Muscle Group	Repetitions			
		Level: A	B	C	D
1. Push-Ups	Triceps	5	10	15	30
2. Sit-Ups (Bent Knee)	Abdominals	10	15	25	40
3. Pull-Ups	Biceps	5	10	15	25
4. Half Squats	Quadriceps	10	15	25	35
5. Side Leg Raises	Tensor Fasciae Latae	10	15	20	30
6. Supine Lifts	Gluteals	10	15	25	35
7. Heel Raises	Gastrocnemius	10	15	25	30

Total Test Time (min.) ——— × 3 = ——— Circuit Target Time

Instructions:
1. Warm-up before beginning the circuit and cool-down after completing the circuit.
2. Begin at an appropriate level (A–D), and complete three sets of exercises at that level.
3. Complete the circuit in a sequential manner (that is, move from station 1 to station 7).
4. Since cardiorespiratory endurance is not the objective of this circuit training program, it is not necessary to adhere to a strict target time. Therefore, complete the circuit by performing the exercises at a comfortable pace. You may rest for 15 to 30 seconds between each exercise and for 2 to 3 minutes between each complete circuit. You may also complete the circuit without resting between each station.

Exercises for the Arm Muscles

Push-up Sequence

1. Knee Push-up (Figure 11.17)

Instructions: Assume a position with both hands and knees on the floor or mat. Keep a straight line between knees and shoulder, with the feet off the floor and the heels close to the buttocks. With a straight body, lower your chest to the floor or mat and push yourself back to the starting position.

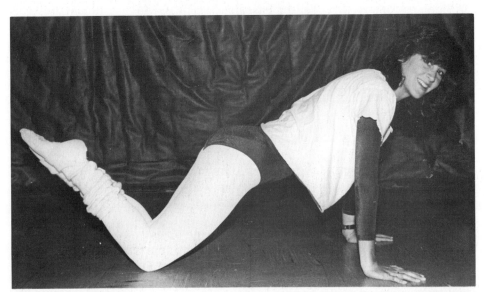

(a)

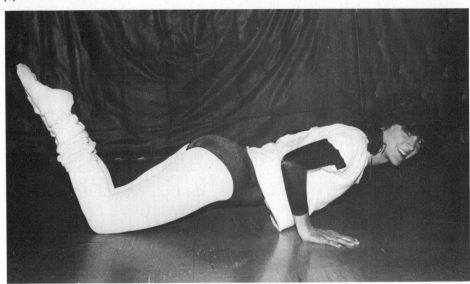

(b)

Figure 11.17
Knee push-ups:
(a) start, (b) finish.

2.   Regular Push-up (Figure 11.18)

Instructions: Assume a prone position with hands and toes on the floor and the body straight. Keeping the body straight, lower your body until your chest touches the floor; then return to the starting position.

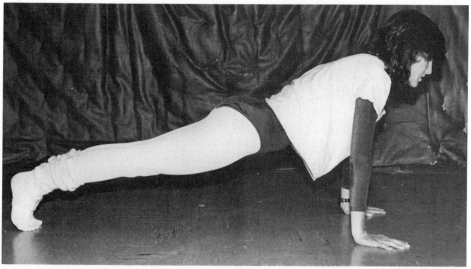

(a)

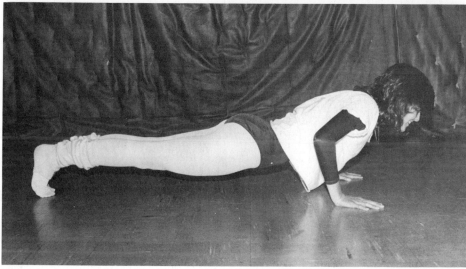

(b)

Figure 11.18
Regular push-up:
(a) start, (b) finish.

3. Push-up with Feet Elevated (Figure 11.19)

Instructions: Place the feet on an elevated surface such as a bench or chair, and perform the push-up as described for the regular push-up.

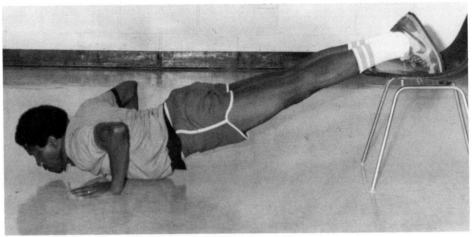

(a)

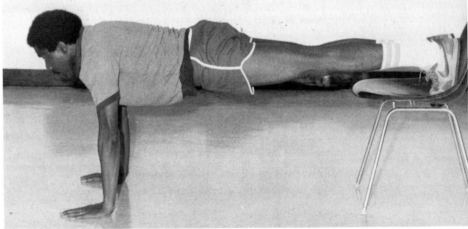

(b)

Figure 11.19
Push-up with feet
elevated: (a) start,
(b) finish.

Pull-up Sequence

4.   Modified Pull-up (Figure 11.20)

Instructions: Use a set of parallel bars or horizontal bar for this
                         exercise. Adjust the bar so that it is about chest high.
                         Assume a backward-leaning position, grasping the
                         bar with both hands (palms facing forward) and the
                         arms fully extended. From this position, pull the
                         body to the bar, touch the chest to the bar, and return
                         to the starting position.

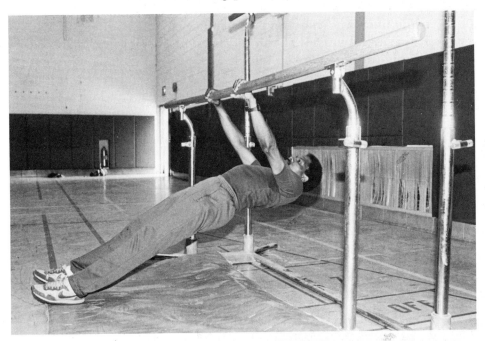

(a)

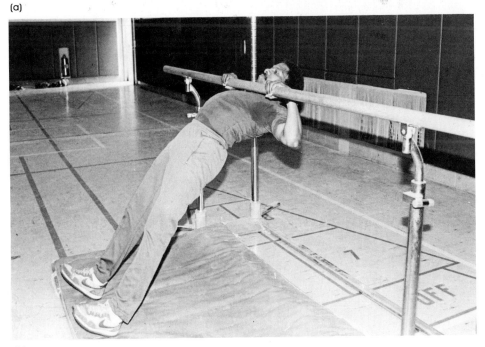

(b)

Figure 11.20
Modified pull-up:
(a) start, (b) finish.

5. Regular Pull-up (Figure 11.21)

Instructions: Assume a hanging position on a horizontal bar with the arms straight and the feet off the floor. Slowly lift the body until the chin is above the bar, and then lower the body until the arms are fully extended. Repeat as many times as possible.

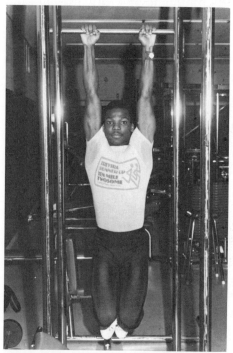

(a)

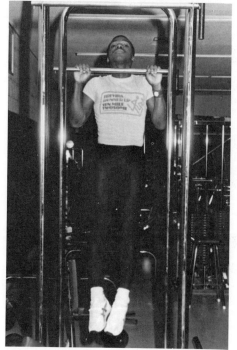

(b)

Figure 11.21
Regular pull-up:
(a) start, (b) finish.

Sit-up Sequence

6. Straight-Arm Bent-Knee Sit-up (Figure 11.22)

Instructions: Assume a position on your back with your knees bent and your feet flat on the floor. Extend your arms straight back beyond your head. From this position, swing your arms up and forward to help pull yourself into a sitting position. (If you cannot perform this exercise, use your hands to grasp your thighs and assist with the sit-up.)

Exercises for the Abdominal Muscles

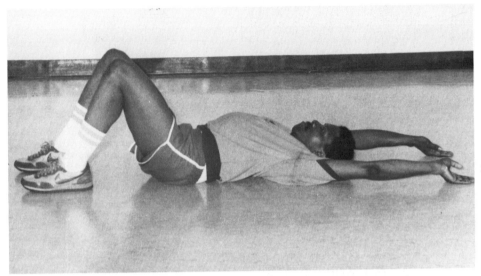

(a)

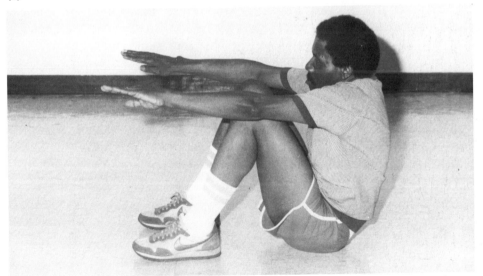

(b)

Figure 11.22
Straight-arm bent-knee sit-up: (a) start, (b) finish.

7. Regular Bent-Knee Sit-up (Figure 11.23)

Instructions: Assume a position on your back with your hands on top of your head, your knees bent, and your feet flat on the floor. From this position, curl your head and upper back and raise your trunk off the floor until your elbows touch your knees. Return to the starting position and repeat the exercise as many times as possible. (Perform the less difficult sit-ups until you develop the abdominal strength to execute the regular sit-up. Use a weight when regular sit-ups become too easy.)

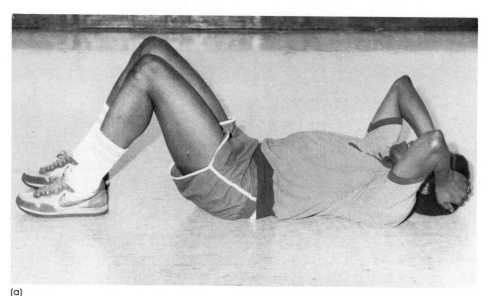

(a)

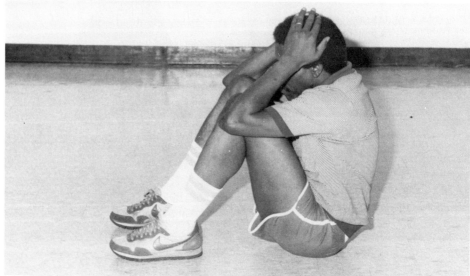

Figure 11.23
Regular bent-knee
sit-up: (a) start,
(b) finish.

(b)

8. "V" Sit-up (Figure 11.24)

Instructions: Assume a sitting position on the floor with knees
                       bent, feet on the floor, and hands on the floor behind
                       your buttocks. From this position, raise your hands
                       up and outward while bringing your legs up to touch
                       your hands (keep the knees locked) to create a "V"
                       while seated on your buttocks. Hold for 3 counts and
                       return to the starting position.

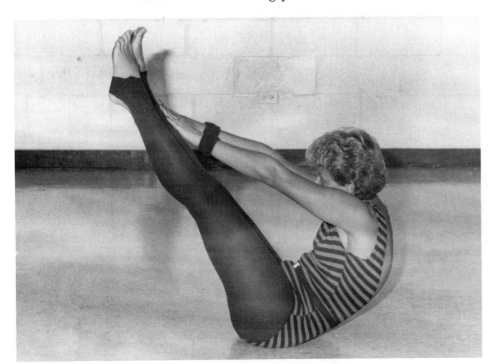

Figure 11.24
"V" sit-up.

Exercises for the Gluteal and Quadriceps Muscles

9. Half Squat (Figure 11.25)

Instructions: Assume a standing position with the body straight and feet less than shoulder-width apart. Slowly lower the body by bending at the knees. Keep the back straight and lower the body until the buttocks are parallel to the floor (do not go beyond this position because you could damage the knee joints). Hold the position for a count of 5, and return to the starting position.

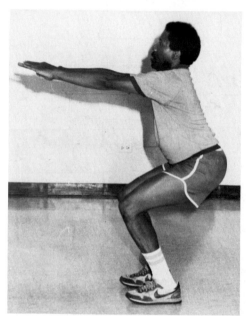

Figure 11.25
Half squat.

10.   Squat Jump (Figure 11.26)

Instructions: Assume a standing position as described for the half squats. Lower yourself to a half-squat position and jump up off the floor, returning to the half-squat position on landing. (Remember not to let the buttocks go beyond the level of the knees!)

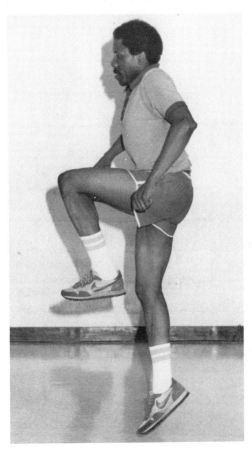

Figure 11.26
Squat jump.

Exercises for the Hip Muscle

11.   Single-Side Leg Raise (Figure 11.27)

Instructions: Lie on one side with head resting on the forearm and legs extended. Slowly raise the top leg as far as possible (keep leg straight and toes pointed). Hold for 2 counts and lower to starting position. Repeat as many times as desired; then perform the exercise on the other side.

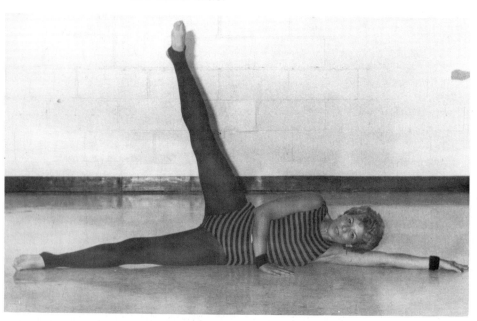

Figure 11.27
Single-side leg raise.

12.   Double Leg Raise (Figure 11.28)

Instructions: Follow the same procedure for the single-side leg raise, except both legs are raised together. Hold for 2 counts and lower to starting position. Repeat as many times as desired; then perform the exercise on the other side.

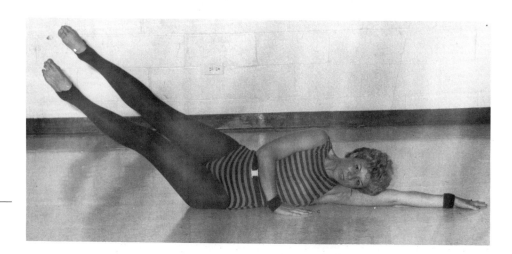

Figure 11.28
Double leg raise.

13. Heel Raise (Figure 11.29)

Instructions: Standing on a block, book, or some other 6-inch-high object, raise the heels off the floor until you are completely on your toes. Hold for 2 counts and then return to the starting position (keep the arms out to the side for balance).

Exercises for the Leg Muscles

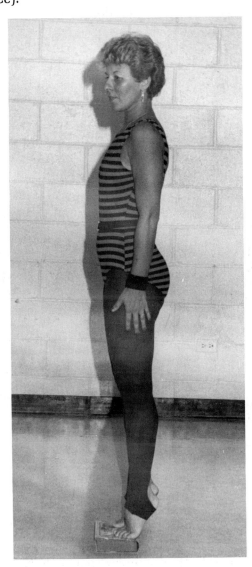

Figure 11.29
Heel raise.

14. Walking Heel Raise (Figure 11.30)

Instructions: Assume the same position as for the heel raise. Raise the heels in an alternating manner while moving the arms back and forth as in walking. (For greater difficulty, do not let the heels touch the floor.)

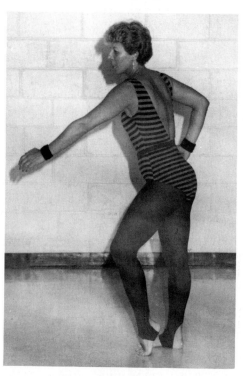

Figure 11.30
Walking heel raise.

Weight Training Exercises.   The basic core of exercises in this weight training section can be performed with either free weights (dumbbells and barbells) or a weight machine. A core of ten exercises using the Universal machine has been chosen for description in this text. Those who wish to use free weights to add variety are urged to do so. In fact, the exercises that are described here can also be performed with free weights.

Before beginning a weight training program, consider the following guidelines and recommendations:

1. For strength development, select a weight that you can lift three or four times in one set to begin with. Arrive at this starting weight by determining the maximum weight you can lift for one repetition (written as 1 RM, for "repetitions maximum"). Use the trial-and-error method to determine your 1 RM (that is, start with the maximum number of pounds you feel you can lift and make necessary adjustments in weight until you reach your 1 RM). You would begin at 40 to 55 percent of the 1 RM. For example, if you were able to bench-press 100 pounds once, your starting weight would be between 40 and 55 pounds.

2. Work up to six repetitions with the maximum weight you can lift

(6 RM). Continue with this weight until you are able to complete ten repetitions. Then add resistance (weight) or overload: 5 pounds for exercises such as arm curls and lateral pull-downs, 10 pounds for the bench press, double leg press, and other large-muscle exercises.

3. For muscular endurance, work with less weight and perform 25 RM or more, depending on the level of endurance desired. See Table 11.2 for a sample prescription for strength and muscular endurance development.

4. Perform three sets three times a week on alternating days.

5. Work alternating muscle groups to avoid placing continual stress on any one muscle group. Arrange the circuit so that different muscles are used from one station to the next: for example, first the arms are exercised, then the abdominal muscles, and so on.

6. Exercise the specific muscle groups that you are endeavoring to develop (principle of specificity).

7. Do not hold your breath when lifting heavy weights. Breath holding places more strain on the heart because of the increased blood pressure. It also restricts blood flow back to the heart and diminishes the blood supply to the brain, often producing dizziness and sometimes fainting.

8. Proper breathing involves exhaling as you lift and inhaling as you lower the weights.

9. Work with a partner for safety and for assistance with the weights, especially if you are using free weights.

10. Warm up by lifting light weights for 10 to 15 repetitions after performing some of the general stretching and calisthenic exercises.

11. Keep accurate records of your progress (weights, repetitions, sets, days exercised, and so on). You might wish to use a weight training record chart like the one in Figure 11.31.

TABLE 11.2 **Prescription for Strength and Muscular Endurance Development**

Objective	Effort	Repetitions	Sets
Strength	Maximum force	6–8 RM	3
Short-term endurance	Persistence with heavy load	15–25 RM	3
Intermediate endurance	Persistence with intermediate load	30–50 RM	2
Long-term endurance	Persistence with light load	Over 100	1

Source: Adapted from Brian J. Sharkey, Physiology of Fitness, *2d ed. (Champaign, Ill.: Human Kinetics Publishers, Inc., 1984), p. 79. Used by permission of the publisher.*

The Weight Training Exercise Core.   As previously stated, the circuit training technique is recommended for weight training workouts. An example of a weight training circuit, designed by Vivian Heyward and adapted for use in this text, appears in Figure 11.32.[2]

Figure 11.31
Example of a weight training record chart. (a) Circle the new weight whenever weight is added; (b) RM indicates the number of repetitions and sets a particular weight is lifted. In performing the bench press on 11/5, for example, three sets of 6, 4, and 4 repetitions, respectively, were completed using 85 pounds of weight

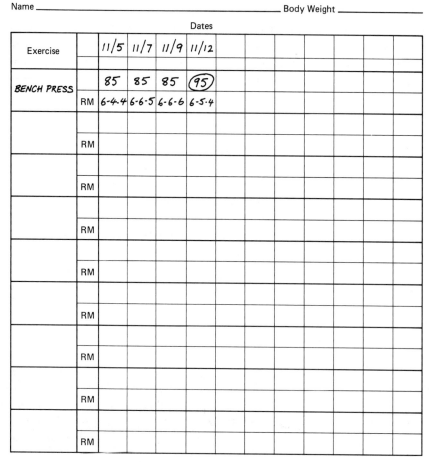

Figure 11.32
Sample circuit training program.

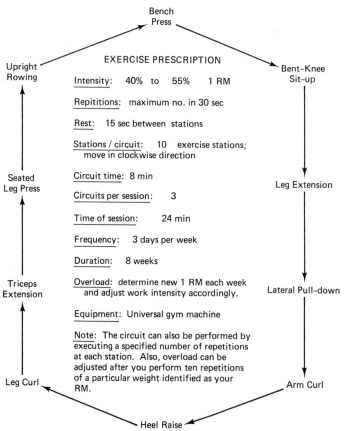

EXERCISE PRESCRIPTION

Intensity: 40%   to   55%   1 RM

Repititions: maximum no. in 30 sec

Rest: 15 sec between stations

Stations / circuit: 10   exercise stations;
   move in clockwise direction

Circuit time: 8 min

Circuits per session: 3

Time of session: 24 min

Frequency: 3 days per week

Duration: 8 weeks

Overload: determine new 1 RM each week
   and adjust work intensity accordingly.

Equipment: Universal gym machine

Note: The circuit can also be performed by executing a specified number of repetitions at each station. Also, overload can be adjusted after you perform ten repetitions of a particular weight identified as your RM.

Information presented for the core of exercises includes the name of the exercise* (and the name of the station for that exercise on Universal's wall charts), the major muscle group or groups affected by the exercise, instructions for performing the exercise, and variations for performing some of the exercises.

1. Bench Press (Chest Press Station) (Figure 11.33)

Major muscle groups: Pectorals, deltoids, triceps

Instructions: Lie on your back on the bench with your head on the bench and feet flat on the floor. Using a pronated grip (hands facing away from the body and thumbs toward each other) on the bar about shoulder-width apart, inhale and press the bar to arm's length while exhaling. Return the bar slowly with control and without allowing the weight to touch completely. Keep your head and back in contact with the bench and your feet in contact with the floor throughout the movement. Repetitions should be continuous and without pause.

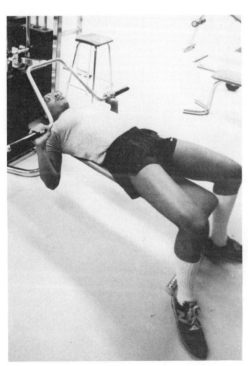

(a)

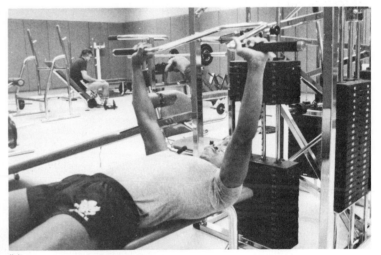

(b)

Figure 11.33
Bench press: (a) start, (b) finish.

---

*The number of repetitions for each exercise must be determined by the individual performing the exercise. Therefore, no suggested number of repetitions is given in the instructions for the various exercises.

2. Bent-Knee Sit-up (Abdominal Conditioner Station) (Figure 11.34)

Major muscle groups:	Abdominals, hip flexors
Instructions:	Lie on your back with your feet hooked under rollers, with your knees bent and your hands behind your neck. Curl up to a sitting position, touching elbows to knees or beyond. Exhale as you sit up and inhale as you lower your body.
Variation:	At the top of the sit-up, twist your body and touch your right elbow outside your left knee and your left elbow outside your right knee. (Perform sit-ups with the abdominal board at the lowest height until you develop sufficient strength to perform sit-ups at higher positions. For those who wish to develop greater abdominal strength, a weight (such as a dumbbell or a plate from a free weight) can be held in the hands and placed behind the head to provide additional resistance during the sit-up.

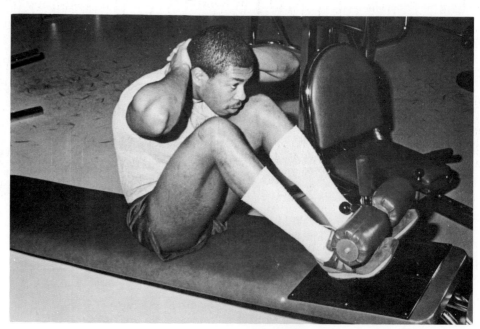

Figure 11.34
Bent-knee sit-up.

3.   Leg Extension (Thigh and Knee Machine) (Figure 11.35)

Major muscle group: Quadriceps

Instructions: Sit on the bench with your feet under the bottom rollers and your back straight. Holding onto the bench with your hands near your buttocks, extend both legs until they are parallel to the floor. Lower the weight slowly to the starting position and repeat. (Do not bend the knees to a point that will allow the weights to touch.)

Variation: Use one leg at a time.

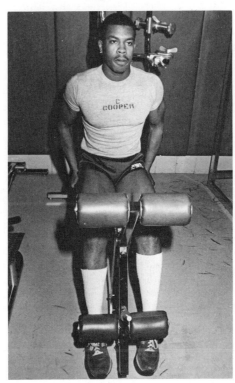 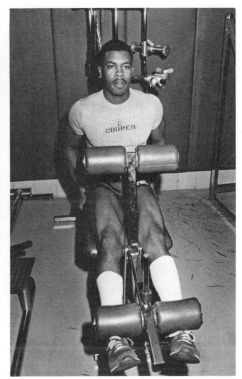

Figure 11.35
Leg extension: (a) start, (b) finish.

(a)   (b)

4. Lateral Pull-down (High Lat Station) (Figure 11.36)

Major muscle groups:	Latissimus dorsi, trapezius, deltoids, triceps
Instructions:	Assume a kneeling position, facing the machine, directly under the bar with back straight. Grasp the bar with a pronated grip (hands more than shoulder-width apart) and pull bar down to the back of the neck. Return the bar slowly back to the starting position.
Variations:	1. From the same position, pull the bar down in front of the body so that the bar touches the sternum. Tilt the head back slightly.
	2. Holding the bar at the back of the neck, bend the head toward the knees.

Figure 11.36
Lateral pull-down:
(a) start, (b) finish.

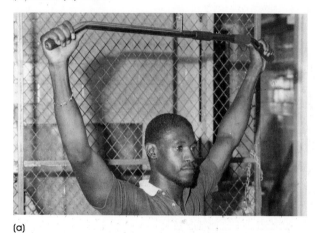
(a)

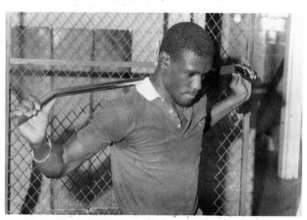
(b)

5. Arm Curl (Low Pulley Station) (Figure 11.37)

Major muscle groups:	Biceps, brachialis
Instructions:	Assume a standing position, erect posture with back straight and hands grasping the bar with a supinated grip (palms facing body with thumbs away from each other), with hands about shoulder-width apart. Curl bar toward shoulders. Slowly lower the bar to the starting position. Keep your elbows at your side and your back straight (the knees can be bent slightly).
Variations:	1. Use a pronated grip (palms away from body with thumbs toward each other).
	2. Using stirrup handles, perform curls with one arm at a time.

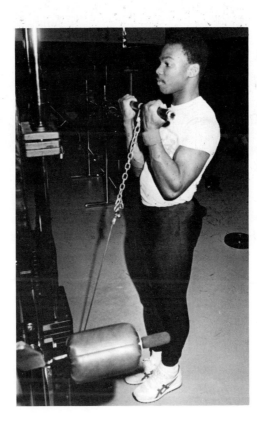

Figure 11.37
Arm curl.

6.   Heel Raise (Leg Press Station) (Figure 11.38)

Major muscle groups: Gastrocnemius, soleus

Instructions: Assume a seated position on the chair with your back flat against the chair back and your feet on the lower pedals. Grasp the handles on both sides of the chair for balance and support. Press with the balls of the feet until the legs are fully extended, and dorsiflex the ankles (bring your toes toward your shins). Then plantarflex the ankles (press the balls of the feet so that the feet move away from you). Make continuous movements with the feet, letting them come back as far as possible and extending them as far as possible.

Variation: Perform this exercise with one leg at a time. (This exercise may also be performed at the shoulder press station. When performing the heel raise at the shoulder press station, use a block or some other object on which to place the balls of the feet.)

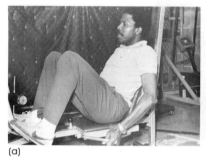
(a)

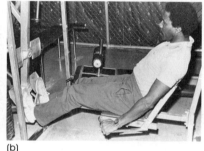
(b)

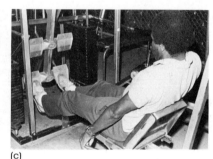
(c)

Figure 11.38
Heel raise: (a) start,
(b) dorsiflex,
(c) plantarflex.

7. Leg Curl (Thigh and Knee Machine) (Figure 11.39)

Major muscle group: Hamstrings

Instructions: Assume a prone (face-down) position on the bench with your legs extended and place your heels under the rollers, with your knees in line with the hinge or pin. Keeping hips flat, chest and head down, and holding on to the bench with the hands, pull the heels as far as possible toward the buttocks, bending at the knees. (If your hips rise during the curl, you probably have too much weight.)

Variation: Perform the exercise with one leg at a time.

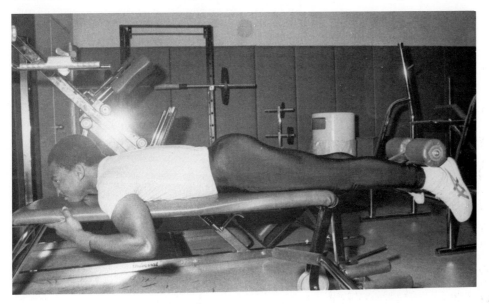

(a)

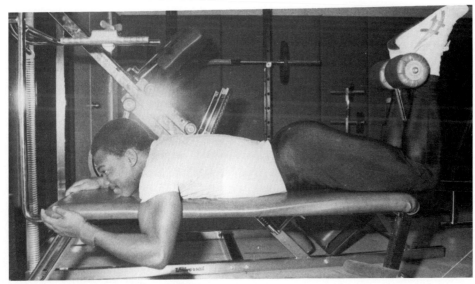

(b)

Figure 11.39
Leg curl: (a) start,
(b) finish.

8. Triceps Extension (High Lat Station) (Figure 11.40)

Major muscle groups: Triceps

Instructions: Assume an erect position close to the bar with your elbows close to your sides. Grasp the bar with a pronated grip and with your hands close together at the center of the bar. Push your hands down until your arms are straight; then return to the starting position. Do not let the weight pull your arms back up; rather, keep tension on the bar so that it slowly goes back up under your control.

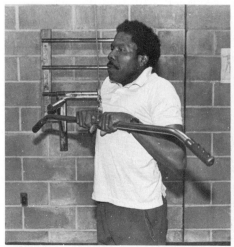 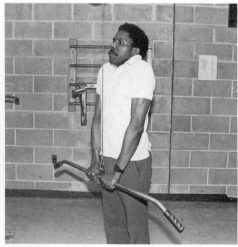

Figure 11.40
Triceps extension:
(a) start, (b) finish.

(a)   (b)

9. Seated Leg Press (Leg Press Station) (Figure 11.41)

Major muscle group: Quadriceps, psoas group, gluteals

Instructions: Adjust the seat so that you can assume a seated position with your back straight and against the chair back, your knees bent (about 90 degrees), and your feet on the pedals. Grasp the handles on both sides of the chair for support and balance. Extend your legs, pushing the pedals until your knees are almost locked, and then return to the starting position (without letting the weight touch). Repeat as many times as desired.

Variation: If your Universal machine has upper pedals, use them to perform the leg press. The upper pedals contain heavier loads, and the angle provides more work for the gluteal muscles.

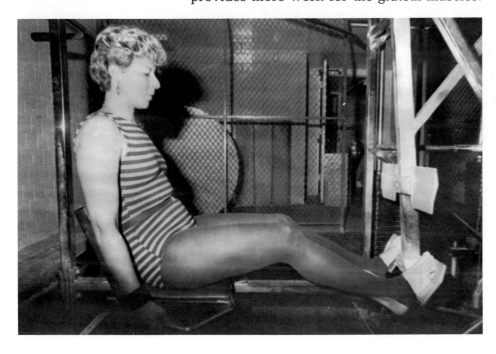

Figure 11.41
Seated leg press.

10.   Upright Rowing (Low Pulley Station) (Figure 11.42)

Major muscle groups: Trapezius, deltoids, rhomboids, biceps, brachialis

Instructions: Stand with your back straight and face the machine. Grasp the bar with your hands close together (about six inches apart) with a pronated grip; pull your elbows high and bring your hands under your chin. Return slowly to the starting position, keeping your back straight (the knees can be slightly bent). (Barbells or dumbbells can be used to perform this exercise.)

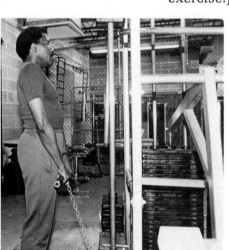 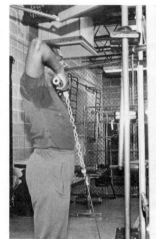 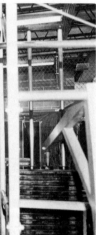

Figure 11.42
Upright rowing:
(a) start, (b) finish.

(a)   (b)

Reminders

1. Start with weights that you can handle comfortably. Chances for injury are increased when you lift weights that are too heavy. Use the trial-and-error method to determine your starting weight. Progress slowly toward your optimal weight to be lifted.
2. Breathe properly. Inhale before the lift or movement and exhale during the movement. Do not hold your breath during a movement! This is especially important when lifting heavy weights because more pressure is built up in the thoracic cavity, causing a physiological condition that can cause dizziness or loss of consciousness.
3. Warm up thoroughly before lifting weights. Besides basic stretching and calisthenic exercises, use light weights to warm up.
4. Practice safety habits: Work with a partner. Check to see that pins are securely in place when using a Universal or Nautilus machine and that the collars are tight when using free weights. Wear good skid-proof shoes to prevent sliding.
5. The exercises presented here are not the only ones that can be used. Feel free to add or substitute other exercises to develop the desired muscle groups.

1. T. L. Hettinger and E. A. Muller, "Muskelleistung und Muskeltraining," *Internationale Zeitschrift füer Angewandte Physiologie* 15 (1953):111.
2. Vivian H. Heyward, *Designs for Fitness* (Minneapolis: Burgess, 1984), p. 97.

Notes

CHAPTER 12

Pathways to Weight Control

basal metabolic rate   food exchange lists
fitcomp   principle of progression

Chapter Highlights

After reading this chapter, you should be able to:
1. Define and/or explain the key words listed above.
2. List the three physical activities that are presented as pathways to weight control and the number of Calories that will be expended by participating in them.
3. List eight additional physical activities that are recommended for a weight control program.
4. Design a weight control program using a combination of Calorie reduction and increased physical activity.

Basic information related to weight control appears in several other chapters of this book. The most comprehensive material is presented in Chapter 4, "Nutrition, Exercise, and Weight Control." This chapter focuses on specific pathways to weight control—both weight loss and weight gain.

Physical Activities plus Calorie Reduction

The caloric costs of walking, jogging, and bicycling are presented in Tables 12.1, 12.2, and 12.3. As with all physical activities, participation in these activities should be combined with caloric reduction to lose weight. Therefore, sample food plans of 1200 Calories for women and 1600 Calories for men also appear in this chapter (see Table 12.5). The number of Calories needed to lose one pound is presented as a combination of Calories resulting from increased physical activity and decreased food intake.

TABLE 12.1   Calories Expended by Males and Females by Walking[a]

| | Body weight | | | | | | | |
| | 64 kg (140 lb) | | 73 kg (160 lb) | | 82 kg (180 lb) | | 91 kg (200 lb) | |
Time/Distance	Per Session	Per 7 Sessions[b]	Per Session	Per 7 Sessions	Per Session	Per 7 Sessions	Per Session	Per 7 Sessions
MEN								
30 min./1.75 miles	144	1008	167	1166	189	1323	207	1449
45 min./2.3 miles	192	1344	223	1561	252	1764	276	1932
60 min./3.5 miles	288	2016	334	2338	378	2646	414	2898
WOMEN								
30 min./1.75 miles	131	914	149	1040	167	1166	185	1292
45 min./2.3 miles	175	1225	199	1393	223	1561	247	1729
60 min./3.5 miles	262	1834	298	2086	334	2338	370	2590

[a]Caloric expenditures were calculated on the basis of the individual walking at a rate of 3.5 mph (which is equivalent to 4.5 METs) for the time periods noted. Persons who are different weights and would like to determine their caloric expenditure should locate their half-hour Calorie count in Table 4.3 and multiply this by 4.5 (the MET value) to get their caloric expenditure for a half hour. From this figure, values for other times can be calculated.

[b]Seven sessions may in fact consist of any combination of times equal to seven times the duration of a single session. All figures are approximate; actual caloric count depends on age, physical condition, and skill in the activity as well as sex and weight.

TABLE 12.2   Calories Expended by Males and Females by Jogging[a]

| | Body weight | | | | | | | |
| | 64 kg (140 lb) | | 73 kg (160 lb) | | 82 kg (180 lb) | | 91 kg (200 lb) | |
Time/Distance	Per Session	Per 7 Sessions[b]	Per Session	Per 7 Sessions	Per Session	Per 7 Sessions	Per Session	Per 7 Sessions
MEN								
30 min./2.5 miles	224	1568	259	1813	294	2058	322	2254
45 min./3.75 miles	373	2613	432	3022	480	3430	537	3757
60 min./5.0 miles	448	3136	518	3626	588	4116	644	4508
WOMEN								
30 min./2.5 miles	203	1421	231	1617	259	1813	287	2009
45 min./3.75 miles	338	2366	385	2695	432	3024	478	3448
60 min./5.0 miles	406	2842	462	3234	518	3626	574	4018

[a]Caloric expenditures were calculated on the basis of the individuals jogging at a rate of 5 mph (which is equivalent to 7 METs) for the time periods noted. Persons who are different weights and would like to determine their caloric expenditure should locate their half-hour Calorie count in Table 4.3 and multiply this by 7 (the MET value) to get their caloric expenditure for a half hour. From this figure, values for other times can be calculated.

[b]Seven sessions may in fact consist of any combination of times equal to seven times the duration of a single session. All figures are approximate; actual caloric count depends on age, physical condition, and skill in the activity as well as sex and weight.

For each of the activities, the approximate caloric expenditure is indicated for participating in the activity for 30, 45, and 60 minutes. Depending on weight goals, fitness level, and interests, a person would choose one or more of the activities to participate in for a sufficient duration to expend a desired number of Calories. Calories expended by physical activity plus caloric reduction through lowered food intake would determine the total weight loss.

The recommended plan is to lose one pound a week until the weight goal is reached. Under certain circumstances (such as being grossly obese) a person might lose 2 pounds a week—the maximum suggested for special cases.

Let's use the information in Table 12.1 together with the menus for one week to illustrate the procedure for weight reduction using the specific activities and food plans in this text. Suppose, for example, that you are a woman who weighs 160 pounds, which is 20 pounds too much for you. To lose the 20 pounds you decided to walk for weight control. By walking for 60 minutes at a pace fast enough to cover 3.5 miles, you would expend 298 Calories. Further, if you were to walk that distance every day, in seven days you would expend 2086 Calories. This means that you would need to reduce your caloric intake by only 1414 Calories for the seven-day period (3500 − 2086), or 200 Calories per day.

The Calorie reduction needed through a lowering of caloric intake will decrease as you increase your energy expenditure. It is recommended that you expend more energy to burn Calories and rely less on lowering the caloric intake. You should try to keep your caloric reduction through decreased food intake to 500 Calories a day or less. Once you have reached your weight goal, maintain your caloric intake at a con-

TABLE 12.3 **Calories Expended by Males and Females by Bicycling**[a]

| | Body weight | | | | | | | |
| | 64 kg (140 lb) | | 73 kg (160 lb) | | 82 kg (180 lb) | | 91 kg (200 lb) | |
Time/Distance	Per Session	Per 7 Sessions[b]	Per Session	Per 7 Sessions	Per Session	Per 7 Sessions	Per Session	Per 7 Sessions
MEN								
30 min./5.0 miles	160	1120	185	1295	210	1470	230	1610
45 min./7.5 miles	213	1491	247	1729	280	1960	307	2149
60 min./10.0 miles	320	2240	370	2590	420	2940	460	3220
WOMEN								
30 min./5.0 miles	145	1015	165	1155	185	1295	205	1435
45 min./7.5 miles	193	1351	220	1540	247	1729	273	1911
60 min./10.0 miles	290	2030	330	2310	370	2590	410	2870

[a]Caloric expenditures were calculated on the basis of the individuals riding a bicycle at a rate of 10 mph (which is equivalent to 5 METs) for the time periods noted. Persons of weights other than those indicated in the table can determine their caloric expenditure by locating their half-hour Calorie count in Table 4.3 and multiplying that by 5 (the MET value). This will reveal the caloric expenditure for a half hour. From this figure, values for other times can be calculated.

[b]Seven sessions may in fact consist of any combination of times equal to seven times the duration of a single session. All figures are approximate; actual caloric count depends on age, physical condition, and skill in the activity as well as sex and weight.

TABLE 12.4   **Combining Calorie Reduction with Walking, Jogging, and Bicycling to Lose One Pound a Week**[a]

Weight	Calories Used per Minute	Minutes per Week in Activity	Calories Used per Week	Daily Calorie Reduction Needed
		Walking		
MEN				
140	4.8	420	2016	212
160	5.6	420	2338	166
180	6.3	420	2646	122
200	6.9	420	2898	86
WOMEN				
140	4.37	420	1834	238
160	4.97	420	2086	202
180	5.57	420	2338	166
200	6.17	420	2598	129
		Jogging		
MEN				
140	7.5	120	900	372
160	8.6	120	1032	353
180	9.8	120	1176	332
200	10.7	120	1284	317
WOMEN				
140	6.8	120	816	383
160	7.7	120	924	368
180	8.6	120	1032	353
200	9.6	120	1152	335
		Bicycling		
MEN				
140	5.3	240	1270	319
160	6.2	240	1448	293
180	7.0	240	1680	260
200	7.7	240	1848	236
WOMEN				
140	4.8	240	1152	335
160	5.5	240	1320	311
180	6.2	240	1488	287
200	6.8	240	1632	267

[a]Weight loss based on walking 60 minutes a day, seven days per week; jogging 30 minutes a day, four days per week; bicycling 60 minutes a day, four days per week; and reducing daily caloric intake.

stant amount while being active enough to expend the necessary Calories to maintain the desired weight.

Table 12.4 provides estimates of combinations of Calories used by walking, jogging, and bicycling and the reduced caloric intake needed to lose one pound in a week. An examination of all four tables will reveal a difference in caloric expenditure for jogging and bicycling even when they are engaged in for the same duration. This difference exists because the caloric expenditures indicated in Tables 12.1 through 12.3 are based on participation in the activities seven days a week, whereas the frequencies of jogging and bicycling noted in Table 12.4 are less than seven days a week. For example, a 140-pound female who jogs for 30 minutes a day, seven days a week will expend 1421 Calories. On the other hand, the same person will expend only 816 Calories by jogging 30 minutes a day, four days a week (Table 12.4).

The recommended frequencies and durations of the three activities for weight control are considered appropriate, according to guidelines established by the American College of Sports Medicine.[1] However, you may prefer to design a program prescription with different combinations of frequencies and durations to suit your personal needs. If you do, please adhere to the principles of training presented in Chapter 9.

Of course, activities other than walking, jogging, and bicycling can be used for weight control. In fact, most of the activities recommended as pathways to cardiorespiratory endurance can be used for weight control. Specifically, the following additional activities are recommended for weight control programs: swimming, skating, cross-country skiing, aerobic dance, racquetball, paddleball, squash, tennis, and basketball. These activities are not presented in greater detail because it is difficult to quantify the number of Calories used while participating in them. However, swimming (using the crawl stroke) at a rate of 30 yards per minute and a vigorous aerobic dance workout are approximate equivalents of jogging at a rate of 5 miles per hour. The caloric costs of theses activities can be estimated by using the information in Tables 4.4 and 4.5 and Appendix F.

Other Activities for Weight Control

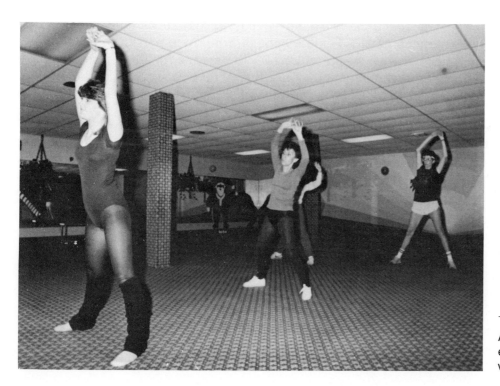

Aerobic dance is an excellent pathway to weight control.

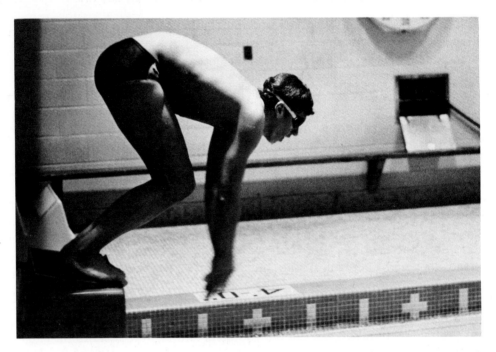

This individual is beginning his lap swimming workout, which is also an excellent pathway to weight control.

The Food Plan

Eating fewer Calories of a nutritionally sound diet along with increased physical activity is the key to weight reduction. Fad diets have been shown in Chapter 4 to be ineffective as weight reduction methods. I advocate the food plan used in the Weight Watchers program. Menus for the year are included in the *Weight Watchers 365-Day Menu Cookbook*.[2] Unfortunately, the Weight Watchers Organization does not permit the use of this information in other books. However, their cookbook is sold in many bookstores.

An overview of the Weight Watchers cookbook is presented here. The menus are arranged according to a weekly menu plan, which consists of a nutritionally sound seven-day intake of food. Further, the weekly menu plan is flexible enough to allow a person to eat the food provided for any week, so long as the menus for the entire week are eaten. For example, you may use the menu plan for Week 5 before that for Week 1. Similarly, you can use the menu for Day 4 on Day 1. The only requirement is that you use the whole day's menu when you make a change.

Besides being well-balanced nutritionally, the Weight Watchers food plan allows one to eat several different kinds of foods and to use a range of cooking methods, including sautéing and stir-frying. Special menus for holiday meals are also included. For example, the sample menu for Week 15 includes meals for Passover and Easter.

Although the menus in the Weight Watchers cookbook are for women, allowances are made so that everyone can use them. The amounts in the menus are for one serving. When a serving-size range is given, men should choose the upper end of the range; the entire range is available to youths (males 11 through 17 and females 11 through 14).

Additions for men and youths are indicated on each menu plan. Other information to make the cookbook more useful is provided by Weight Watchers in the book.

Food Exchange Lists.   Food exchange lists, which list food servings of similar nutrient content and caloric value, are designed to provide flexibility in menu planning. You may exchange any item on an exchange list for any other item on the list. A person who does not eat pork, for example, may substitute fish, beef, liver, cheese, or any other item listed as Lean Meat, Protein Rich Exchanges.

All exchange lists contain foods of similar nutrient content and are grouped according to recognized food groups. Here they are presented for the following six food groups: milk, vegetables, fruit, bread, lean meat (protein), and fat. The exchange lists show the number of grams of carbohydrate, protein, and fat and the number of kilocalories in one exchange, among other descriptive information. They also explain the kinds and amounts of food to use for one exchange. For instance, in the Nonfat Milk Exchanges, 1 cup of skim or nonfat milk, or ⅓ cup of powdered (nonfat dry) milk should be used for one exchange.

The exchange lists might seem confusing to someone who has not used them before. So in Table 12.5 we present an 1800-kilocalorie daily diet translated into food exchanges and distributed among three meals and snacks.

To demonstrate further how the exchange lists can be used, here is a menu for breakfast developed from the recommended caloric distribution for breakfast.

Breakfast menu using exchange lists

Milk, skim: 1 Exchange	Skim milk, ½ cup
Fruit: 3 Exchanges	Grapefruit, ½
	Blueberries, ½ cup
	Apple juice, ⅓ cup
Bread: 2 Exchanges	Whole-wheat bread, 2 slices
Meat, medium fat: 1 Exchange	Egg, 1
Fat: 3 Exchanges	Margarine, 1 tsp.
	Avocado, ⅛
	Crisp bacon, 1 slice

Innumerable menus for breakfast and other meals are possible using the exchange lists. Food preferences, seasonality, financial ability to purchase different foods, and other factors will dictate the menus that different people will prepare. Whatever the personal situation, however, food should be prepared and eaten following sound nutritional practices.

TABLE 12.5   **An 1800-Kilocalorie Daily Diet Translated into Food Exchanges and Distributed by Meals and Snacks**

(1800-Kcal diet: 90 g protein, 60 g fat, 225 g carbohydrate)
Translation into Food Exchanges

Food	Total for day (exchanges)	Carbohydrate (g)	Protein (g)	Fat (g)
Milk, skim	2	24	16	0
Vegetables	2	10	4	0
Fruit	7	70	0	0
Bread	8	120	16	0
Meat, lean	6	0	42	18
Meat, medium fat	2	0	14	11
Fat	6	0	0	30
Total distribution	—	224	92	59

Distribution by Meals and Snacks

Food	Breakfast	Lunch	Dinner	Snacks
Milk, skim	½ cup	½ cup	½ cup	½ cup
Vegetables	0	1	1	0
Fruit	3	3	1	0
Bread	2	2	3	1
Meat, lean	0	3	3	0
Meat, medium fat	1	0	0	1
Fat	3	2	1	0
Total carbohydrate	66	71	66	21
Total kilocalories	513	580	520	218
Fractional distribution	3/10	3/10	3/10	1/10

Note: Many variations are possible for diabetics, depending on the individual's needs and preferences and the dosage and type of insulin administered.

Source: The exchange lists, from the Exchange Lists for Meal Planning, *were prepared by committees of the American Diabetes Association, Inc., and The American Dietetic Association in cooperation with the National Institute of Arthritis, Metabolism and Digestive Diseases and the National Heart and Lung Institute, National Institutes of Health, Public Health Service, U.S. Department of Health, Education and Welfare. Copyright © American Diabetes Association, Inc., and The American Dietetic Association, 1976.*

LIST 1
Nonfat Milk Exchanges

One Exchange of nonfat milk contains 12 grams of carbohydrates, 8 grams of protein, a trace of fat, and 80 kilocalories.

Milk is the leading source of calcium. It is a good source of phosphorus, protein, some of the B-complex vitamins, including folacin and vitamin B_{12}, and vitamins A and D. Magnesium is also found in milk.

Whole milk contains 12 grams of carbohydrate, 8 grams of protein, 9 grams of fat, and 160 kilocalories.

Milk can be used to drink, to add to cereal, in coffee or tea, or with other foods.

This list shows the kinds and amounts of milk or milk products to use for one Nonfat Milk Exchange:

Nonfat fortified milks	Amount to Use
	LIST 1 (*Continued*)
Skim or nonfat milk	1 cup
Powdered (nonfat dry)	1/3 cup
Canned, evaporated—skim	1/2 cup
Buttermilk made from skim milk	1 cup
Yogurt made from skim milk (plain, unflavored)	1 cup
1% skim	1 cup
2% fortified skim (omit 1 Fat Exchange)	1 cup

Whole milks (omit 2 Fat Exchanges)

Whole milk	1 cup
Canned, evaporated	1/2 cup
Buttermilk made from whole milk	1 cup
Yogurt made from whole milk (plain, unflavored)	1 cup

One Exchange of most vegetables on this list is 1/2 cup and contains about 5 grams of carbohydrate, 2 grams of protein, and 25 kilocalories.

**LIST 2
Vegetable
Exchanges**

Dark green and deep yellow vegetables are leading sources of vitamin A. Some vegetables such as asparagus, broccoli, brussels sprouts, cauliflower, cabbage, green peppers, greens, and tomatoes contain vitamin C. Green leafy vegetables contain folacin; and broccoli, cabbage, carrots, spinach, and tomatoes are good sources of vitamin B_6. Brussels sprouts, greens, tomatoes, and broccoli contain potassium. Spinach is a source of zinc, and magnesium is found in green beans, broccoli, and tomatoes. Vegetables are good sources of fiber.

Serve vegetables cooked or raw. If fat is added in preparation, omit the equivalent number of Fat Exchanges.

Asparagus
Bean sprouts
Beets
Broccoli
Brussels sprouts
Cabbage
Carrots
Cauliflower
Celery
Cucumbers
Eggplant
Green pepper
Greens:
  Beet
  Chards
  Collards
  Dandelion
  Kale

Greens
  Mustard
  Spinach
  Turnip
Mushrooms
Okra
Onions
Radishes
Rhubarb
Rutabaga
Sauerkraut
String beans, green or yellow
Summer squash
Tomatoes
Tomato juice
Turnips
Vegetable juice cocktail
Zucchini

Raw celery, chicory, chinese cabbage, cucumbers, endive, escarole, lettuce, and watercress can be used as desired.

Starch vegetables are found in the **Bread Exchanges.**

One Exchange of fruit contains 10 grams of carbohydrate and 40 kilocalories.

Fruits are valuable for vitamins and minerals and fiber. Oranges, tangerines, grapefruit, strawberries, cantaloupe, and honeydew melon are good sources of vitamin C. Apricots and peaches contain vitamin A. Mangoes and papaya contain both vitamin A and vitamin C. Bananas, nectarines, oranges, plums, and dried fruits are sources of potassium. Cantaloupe, oranges, and strawberries contain folacin. Magnesium and vitamin B_6 are found in bananas.

Fruit may be used fresh, dried, canned or frozen, cooked or raw, as long as no sugar is added. Read the label on the can or package to be certain no sugar or sorbitol has been added.

This list shows the kinds and amounts of fruits to use for one Fruit Exchange:

	Amount to use		Amount to use
Apple	1 small	Grape juice	1/4 cup
Apple juice	1/3 cup	Mango	1/2 small
Applesauce (unsweetened)	1/2 cup	Cantaloupe	1/4 small
		Honeydew	1/8 medium
		Watermelon	1 cup
Apricots, fresh	2 medium	Nectarine	1 small
Apricots, dried	4 halves	Orange	1 small
Banana	1/2 small	Orange juice	1/2 cup
Berries		Papaya	3/4 cup
Blackberries	1/2 cup	Peach	1 medium
Blueberries	1/2 cup	Pear	1 small
Raspberries	2/3 cup	Persimmon,	
Strawberries	3/4 cup	native	1 medium
Cherries	10 large	Pineapple	1/2 cup
Cider	1/3 cup	Pineapple juice	1/3 cup
Dates	2	Plums	2 medium
Figs, dried	1	Prunes	2 medium
Figs, fresh	1	Prune juice	1/4 cup
Grapefruit	1/2	Raisins	2 tbsp
Grapefruit juice	1/2 cup	Tangerine	1 medium
Grapes	12		

For variety serve fruit as a salad or in combination with other foods as desert.

Cranberries may be used as desired if no sugar is added.

One Exchange contains 15 grams of carbohydrate, 2 grams of protein, and 70 kilocalories.

Whole grain or enriched breads and cereals are good sources of iron and some of the B vitamins, as are dried beans and peas and the vegetables on this list. Magnesium is found in dried cooked beans and whole grain cereals. Dried beans, peas, and lentils are sources of zinc. Dried peas and beans and whole grain breads and cereals are excellent sources of fiber.

This list shows the many kinds and amounts of breads, cereals, and starchy vegetables to use for one Bread Exchange:

Amount to use

BREAD

White (including French and Italian)	1 slice
Whole wheat	1 slice
Rye or pumpernickel	1 slice
Raisin	1 slice
Bagel, small	1/2
English muffin, small	1/2
Plain roll, bread	1
Frankfurter roll	1/2
Hamburger bun	1/2
Dry bread crumbs	3 tbsp
Pancake, 5″	1
Waffle, 5″	1
Tortilla, 6″	1

CEREAL

Bran flakes	1/2 cup
Other ready to eat unsweetened cereal	3/4 cup
Puff cereal, unfrosted	1 cup
Cereal, cooked	1/2 cup
Grits, cooked	1/2 cup
Rice or barley, cooked	1/2 cup
Pastas, cooked spaghetti, noodles, macaroni	1/2 cup
Cornmeal, dry	2 tbsp
Flour	2½ tbsp
Wheat germ	1/4 cup

CRACKERS

Arrowroot	3
Graham 2½″	2
Matzoth, 4″ × 6″	1/2
Oyster	20
Pretzels 3″ long, 1/8″ dia.	25

Amount to use

DRIED BEANS, PEAS, AND LENTILS

Beans, peas, lentils, dried and cooked	1/2 cup
Baked beans, no pork	1/4 cup

STARCHY VEGETABLES

Corn	1/3 cup
Corn on cob	1 small
Lima beans	1/2 cup
Parsnips	2/3 cup
Peas, green—canned or frozen	1/2 cup

LIST 4 (*Continued*)

	Amount to use
Potato, white	1 small
Potato, mashed	½ cup
Pumpkin	¾ cup
Winter squash, acorn or butternut	½ cup
Yam or sweet potato	¼ cup

MISCELLANEOUS

Biscuit 2″ dia. (Omit 1 Fat Exchange)	1
Corn muffin 2″ dia. (Omit 1 Fat Exchange)	1
Crackers, round butter type (Omit 1 Fat Exchange)	5
Muffin, plain small (Omit 1 Fat Exchange)	1
Popcorn, popped	3 cups
Potatoes, French fried, length 2 to 3½″ (Omit 1 Fat Exchange)	8
Potato or corn chips (Omit 2 Fat Exchanges)	15

CRACKERS

Rye Wafers, 2″ × 3½″	3
Saltines	6
Soda 2½″ sq.	4

LIST 5
Lean Meat, Protein Rich Exchanges

One Exchange of meat (1 oz) contains 7 grams of protein, 3 grams of fat, and 55 kilocalories.

Meat, poultry, fish, cheese, and eggs are important sources of protein, iron, vitamin B_{12}, and other B-complex vitamins. Liver and eggs also contain vitamin A. Oysters and peanut butter contain magnesium. Liver is a good source of iron and both liver and peanut butter contain folacin. Zinc is found in lean beef, cheddar type cheese, crab, liver, peanut butter, oysters, and the dark meat of turkey.

Cholesterol is of animal origin; therefore, peanut butter and dried peas and beans contain no cholesterol.

To plan a diet low in saturated fat and cholesterol, choose only those exchanges listed in the first group—Low Fat Meat Exchange.

You may use the meat, fish, etc., that is prepared for the family when no fat or flour has been added. If meat is fried, use the fat included in the meal plan. Meat juices with the fat removed may be used with your meat or vegetables for added flavor. Be certain to trim off *all* visible fat and measure meat after it has been cooked. A 3-oz serving of cooked meat is about equal to 4 oz of raw meat.

This list shows the kinds and amounts of meat and protein rich foods to use for one Low Fat Meat Exchange:

Beef:	Baby beef; chipped beef; chuck; flank steak; tenderloin; plate ribs; plate skirt steak; round (bottom, top); all cuts rump; spare ribs; tripe	1 oz	**LIST 5** (*Continued*)
Lamb:	Leg; rib; sirloin; loin (roast and chops); shank; shoulder	1 oz	
Pork:	Leg (whole rump, center shank); ham, smoked (center slices)	1 oz	
Veal:	Leg; loin; rib; shank; shoulder; cutlets	1 oz	
Poultry:	Meat without skin of chicken, turkey, cornish hen, guinea hen, pheasant	1 oz	
Fish:	Any fresh or frozen Canned salmon, tuna, mackerel, crab, and lobster	1 oz	
		¼ cup	
	Clams, oysters, scallops, shrimp	5 or 1 oz	
	Sardines, drained	3	
Cheeses containing less than 5% butterfat		1 oz	
Cottage cheese, dry and 2% butterfat		¼ cup	
Dried peas and beans (Omit 1 Bread Exchange)		½ cup	

Medium Fat Meat and Protein Rich Exchanges contain 7 grams of protein, 5 grams of fat, and 75 kilocalories (1 oz).

This list shows the kinds and amounts of meat and protein rich foods to use for one Medium Fat Meat Exchange:

Beef:	Ground, 15% fat; corned beef, canned; rib eye; round, ground (commercial)	1 oz
Pork:	Loin (all cuts); tenderloin; shoulder arm, picnic; shoulder blade (Boston butt); Canadian bacon, boiled ham; loin, shoulder, picnic ham	1 oz
Liver, heart, kidney, and sweetbreads (these are high in cholesterol)		1 oz
Cottage cheese, creamed		¼ cup
Cheese, mozzarella, ricotta, farmer's cheese, Neufchâtel		1 oz
Cheese, Parmesan		3 tbsp
Egg (high in cholesterol)		1
Peanut butter (Omit 2 Fat Exchanges)		2 tbsp

LIST 5 (*Continued*) High Fat Meat and Protein Rich Exchanges contain 7 grams of protein, 8 grams of fat, and 100 kilocalories (1 oz).

This list shows the kinds and amounts of meat and protein rich foods to use for one High Fat Meat Exchange:

Beef:	Brisket; corned beef (brisket); ground beef, more than 20% fat; hamburger (commercial); chuck, ground (commercial); roasts, rib; steaks, club and rib	1 oz
Lamb:	Breast	1 oz
Pork:	Spare ribs; loin (back ribs); pork, ground; country style ham; deviled ham; spare ribs	1 oz
Veal:	Breast	1 oz
Poultry:	Capon, duck (domestic); goose	1 oz
Cheese, cheddar type		1 oz
Cold cuts		4½″ × ⅛″ slice
Frankfurter		1

LIST 6
Fat Exchanges

One Exchange of fat contains 5 grams of fat and 45 kilocalories.

Since all fats are high in kilocalories, foods on this list should be measured carefully to control weight. Margarine, butter, cream, and cream cheese contain vitamin A. Use the fats on this list in the amounts on the meal plan.

To plan a diet low in saturated fat select only those exchanges which appear in **bold type** and are polyunsaturated.

This list shows the kinds and amounts of fat containing foods to use for one Fat Exchange:

	Amount to use
Margarine, soft, tub or stick*	1 tsp
Avocado (4″ in diameter)†	⅛
Oil, corn, cottonseed, soy, sunflower	1 tsp
Oil, olive†	1 tsp
Oil, peanut†	1 tsp
Walnuts	6 small
Nuts, other†	6 small
Olives†	5 small
Margarine, regular stick	1 tsp
Butter	1 tsp
Bacon fat	1 tsp
Bacon, crisp	1 strip

Amount to use

Cream, light	2 tbsp
Cream, sour	2 tbsp
Cream, heavy	1 tbsp
Cream cheese	1 tbsp
French dressing‡	1 tbsp
Italian dressing‡	1 tbsp
Lard	1 tsp
Mayonnaise†	1 tsp
Salad dressing, mayonnaise type‡	2 tsp
Salt pork	¾" cube

*Made with corn, cottonseed, safflower, soy, or sunflower oil only.

†Fat content is primarily monounsaturated.

‡If made with corn, cottonseed, safflower, or soy oil, can be used on fat-modified diet.

Sources: The exchange lists, from the Exchange Lists for Meal Planning, *were prepared by committees of the American Diabetes Association, Inc., and The American Dietetic Association in cooperation with the National Institute of Arthritis, Metabolism and Digestive Diseases and the National Heart and Lung Institute, National Institutes of Health, Public Health Service, U.S. Department of Health, Education and Welfare. Copyright © American Diabetes Association, Inc., and The American Dietetic Association, 1976.*

Adjusting Caloric Intake and Energy Expenditure

It has been stressed repeatedly that Calories consumed and energy expenditure must be coordinated to produce the weight loss you desire. You must burn up 3500 more Calories than you consume to lose one pound. The food plan and exercise program should be designed so that you will lose no more than 2 pounds in one week. Also, a *minimum* of 1200 Calories for women and 1600 Calories for men is necessary to meet the body's need for protein, vitamins, and minerals.

To balance caloric intake with energy expenditure to ensure proper weight loss it might be necessary for some to consume more Calories than are provided in the sample menus. A female who loses more than 2 pounds a week by bicycling for 240 minutes a week, for example, will need to consume more than 1200 Calories. (A menu planned from the 1860-kilocalorie diet in Table 12.2 might be sufficient.) Conversely, a woman who does not lose one pound a week on the combination 1200 Calorie-a-day food plan will need to increase her energy expenditure through more exercise. Lowering the caloric intake beyond 1200 Calories a day is considered nutritionally unsound.

Use Table 4.3 to determine your energy expenditure. To this figure must be added the energy expenditure of the physical activity that you engage in on a daily basis. Following a food plan such as Weight Watchers (which is highly recommended) will also simplify the determination of your caloric intake. If you have a problem adhering to the eating and exercise plan after determining what it should be, consult Chapter 8 for behavior modification strategies to aid you in your endeavor. If you still find that you can't quite stick to your program, you might wish to check with the Weight Watchers organization in your local community. This organization provides the necessary group support for people who want to lose weight but cannot do it alone.

Gaining Weight

People who need to gain weight should consume more Calories than they expend. Though simple to say, the practice of coordinating caloric intake with energy expenditure to gain weight is as difficult as balancing the Calorie-energy equation for weight loss. But weight gain is possible if certain guidelines are adhered to.

As was mentioned in Chapter 4, the first step in establishing a weight gain program is to have a complete medical examination to determine your present health status. The findings of the medical examination should help to guide future plans regarding the development of a specific weight gain program. However, certain guidelines should be followed by all who are desirous of gaining weight. These recommendations are presented as a summary of and supplement to the guidelines contained in Chapter 4. They are offered for underweight individuals who are otherwise healthy.

1. Determine your caloric intake and energy expenditure for a week or two to get some idea of the disparity between these measures. Use the procedures outlined in Chapter 4.
2. Increase your caloric intake according to the disparity between Calories consumed and energy expended. (Remember that a pound of lean body weight is equal to about 2500 Calories.) While eating a well-balanced diet with foods from each of the Basic Four Food Groups, gradually increase the caloric intake until it is about 1000 Calories more than caloric (energy) expenditure. The increased caloric intake can be gotten by eating four or five small meals with high-Calorie snacks between meals.
3. The increased caloric intake should be mainly complex carbohydrates and some protein, with a slight increase in polyunsaturated fat.
4. Get adequate exercise and rest. Engage in high-intensity weight training workouts consisting of four to six exercises for the lower body and six to eight exercises for the upper body. Limit the workouts to 30 minutes or less. Allow at least 48 hours between workouts but no more than 96 hours. (Also perform aerobic exercises to keep the cardiorespiratory system at an optimal level of development.)
5. Get at least 8 to 10 hours of sleep every night with periods of rest during the day. Help to control nervous energy with yoga, meditation, massage, or soft music. A cup of warm milk might help to make you sleep better at night.
6. Avoid caffeinated foods such as colas, coffee, tea, and cocoa if you are caffeine-sensitive; and use them sparingly even if you are not caffeine-sensitive. Tobacco, an appetite suppressant, should also be avoided.[3]
7. Use the self-modification-of-behavior techniques presented in Chapter 8 to help you develop positive and desirable behaviors as you attempt to gain weight. Reward yourself for any gains you make.

8. Be realistic in your weight gain goals. Plan to gain no more than one or two pounds per week.

9. Use protein and vitamin supplements only under the direction of your physician. A well-balanced diet should provide ample vitamins. However, some underweight individuals might be advised to get extra amounts of vitamins and protein by physicians who are aware of their personal medical histories.

A Computer-assisted Nutrition and Exercise Plan

For individuals who are weary of counting Calories, working with food exchange lists, and calculating the caloric costs of physical activities, computer technology may provide welcome relief. Using FITCOMP (acronym for "fitness by computer"), a computer assessment system, a person can have a nutrition and exercise plan developed on an individual basis. The uniqueness of the application of computer technology to nutrition management, according to a description of the plan in *Preventive Medicine*,[4] is that individuals can select the foods they will eat from a list of preferred choices from the basic food groups. The menus are designed to provide an optimal blend of nutrients aimed at achieving ideal body mass and fat percentage.

The overall nutrition plan is based on guidelines formulated by the American Dietetic Association. Foods are arranged as exchanges within a given food category (breads, dairy products, fruits, meats, fats, vegetables, alcohol, and "treats"), and each exchange is assigned a specific Calorie value. Like other food exchange plans, food can be exchanged within any food category. The basic food list includes 11 food choices from the milk category, 35 each from breads and fruits, 42 from meats, 17 from fats, 28 from vegetables, 7 from low-Calorie vegetables, 12 from treats, and 7 from alcoholic beverages. The current list of 194 foods was based on those most frequently chosen by approximately 13,000 individuals throughout the United States who responded to a questionnaire that included 234 food items.

The exercise plans are geared for the beginner, intermediate, or advanced participant and are designed to enable individual users to expend about 300 to 500 Calories per exercise session. Individuals are assigned to one of the three program levels based on their response to a questionnaire, their age, and their sex. The three main aerobic activities are walking, jogging or running, and swimming or cycling. Selections can also be made from nine other popular choices: racquetball, circuit training, squash, badminton, basketball, downhill skiing, tennis, golf, and aerobic dancing.

A computerized meal and exercise plan can be purchased. Interested persons should contact sponsors of the computer meal and exercise plan at the following address: Computer Meal and Exercise Plan, P.O. Box

431, Amherst, MA 01004. A questionnaire will be sent to you to be completed to get the information to design your meal and exercise plan. Questionnaires are processed within 48 hours, and the printout should be received, under normal conditions, within 10 days. For more information, write to the address indicated above or review the article by Katch and Katch in Note 4.

Notes

1. American College of Sports Medicine, "Proper and Improper Weight Loss Programs," *Medicine and Science in Sports* 15 (1983):ix–xiii.
2. *Weight Watchers 365-Day Menu Cookbook* (New York: New American Library, 1983).
3. Jeannette Pichulik, "Weight Gain: A Sensible Approach," *Sports Medicine* 1 (1984):1, 11–12.
4. Frank I. Katch and Victor L. Katch, "Computer Technology to Evaluate Body Composition, Nutrition, and Exercise," *Preventive Medicine* 12 (1983):619–631.

CHAPTER 13

Pathways to Fitness for Individuals with Handicapping Conditions

asthma
cystic fibrosis

diabetes
epilepsy

Chapter Highlights

After reading this chapter, you should be able to:
1. Define and/or explain the key words listed above.
2. Design an exercise program for a person who has had a heart attack.
3. Identify the medical problems that would cause a person not to engage in a strenuous exercise program.
4. Explain the phenomenon of exercise-induced asthma (EIA).
5. List the recommended activities for people with asthma.
6. Develop an exercise program for a person with asthma.
7. Differentiate between cystic fibrosis and asthma, including the different exercise prescriptions that would be developed.
8. Compare and contrast juvenile-onset diabetes and maturity-onset diabetes.
9. Identify the symptoms of both juvenile-onset diabetes and maturity-onset diabetes.
10. Discuss the role of exercise in a therapeutic program for diabetics.
11. Identify the recreational activities most often participated in by the amputees in the study cited in the chapter.
12. Discuss the role of exercise in the life of an epileptic.
13. Identify an appropriate organization with programs that would aid a person with a visual, auditory, or physical handicap.

Until now information in this text has been presented for the "average" individual, including information designed to serve as the foundation for physical fitness, to motivate people to exercise, and to promote the development of proper exercise prescriptions for various fitness components. Persons with handicapping conditions can be guided by much of the information previously presented. However, more specific information and guidelines are needed for persons with specific handicapping conditions.

This chapter will provide specific information and guidelines to help develop pathways to fitness for persons with cardiovascular disease, asthma, cystic fibrosis, diabetes, epilepsy, and physical handicaps. This chapter emphasizes the modification and adaptation of activities to suit the needs of the person with a particular handicap. Some form of physical activity is advocated for individuals with any handicapping condition.

Exercise for Persons with Cardiovascular Disease

Exercise is recommended as both a preventive and rehabilitative measure for persons with cardiovascular disease. The type of exercise prescription that is designed for a person with heart disease should be based in part on the results of an exercise tolerance (or stress) test. Remember that exercise is a form of therapy and as such is designed to

TABLE 13.1   **Contraindications for Physical Activity**

General Disease Category	Specific Medical Problem
Acute illness	Recent myocardial infarction; respiratory, G.I., or other febrile illness; phlebitis and embolism
Active, chronic, systemic disease (uncontrolled)	Thyroid, renal, hepatic, rheumatic disease, gout, etc.
Anatomic abnormalities	Uncompensated valvular heart disease; gross cardiomegaly[a]
Functional abnormalities	Dysrhythmia: ventricular tachycardia,[b] uncontrolled atrial fibrillation; second- and third-degree heart block

[a]Abnormal enlargement of the heart.

[b]Excessively rapid heartbeat.

Source: © *Reproduced with permission.* Exercise Testing and Training of Individuals with Heart Disease or at High Risk for Its Development: A Handbook for Physicians. *American Heart Association. p. 41.*

promote cardiovascular functioning in persons with heart disease. Be aware, however, that a cardiac patient or an extremely deconditioned person might experience adverse reactions to exercise.

Sometimes exercise therapy is contraindicated, particularly in cases of acute illness, uncontrolled systemic illness such as congestive heart failure, precipitation of life-threatening dysrhythmias during exercise, and symptoms or signs at minimal exercise stress levels.[1] Specific contraindications to physical activity are indicated in Table 13.1.

As was stated, the exercise prescription should be based on the results of the exercise stress test. Table 13.2 shows the information from the stress test that is needed to develop an exercise prescription.

Although the intensity and duration of the exercise program for the heart patient would vary according to the severity of the disease, the frequency would be three or four times a week. Care must be exercised in recommending physical activities for heart patients. Walking is an especially good activity for heart patients who engage in an unsupervised physical activity program. An example of an unsupervised walking program is presented in Table 13.3.

The unsupervised walking program was developed according to the principles of training that should guide the development of a physical fitness program. A heart patient who is given permission to engage in the unsupervised walking program (Table 13.3) should exercise at each prescription level for three weeks before beginning the next exercise prescription.

It cannot be emphasized too strongly that persons with symptoms of cardiovascular disease or on a rehabilitation program should be guided

The Exercise Prescription

TABLE 13.2   **Information from Stress Test Needed for Exercise Prescription**

Data	Reason
Maximum oxygen uptake (may be directly measured or estimated reliably from tables under certain circumstances)	Exercise intensity can be prescribed as 60% to 85% of maximum oxygen uptake to achieve a training effect.
Maximum attainable heart rate	Exercise is most conveniently prescribed at a target heart rate in the range of 70% to 85% of maximum attainable heart rate.
Limiting symptoms and their physiologic accompaniments	Exercise should be prescribed below this level, preferably as a percentage of it.
Occurrence of asymptomatic ischemic ECG changes, dysrhythmia, or excessive blood pressure responses	Prescription must provide a method by which the patient can avoid these asymptomatic abnormalities during exercise.

Source: The Committee on Exercise, American Heart Association, Exercise Testing and Training of Individuals with Heart Disease or at High Risk for Its Development: A Handbook for Physicians. *(Dallas: 1975), p. 24. Reproduced with permission.*

TABLE 13.3   **Unsupervised Walking Program Prescriptions**[a]

Prescription Number	Exercise Phase	Speed	Intensity (METs)	Intensity (ml O$_2$/kg/min)	Distance (miles)	Time Goal (minutes)	Times per Week
	Warm-up	2 mph	2–3	7–11	0.25	7:30	
1	Conditioning bout	3 mph	4.5[b]	14–18	1.00	20:00	7
	Cool-down	2 mph	2–3	7–11	0.25	7:30	
	Warm-up	2 mph	2–3	7–11	0.25	7:30	
2	Conditioning bout	3 mph	4.5	14–18	2.00	40:00	7
	Cool-down	2 mph	2–3	7–11	0.25	7:30	
	Warm-up	2 mph	2–3	7–11	0.25	7:30	
3	Conditioning bout	3.5 mph	6.5	21–23	2.00	35:00	7
	Cool-down	2 mph	2–3	7–11	0.25	7:30	
	Warm-up	2 mph	2–3	7–11	0.25	7:30	
4[c]	Conditioning bout	3.5 mph	6.5	21–23	3.00	51:00	7
	Cool-down	2 mph	2–3	7–11	0.25	7:30	

[a]This exercise prescription is based on the following exercise tolerance test information: A patient is stopped by 3+ angina (heart rate 130) after 2.5 minutes at 3 mph on a 10% upgrade on the treadmill. Angina and ST segment depression began at 2.5 mph at a heart rate of 120. Exercising at a rate of 2.5 mph at 10% grade = 6 METs = 21 ml O$_2$/kg/min, which is the angina threshold.
[b]This represents an intensity of 75% of the angina threshold (0.75 × 6 METs = 4.5).
[c]Prescription 4 would be undertaken if, on retest, the patient completes the 4-mph stage at 10% grade on the treadmill with 3 mm ST depression (8 METs = 28 ml O$_2$/kg/min) and develops 1+ angina at the 3.5-mph stage. (The patient should gradually increase the distance from 2 miles in 35 minutes to 3 miles in 51 minutes within three weeks.)

Source: Adapted from The Committee on Exercise, American Heart Association, Exercise Testing and Training of Individuals with Heart Disease or at High Risk for Its Development: A Handbook for Physicians. (Dallas: 1975), pp. 55–56. Reproduced with permission.

by their physician before beginning an exercise program, even unsupervised walking.

The walking program presented in Table 13.3 is but one example of an excellent activity that can be used for the prevention of cardiovascular disease or the rehabilitation of persons recovering from heart disease. Other aerobic activities such as jogging, stair climbing, bicycling, dancing, and swimming are also recommended for heart patients. The exercise prescription would be an individual prescription, based on the results of the exercise stress or tolerance test, the patient's medical history, and present physical condition. Physicians who are not specialists in the area of sports medicine or cardiac care might wish to examine the handbook on exercise testing and training of individuals with heart disease developed by the American Heart Association's Committee on Exercise (see note 1).

High-intensity, strenuous, anaerobic-type activities such as weight training, isometric training (push-ups, pull-ups, and the like) are not recommended for the heart patient. These type of activities do not improve cardiovascular fitness. Furthermore, they often place unusually high demands on an already impaired cardiovascular system.

In summary, it can be stated with confidence that exercise can be used to reduce the risk of cardiovascular disease (see Chapter 6). Individualized exercise programs can also be used effectively in the rehabilitation of individuals who have heart disease.

Proper guidelines for an exercise program for cardiac patients must be established. Here is a summary:

1. Get the patient active as early in the rehabilitative process as practicable. Having the patient sit on the side of the bed or walking with the assistance of a nurse in the hospital room can be done a day or two following a heart operation, for example.
2. Before designing the exercise prescription, perform an exercise tolerance test to study the patient's response to increased levels of stress (starting with mild intensities).
3. Base the exercise prescription on the results of the exercise tolerance test, among other factors.
4. Design the program according to the principles of training discussed in Chapter 9.

Exercise for the Asthmatic

Bronchial asthma, a chronic illness of childhood, is a main category of respiratory diseases. Emphysema and chronic bronchitis are two other lung diseases. This section focuses on exercise for the asthmatic because, unlike chronic bronchitis and emphysema, which are irreversible, asthma sometimes lessens in severity or disappears completely as a person grows older.

Bronchial asthma is a generalized condition of the lungs characterized by bronchospasm, mucosal edema, and thick mucus that can lead to ventilatory insufficiency.[2] Bronchial asthma is an allergic reaction to foreign substances such as house dust, animal hair, and pollen and is characterized by attacks of wheezing and labored breathing.

Asthma attacks might also be precipitated by participation in strenuous physical activities. Such asthmatic attacks are referred to as exercise-induced asthma (EIA) or exercise-induced bronchospasm (EIB). Although the underlying causes of EIA are not fully understood, it has been observed that the increased airway obstruction often occurs 5 to 20 minutes after a short period of strenuous exercise. It may also occur during prolonged physical activity. The reaction to asthma is widely variable; some children might complain of asthmatic attacks during exercise, whereas others can participate without incident.

Reactions to medication to block EIA are as variable as the asthmatic attacks themselves. Some asthmatic individuals can be relieved by a single medication such as cromolyn sodium, while others might need a combination of medications. In a study of 53 children with moderately severe asthma, for example, Cummings and Strunk reported that EIB was completely blocked in 47 children by an inhaled metaproterenol 10 minutes before exercise, in combination with theophyline. In six children, however, EIB was only partially blocked when either metaproterenol or cromolyn was added to the theophyline but was completely blocked when all three drugs were used.[3]

Swimming* is the activity most often recommended for asthmatics. Other recommended activities, in order of preference, are walking, cycling, and jogging. The specific exercise prescription should be based on the results of an evaluation of the patient, including a complete history, a physical examination, and an exercise tolerance test to define the patient's functional capacities and limitations.

It is important to include a 10- to 15-minute warm-up in an exercise program for asthmatics. The warm-up has proved to be an effective way to improve lung ventilation, enabling the asthmatic to engage in more strenuous activity with less wheezing and discomfort. Robert Kersee, assistant track coach at UCLA, reports on the preworkout procedure of Janet Bolden, an outstanding track performer at UCLA. According to the coach, Bolden takes an oral medication 1 to 1½ hours before her warm-up. The warm-up itself consists of 10 to 15 minutes of jogging, stretching, and some flexibility drills. After the warm-up Bolden often wheezes and is short of breath. During such times she takes an aerosol bronchodilator, which relieves the discomfort in about five minutes.[5]

Normally cardiorespiratory endurance is developed by participation in aerobic activities for a minimum of 30 minutes. However, the interval training technique is recommended for people with asthma because of the impairment of the respiratory passageways. Bouts of two to three minutes of jogging, for example, should be followed by three to five minutes of rest or slow walking.[6]

This is not to suggest that the intervals of jogging should be at a high intensity level. On the contrary, the jogging should be performed at a slow to moderate pace, with an interval of rest or slow walking to allow time for the body to recover for the next conditioning bout. Since asthmatics' responses to exercise are so variable, determination of intensity level should be made on an individual basis.

Some well-conditioned asthmatics can tolerate longer intervals or intense exercise bouts. For instance, Bolden engages in intervals of 20 to 30 minutes of running 200 to 300 meters with a controlled rest period between the exercise bouts.

The asthmatic should develop a positive attitude toward exercise. People tolerate asthma attacks differently, and the severity of the asthmatic condition varies widely from one person to another. Therefore, not all asthmatics can hope to excel in track and field like Janet Bolden. However, each asthmatic should attempt to participate in physical activity with the objective of maintaining a physically healthy body.

---

*Although the data on swimming as a recommended activity for asthmatics are limited, it has been reported that swimming reduces the incidence and severity of postexercise bronchoconstriction. Possible factors for the favorable effect of swimming on asthmatics include the horizontal position of the exercise and the effects of hydrostatic pressure. Another hypothesis is that the warm humid air reduces and sometimes abolishes EIA.[4]

Exercise and Cystic Fibrosis

Cystic fibrosis (CF) is an inherited generalized body disease that first appears in children and is characterized by chronic lung disease, a deficiency of pancreatic enzymes, and an abnormally high concentration of salt in the sweat.[7] The disease is life-threatening.

Cystic fibrosis patients can safely engage in exercise programs and can increase the endurance of their respiratory muscles. However, their pulmonary function will not be significantly improved through exercise. Exercise may be as good as traditional chest physical therapy for removing mucus from the lungs.

Like persons with asthma, the variability of individuals with CF is large, and there is a high correlation between exercise tolerance and the resting maximum oxygen ventilation. In one study it was found that the resting oxygen level lowered in relationship to the severity of the disease, but there was an increase in oxygenation during exercise.[8]

Because of variability in oxygenation and carbon dioxide elimination among patients with cystic fibrosis, extreme care should be used in planning exercise programs for these persons. It is recommended that a supervised exercise tolerance test be administered to CF patients to determine their exercise prescriptions.

When exercising in hot weather, CF patients should ingest ample fluids and increase their salt intake. These patients should avoid exercising during the hottest part of the day during extremely hot weather. One study in which CF patients exercised on a bicycle ergometer at 100° F and 50 percent vO_2 max demonstrated that their thermoregulatory mechanisms were not adversely affected. However, they lost significantly more salt in their sweat than normal subjects.[9]

The exercise prescription for patients with cystic fibrosis should be developed on an individual basis. In one study, 21 CF patients engaged in a walking and jogging program for ten minutes (three times per week) the first week and slowly increased both the intensity and the duration of the exercise until they were all jogging continuously for 30 minutes by the twelfth week. The walking and jogging were performed at an intensity level of between 70 and 85 percent of their heart rate maximum. The exercise group improved in all the important cardiorespiratory parameters. However, there was no significant change in pulmonary function during the study.[10]

Besides increasing their tolerance for physical activity, cystic fibrosis patients can also use exercise as pulmonary therapy. Specific upper-body exercises such as swimming, canoeing, and running have been shown to increase the endurance of the respiratory muscles. So although persons suffering from cystic fibrosis are likely to be less fit than their normal peers, the vast majority can exercise safely.

Exercise and Diabetes

Diabetes mellitus, caused by an absolute or relative deficiency of insulin that results in an abnormally high concentration of blood sugar (hyperglycemia), affects some 10 million Americans.

There are two major types of diabetes: insulin-dependent diabetes mellitus (IDDM), also called Type I or juvenile-onset diabetes, and non-insulin-dependent diabetes mellitus (NIDDM), also called Type II or maturity-onset diabetes. Neither type should be used as an excuse for inactivity. In fact, proper diet, insulin for insulin-dependent diabetics, and exercise are prescribed as components of a diabetic management program.

IDDM develops in people under the age of 20. It is generally more severe than maturity-onset diabetes and usually requires the patient to take insulin for the regulation of the blood sugar level. However, there is a risk of blood sugar levels becoming too low (hypoglycemia), causing insulin shock. An extremely low level of glucose (blood sugar) can cause nausea, dizziness, and fainting. To protect against such occurrences, insulin-dependent diabetics should keep candy or some other sugar-rich food handy to elevate their blood sugar when the symptoms of hypoglycemia appear.

NIDDM most often occurs in people who are over 40 and overweight and accounts for 90 percent of all diabetes cases. It has been demonstrated that diabetes can be controlled with a program of regular vigorous, rhythmic endurance exercise. Since obesity appears to be the major environmental factor contributing to NIDDM, exercise would seem to be a logical modality. Besides helping to control weight, exercise also aids the entry of glucose into muscle cells (persons with this type of diabetes have high insulin levels, but insufficient amounts reach the muscles and other target organs). Exercise also helps to control cholesterol and triglycerides.

In one study of the energy metabolism in diabetic distance runners, it was concluded that the diabetic must have some active insulin available to facilitate glucose intake. It was suggested that the insulin-dependent diabetic administer part of the daily dose the evening before the run if intending to run in the early morning. Alternatively, 25 to 50 percent of the daily dose of insulin can be administered (in the abdomen or the arm) 2½ to 3 hours before the exercise.[11]

Here are some tips for the diabetic who exercises:[12]

1. Be aware of your state of control before beginning a running program.
2. Older diabetics should check with a physician regarding cardiac status before running.
3. Begin slowly and build gradually.
4. Diabetics with poor circulation and decreased sensation must take special precautions regarding their feet to avoid injuries that can lead to infection and more serious complications such as gangrene.

Allow ample room for edema or swelling if that is a problem. If there are points of abrasion, be sure they are cushioned. Check with a podiatrist if you have questions about proper foot care.

5. Wear or carry an indication that you are a diabetic.
6. Exercise with at least one other person.
7. Carry sugar or a sugar-containing liquid when you exercise.
8. Consult with your physician about adjusting your diet or insulin regimen to take your increased activity into account.
9. Be aware that you may have an increased need for liquids.
10. To increase the efficiency of your diabetic management program (diet, exercise, insulin), try to schedule your workout at the same time each day. Also try to engage in exercise of the same intensity and duration each day.
11. When engaged in extensive training, test your blood using one of the new portable devices and strips to get prompt assessment of your diabetic control.
12. Carry small change for candy, drinks, or phone calls.

Are you diabetic? The American Diabetic Association cites the following signs of diabetes:

Juvenile-onset diabetes	Adult-onset diabetes
Frequent urination	Excess weight
Excessive thirst	Drowsiness
Unusual hunger	Blurred vision
Weight loss	Tingling, numbness in hands and feet
Irritability	Skin infections
Weakness and fatigue	Slow healing of cuts (especially on the feet)
Nausea and vomiting	Itching

If you notice some of the warning signs of diabetes, check with your physician immediately. Detection of diabetes in its early stages will enable you to develop an appropriate diabetic management program.

Fitness for the Physically Handicapped

Physically handicapped people need to develop their fitness to an optimal level, just like able-bodied people. In fact, people with handicaps that are permanent, most notably those who have lost one or more limbs or are confined to wheelchairs, are especially in need of a program of physical fitness to prevent regression of basic body functions. A program aimed at developing minimal strength, muscular endurance, flexibility, and cardiorespiratory endurance should be designed for the physically handicapped to increase the fitness components and prevent the increased body weight (and all the health problems associated therewith) that usually accompanies inactivity.

Besides the regular physiological benefits that accrue from participation in physical activity, such participation will provide an outlet for the physically handicapped to socialize with other individuals, both handicapped and able-bodied. Often participation in physical activities will result in the disabled person's spending less time thinking about the handicap and more time enjoying the activities.

What Kinds of Activities Can the Physically Handicapped Participate In?

The physically handicapped who is physically fit can safely participate in a variety of sports and recreational activities. Depending on the type of handicap, some activities will require adaptation or special equipment. The staff at the Army Fitzsimons General Hospital in Denver say, "The sky's the limit—literally," when speaking of the activities that the physically handicapped can participate in. Patients at their hospital participate in virtually all sports, from horseback riding to skydiving.[13] In a study of the recreational activities of 134 lower-extremity amputees it was revealed that these disabled persons participated in a wide variety of activities (see Table 13.4).[14]

Another activity in which the disabled can participate is weight training. Weight training can be used as a therapeutic modality as well as a recreational activity. In fact, weight training is often prescribed for people who are recuperating from an injury to a limb to prevent atrophy or to build up a limb that has lost muscle mass and strength. In one study of the effects of therapeutic exercises on the peripheral circulation of normal and paraplegic individuals, for example, it was concluded that "when exercise of one upper extremity consisted of a heavy weight (40 pounds), the contralateral unexercised upper extremity showed a good

TABLE 13.4   **Avocational Activities for Amputees**

	Below-knee	Above-knee	Bilateral	Total
Fishing	46	11	5	62
Swimming	29	11	4	44
Dancing	28	8	5	41
Hunting	19	4	1	24
Bowling	15	5	0	20
Golf	15	5	0	20
Hiking	11	3	1	15
Baseball	9	3	2	14
Basketball	7	3	1	11
Running	6	2	1	9
Skiing	4	3	0	7
Football	4	2	1	7
Skating	4	1	1	6
Horseback riding	0	3	1	4
Gardening	3	0	1	4
Miscellaneous[a]	6	6	1	13

[a]Miscellaneous includes waterskiing, motorcycling, soccer, flying a sailplane, throwing a Frisbee, cutting wood, cheerleading, boating, playing table tennis, and using uneven parallel bars.

Source: B. Kegel, M. L. Carpenter, and E. M. Burgess, "Functional Capabilities of Lower Extremity Amputees," Archives of Physical Medicine and Rehabilitation 59 (1978): 115. Used by permission.

increase in blood flow immediately after the exercise."[15] Several studies were cited to demonstrate that progressive resistance exercises might be used to reduce atrophy of disuse and loss of power in immobilized extremities and maintain a better general physical condition in disabled individuals.

Proper supervision is important for the handicapped person who engages in a weight training program for therapeutic purposes. A physical therapist or some other member of the health care team should supervise the weight training program. Special care should be accorded the principles of progression and overload. The weight of resistance should be commensurate with the patient's ability and physical condition, and the degree of overload should be small and increased gradually.

Principles and Guidelines

The handicapped person should be guided by the basic principles and guidelines of program development that are discussed in Chapter 9. Besides the normal considerations, such as choosing the appropriate type of activity for a person with a particular disability, practical matters such as availability of the activity to the handicapped should be considered. An activity such as skiing, for example, is excellent for the development of cardiorespiratory endurance. However, special skiing equipment would be needed for the amputee. The cost factor must also be considered. Skiing might be too expensive for many people to participate in as a recreational activity.

One difficult problem for the physically handicapped person in developing and engaging in a fitness program is the accessibility of facilities. Although laws in the interest of the handicapped have resulted in improvements in this area, many obstacles to full participation in physical fitness programs remain. Many organizations and associations have been organized to foster increased participation by the handicapped in recreational and sports activities. A list of these organizations is presented at the end of this chapter. Although you might be able to plan your own program using the principles and guidelines in this book, as a handicapped individual you should become acquainted with the various organizations devoted to activities related to your specific disability. (If an organization dealing with your particular handicap does not appear in the table, consult the table source.)

Competition for the Handicapped

Handicapped individuals who have developed the necessary physical fitness and skill should not be discouraged from participating in competitive sports and games. There are increasingly more competitions for the handicapped person in a variety of sports. Paraplegics, for instance, can participate in competitions in sports such as basketball, badminton, bowling, croquet, darts, fencing, golf, pool, riflery, track and field, and road races, including marathons. Special wheelchairs are required for participants engaged in such competitions. The National Wheelchair Athletic Association is one organization that is dedicated to stimulating participation in competitive sporting events in wheelchairs by athletes with significant permanent neuromuscular and skeletal disabilities.

Exercise for the Epileptic

Epileptics should be encouraged and assisted to live as normal a life as possible. Participation in various physical activities is recommended under certain conditions, which will be identified shortly.

Epilepsy is a symptom of nervous system dysfunction within the brain and is characterized by brief, periodic episodes of motor, sensory, or psychological malfunction. The usual classifications of epilepsy, according to the type of seizure, are grand mal, petit mal, and psychomotor. Presently, the International Classification System is being used to describe seizures in relation to the area of the brain involved. In this system seizures are divided into two main groups: partial and generalized. Generalized seizures involve the entire brain, and partial seizures affect only part of the brain.[16]

Not only is exercise recommended for the epileptic as a means of increasing general fitness, but research findings suggest that exercise may temporarily ward off seizures.[17] Physical activities such as walking, bowling, golf, tennis, and table tennis are recommended for epileptics.

Swimming should be participated in only if an epileptic's seizures are medically controlled and if the following safety precautions are respected:

1. Swim only on the advice of your doctor.
2. Always swim with one or more persons who are aware of your epileptic condition.
3. Inform the proper authorities (teachers, camp directors or counselors, lifeguards, and so on) of your condition if you have the doctor's permission to swim.
4. Don't swim if you have not taken your medication at the scheduled time or if you have stopped taking the medication on a regular basis.

Is Participation in Competitive Sports Recommended?

This question has received mixed answers over the past few decades. For example, the American Medical Association's Committee on the Medical Aspects of Sports recommended in 1974 that an epileptic whose seizures are under control could safely participate in any sport, including contact football. This recommendation was revised in 1976 to exclude epileptics from participation in contact sports and noncontact sports such as crew, cross-country running, swimming, tennis, track, and volleyball. Amid much adverse reaction to the 1976 recommendations, the guidelines were again revised to include the sanction that epileptics should be able to participate in the sports that were recommended in the 1974 guidelines. In the revised guidelines it was recommended that epileptics whose seizures are not completely controlled by medication should not be permitted to participate in archery; the track and field activities of discus, javelin, and shot put; and riflery.[18]

Here are some cogent points that should be considered when trying to decide whether to recommend sports participation for people with epilepsy.

1. Epilepsy is not a homogeneous disease but a symptom, and therefore the underlying etiology must be considered in an evaluation of the individual's participation in contact sports as well as other activities.
2. Participation in sporting events may result in metabolic or psychological triggering mechanisms regardless of the factor of trauma.
3. Youngsters with posttraumatic epilepsy should not be subjected to repeated head trauma, which may lead to progressive neuron loss.
4. Younger epileptics have a significantly greater susceptibility to seizures than older persons.
5. The psychological trauma of nonparticipation by the child with idiopathic epilepsy must be balanced against the risk of triggering seizures in a public and embarrassing setting plus the hazard of further neurologic damage.[19]

Athletic and Sports Organizations for the Handicapped[20]

American Blind Bowling Association
300 Terry Dr.
Norfolk, VA 23518

Phone: (502) 896-8039
Gilbert A. Bagai, Secretary-Treasurer

Visually impaired

Open to legally blind men and women 18 years of age and older competing in organized tenpin bowling. Promotes bowling as a recreational activity for adult blind persons; sanctions member leagues; runs a yearly "mail-o-graphic"; sponsors annual championship blind bowling tournament.

American Blind Skiing Foundation
610 William Street
Mt. Prospect, IL 60056

Phone: (312) 253-4292
Sam Skobel, Executive Director

For volunteers who teach downhill and cross-country recreational and competitive skiing to the blind and visually handicapped. Holds races including giant slalom, downhill, and cross-country. Travels with blind skiers to skiing areas in Colorado, Wisconsin, and Michigan. Sponsors international races in Canada, World Cup for the Disabled in Switzerland, and Olympics for the Disabled in Austria.

Blind Outdoor Leisure Development
533 East Main Street
Aspen, CO 81611

Phone: (303) 925-8922
Muriel Frei, President

Operates on the "can-do" theory for blind people. Aids in the establishment of local clubs in order to enable the blind to experience the out-of-doors by skiing, skating, hiking, fishing, horseback riding, golfing, swimming, camping, and biking. Designs and conducts training courses for activity leaders; has designed distinctive jackets and bibs to identify participants as blind or as guides; provides insurance program for participants. Local clubs solicit reduced costs for or free use of sports equipment and facilities.

Blind Sports   Phone: (415) 681-1939
1939 16th Avenue   Ralph Rock, President
San Francisco, CA 94116

Represents service clubs, businesses, and corporations promoting sports leagues for the blind throughout the world. Equips and trains blind children and adults in sports. Conducts charitable programs. Publishes rule books for games for the blind.

Ski for Light   Phone: (612) 827-3232
1455 West Lake Street   Dr. Raymond Keith, President
Minneapolis, MN 55408

Dedicated to encouraging and assisting interested groups in conducting cross-country skiing programs and other health sports activities for visually and other physically disabled people. Brings together disabled and nondisabled people from the United States, Canada, Norway, and other countries. Sponsors physically demanding health sports events throughout the year in North America, including the Ski for Light International Program, Vinland Skiathons (fund-raisers), and Sports for Health programs during the summer.

U.S. Association for Blind Athletes   Phone: (609) 492-1017
55 West California Avenue   Arthur E. Copeland, President
Beach Haven, NJ 08008

Open to visually impaired athletes; fully sighted physical educators, coaches, special education teachers; and interested volunteers. Goal is "to develop individual independence through athletic competition without unnecessary restrictions." Promotes sports for the blind and visually impaired, organizes regional and national competitions, and works with other international organizations to promote goodwill and independence through friendly competition. Has sponsored national championships and conducted the first North American Games for the Blind between Canada and the United States. Sponsors coaches' training, seminars, panel discussions, and training groups.

Deaf

American Athletic Association for the Deaf   Phone: (816) 765-5520
10604 East 95th Street Terra   Lyle Mortenson, Secretary-Treasurer
Kansas City, MO 64134

Fosters athletic competition among the deaf and regulates uniform rules governing such competition; provides adequate competition for members who are primarily interested in interclub athletics; provides a social outlet for deaf members and their friends. Sanctions and promotes state, regional, and national basketball tournaments, softball tournaments, and participation in activities of the Comité International des Sports Silencieux and in World Games for the Deaf. Sponsors World Games for Deaf.

International Committee of Sports for the Deaf   Phone: (202) 651-5114
Longaavej 41   Knud Sondergaard,
DK-2650 Hvidorve, Denmark   Secretary-General/Treasurer

Membership composed of athletic organizations for the deaf in 43 countries. Provides an international sports competition for the deaf, patterned after the International Olympic Games. Seeks to promote and develop physical education in general and the practice of sports in particular among the deaf, encourages friendly relations between countries with programs in silent sports, and seeks to form silent sports programs in countries not yet participating. Holds

Summer World Games and Winter Games alternately at two-year intervals. All competitors must have suffered severe hearing loss.

National Deaf Bowling Association   Phone: (303) 771-9018
9244 East Mansfield Avenue   Don G. Warnick, Secretary-Treasurer
Denver, CO 80237

Open to individuals, clubs, and organizations of hearing-impaired bowlers. Conducts bowling tournaments including the World's Deaf Bowling Championship, National Deaf Team Doubles-Singles, and National Deaf Master Tournament.

United States Deaf Skiers Association   Phone: (415) 689-8379
5053 Kenmore Drive   Don Dickerson, President
Concord, CA 94521

Promotes skiing, both recreational and competitive, among the deaf and hearing-impaired in the United States. Provides deaf skiers with benefits, activities, and opportunities that will increase their enjoyment of the sport. Encourages ski racing among the deaf and sponsors national and regional races for deaf skiers.

American Wheelchair Bowling Association   Phone: (414) 781-6876
N54 W15858 Larkspur Lane   Daryl L. Pfister,   **Physically**
Menomonee Falls, WI 53051   Executive Secretary and Treasurer   **Disabled**

Open to male and female athletes with permanent disabilities who are confined to wheelchairs. Organizes and promotes wheelchair bowling and regulates rules. Provides information about wheelchair bowling through a book published by a wheelchair bowler in California (available for a fee upon request). Conducts state and national wheelchair bowling tournaments.

National Amputee Golf Association   Phone: (619) 479-4578
5711 Yearling Court   Bob Wilson, Executive Secretary
Bonita, CA 92002

Open to amputees who have lost a hand or a foot. Established to promote the mental and physical rehabilitation of amputees through the outdoor sport of golf. Sponsors prosthetic seminars and assists in the professional training of members.

National Association for Disabled Athletes   Phone: (201) 569-6627
80 Huguenot Avenue, Suite 11-B   Thomas Scaglione, Executive Director
Englewood, NJ 07631

Organized for individuals dedicated to promoting sports safety and assisting amateur and professional athletes who have become disabled as a result of athletic injuries. Designed to help the disabled athlete regain a sense of self-worth and ensure that all disabled athletes have a chance to contribute on a meaningful and productive level regardless of the severity of the physical handicap. Provides family counseling, educational and vocational guidance, and assistance in health care and education expenses.

National Foundation for Happy Horsemanship for the Handicapped
P.O. Box 462   Phone: (215) 644-7414
Malvern, PA 19355   Maudie Hunter-Warfel, Adviser

Organized by individuals to assist handicapped persons in their involvement with horses as a form of therapy and rehabilitation. Seeks to encourage and unify the teaching of riding or driving horses to the disabled through training of personnel and exchange among those who have experience in the field. Provides films and sponsors how-to clinics for volunteers; offers vocational rehabilitation programs to promote employment of the handicapped in horse industry jobs.

National Foundation of Wheelchair Tennis   Phone: (714) 851-1707
4000 Macarthur Boulevard, Suite 420E   Bradley Parks, Executive Director
Newport, CA 92660

Open to individuals with an orthopedic disability that prevents participation in regular tennis. Organizes, promotes, and encourages enthusiasm for wheelchair tennis throughout the world. Conducts symposia, camps, and consultation programs for schools, parks, and recreation administrators, tennis professionals, and physical or recreational therapists, including exhibitions, basic and advanced clinics, junior programs, and rehabilitative disability information. Holds National Wheelchair Tennis Championships annually.

National Handicapped Sports and Recreation Association
P.O. Box 33141, Farragut Station   Phone: (202) 783-1441
Washington, DC 20033   Rodney Hernley, President

Open to physically handicapped persons who are interested in participating in all kinds of sports. Provides handicapped persons with an opportunity to experience sports and participatory recreational activities. Conducts National Handicap Ski Championships, Adaptive Ski Technique clinics, and physical fitness and general recreation programs for disabled skiing instructors. Sponsors U.S. Handicap Ski Team.

National Wheelchair Athletic Association   Phone: (303) 632-0698
2107 Templeton Gap Road, Suite C   Craig Brown, Executive Director
Colorado Springs, CO 80907

Open to men and women athletes with significant permanent neuromuscular and skeletal disability (spinal cord disorder, poliomyelitis, amputation) who compete in various amateur sports events in wheelchairs. Members compete in regional events and in the annual National Wheelchair Games, which include competitions in track and field (including pentathalon), swimming, archery, table tennis, slalom, and weight lifting. Qualifying rounds are held in each region to select competitors for the national competition. Selection is made at the completion of the nationals to represent the U.S. team in annual international competition.

National Wheelchair Basketball Association   Phone: (606) 257-1623
110 Seaton Building   Stan Labanowich, Commissioner
University of Kentucky
Lexington, KY 40506

Organized for wheelchair basketball teams made up of individuals with severe permanent physical disabilities of the lower extremities. Seeks to provide opportunities on a national basis for the physically disabled to participate in the sport of wheelchair basketball, with its adjunct psychological, social, and emotional benefits, and to maintain a high level of competition through continuing refinement and standardization of playing rules and officiating.

National Wheelchair Softball Association   Phone: (605) 334-0000
P.O. Box 737   David Van Buskirk, Commissioner
Sioux Falls, SD 57101

One-Arm Dove Hunt Association   Phone: (817) 564-2101
P.O. Box 582   Jack Northrup, Cofounder
Olney, TX 76374

Open to hand or arm amputees and nonamputees who enjoy the sport of shotgun shooting. Seeks to help amputees accept their handicap and to provide fellowship and shooting competitions. Activities include dove hunt, One-Arm Tales, One-Arm Talent, and dove dinner.

Wheelchair Motorcycle Association   Phone: (617) 583-8614
101 Torrey Street   Dr. Eli Factor, President
Brockton, MA 02401

Open to handicapped persons confined to wheelchairs who are interested in rediscovering the outdoors and to institutional and individual supporters. Researches, develops, and tests off-road vehicles for quadraplegics and other severely handicapped persons.

American Diabetes Association   Phone: (703) 549-1500
National Service Center   Robert S. Bolan, Executive Vice President
P.O. Box 25757
1660 Duke Street
Alexandria, VA 22313

Health-disabled

National Association of Sports for the Cerebral Palsied
66 East 34th Street   Phone: (212) 481-6359
New York, NY 10016   Raphael Bieberg, Executive Officer

Special Olympics   Phone: (202) 628-3630
1350 New York Avenue, N.W., Suite 500   Eunice Kennedy Shriver, President
Washington, DC 20006

Created and sponsored by the Joseph P. Kennedy, Jr., Foundation to promote physical fitness, sports training, and athletic competition for retarded children and adults. Seeks to contribute to the physical, social, and psychological development of the mentally retarded. Local, area, and chapter games are conducted in all 50 states, the District of Columbia, Puerto Rico, American Samoa, Guam, the Virgin Islands, and more than 50 foreign countries. Participants range in age from 8 years to adult and compete in track and field, swimming, gymnastics, bowling, ice skating, basketball, and other sports. Information materials are available on organization of programs and participation of athletes.

Notes

1. The Committee on Exercise, American Heart Association, *Exercise Testing and Training of Individuals with Heart Disease or at High Risk for Its Development* (Dallas: 1975), p. 24.
2. Joseph A. Bellanti, *Immunology H* (Philadelphia: Saunders, 1978), p. 491.
3. Nancy P. Cummings and Robert C. Strunk, "Combination Drug Therapy in Children with Exercise-induced Bronchospasm," *Annals of Allergy* 53 (1984):395.
4. K. D. Fitch and A. R. Morton, "Specificity of Exercise in Exercise-induced Asthma," *British Medical Journal* 4 (1971):580; Simon Godfrey, "Exercise-induced Asthma," *Archives of Disease in Childhood* 58 (1983):1.
5. "Exercise and Asthma," *Physician and Sportsmedicine* 12 (1984):59–73.
6. Simon Godfrey, "Exercise-induced Asthma," *Archives of Disease in Childhood,* 58:1, 1983; R. P. Schnall and L. I. Landau, "Protective Effects

of Repeated Short Sprints in Exercise-induced Asthma," *Thorax,* 35:382, 1980.

7. Paul A. Di Sant'Agnese, "Cystic Fibrosis of the Pancreas," *Encyclopedia Americana,* vol. 8 (Danbury: Grolier, Inc., 1983), p. 388.

8. David M. Orenstein, Kathe G. Henke, and Frank J. Cerny, "Exercise and Cystic Fibrosis," *Physician and Sportsmedicine* 11 (1983):59–60.

9. Ibid., 61.

10. Ibid., 61–62.

11. David L. Costill, J. M. Miller, and W. J. Fink, "Energy Metabolism in Diabetic Distance Runners," *Physician and Sportsmedicine* 8 (1980): 71.

12. "Diabetes and Exercise," *Physician and Sportsmedicine* 7 (1979):49–61; Ann Kershnar and Bill Carlson, "Exercise: It Can Add a Sweet Spice to Life for Diabetics," *Runner's World* 18 (1980):40.

13. J. P. Smith, "In What Sports Can Patients with Amputations and Other Handicaps Successfully Participate?" *Physical Therapy* 50 (1970):121.

14. B. Kegel, M. L. Carpenter, and E. M. Burgess, "Functional Capabilities of Lower Extremity Amputees," *Archives of Physical Medicine and Rehabilitation* 59 (1978):115.

15. K. G. Wakim et al., "The Effects of Therapeutic Exercise on Peripheral Circulation of Normal and Paraplegic Individuals," *Archives of Physical Medicine and Rehabilitation* 30 (1949):86–95.

16. Harry Sands and Frances C. Minters, *The Epilepsy Fact Book* (New York: Scribner, 1979), pp. 7–8.

17. Ibid., p. 61.

18. Samuel Livingston, Lydia L. Pauli, and Irving Pruce, "Epilepsy and Sports," *Journal of the American Medical Association* 239 (1978):22.

19. Phillip Harris and Clifford Mawdsley, eds., *Epilepsy* (Edinburgh, London: Longman, 1974), p. 305.

20. Excerpted from *Encyclopedia of Associations: 1987,* edited by Katherine Gruber (Copyright © 1986 by Gale Research Company; reprinted by permission of the publisher; all rights reserved), 21st edition, Gale Research, 1986; also excerpted from *Encyclopedia of Associations: International Organizations 1987,* edited by Karin E. Koek (Copyright © 1987 by Gale Research Company; reprinted by permission of the publisher; all rights reserved), 21st edition, Gale Research, 1986.

CHAPTER 14

Special Considerations and Concerns

acclimatization	hypoxia
bursitis	sprain
frostbite	strain
hyperthermia	wind-chill factor
hypothermia	

Key Words

After reading this chapter, you should be able to:

1. Define and/or explain the key words listed above.
2. Summarize the latest research findings on the effects of exercise on menstruation.
3. Provide a rationale for exercising during pregnancy and list ten recommendations for women who wish to do so.
4. Discuss the findings of the U.S. Department of Health and Human Services study *Promoting Health/Preventing Disease* as it relates to the low level of fitness of America's youth and indicate what is needed to improve the situation.
5. Develop a program of exercises for the chairbound elderly.
6. List and discuss five recommendations and/or precautions for exercising in urban environments.
7. List and discuss the four processes by which the body loses heat.
8. List and discuss three health hazards associated with exercising in extremely hot climates and indicate the appropriate first aid treatment for each health hazard.
9. Discuss five precautions and/or recommendations for persons who run distance races during hot weather.
10. Discuss the symptoms of frostbite and hypothermia and indicate the first aid treatment for each.

Chapter Highlights

11. Discuss seven recommendations and/or guidelines for exercising during extremely cold weather.
12. Discuss the health hazards of exercising at high altitude and indicate the precautions that should be taken when doing so.
13. List and discuss the proper attire needed for exercising during extremely hot and extremely cold weather.
14. List and describe ten exercise-related injuries and cite the causes, treatment, and preventive measures for each.
15. Identify and discuss the phases or steps of the ICE treatment procedure for athletic injuries.

This final chapter deals with topics that need special consideration: the relationship between exercise and menstruation in women, exercise during pregnancy, physical fitness for children, exercising under extreme weather conditions, proper training attire, and care and prevention of exercise-related injuries.

Special Considerations for Women

The basic principles and procedures for developing and engaging in a fitness program are the same for males and females. However, women must pay special attention to the effects of exercise on menstruation and on pregnancy.

Exercise and Menstruation

Menstruation is a discharge of blood, tissue debris, and other secretions from the uterus at regular intervals in nonpregnant women of reproductive age. An average menstrual interval is 28 days, and the discharge phase usually lasts for five days.

Without discussing the delicate interactions of the hypothalamus, the pituitary, and the ovaries that are necessary for normal and uncomplicated ovulation and menstruation, it can be stated that many women do have normal 28-day cycles. However, some experience menstrual dysfunctions. These menstrual problems include delayed menstruation, absence of menstruation (amenorrhea), and painful menstruation (dysmenorrhea). What is the relationship of exercise to each of these menstrual problems?

There is some research evidence to associate strenuous exercise to the problem of amenorrhea. However, since several variables have been indentified in these menstrual aberrations, no cause-and-effect relationship has been established. For example, an absence of menstruation in athletes has been associated with low body weight and body fat as well as with strenuous exercises. It has also been demonstrated that loss of body weight and body fat may lead to amenorrhea even in the absence of exercise, and vice versa.

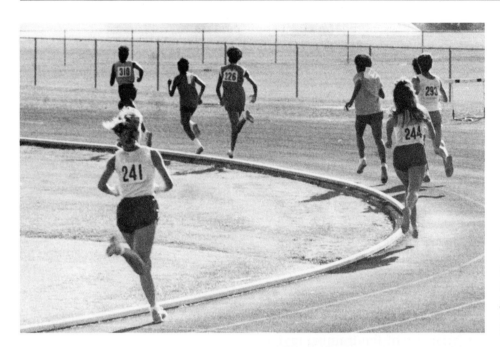

Girls and women can participate in an activity such as track and field without any harmful effects.

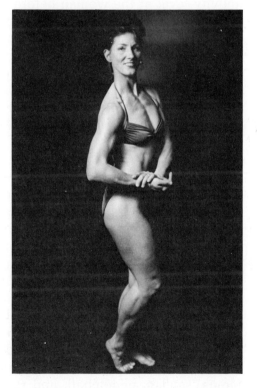

Some women prefer to train with weights to establish muscle definition, as this bodybuilder has.

The threshold level of body fat that will predispose women to amenorrhea varies. Amenorrheic runners tend to be thinner than runners who menstruate regularly. In a study of ballet dancers it was also concluded that dancers with amenorrhea and with irregular cycles were significantly leaner than dancers with regular cycles.[1] It was also reported that amenorrhea and late onset of menstruation in girls and women with average activity levels are associated with undernutrition and with a weight loss of 10 to 15 percent of normal weight for height.[2]

Although the reasons are not completely understood, exercise reduces dysmenorrhea (painful menstruation). Dr. Mona Shangold, Director of the Sports Gynecology Center at the Georgetown University Hospital in Washington, D.C., speculates that the relief of dysmenorrhea may be due to exercise-induced production of endorphins or vasodilating prostaglandins. Another hypothesis is that the self-discipline of the athletes during training may enable them to tolerate more pain, and the distraction of physical exercise may decrease the awareness of pain.[3]

In summary, a program of regular exercise will not of itself cause any problems associated with menstruation, and such a program might reduce painful menstruation in some women. Therefore, it is recommended that women engage in a regular program of physical fitness that is developed according to the principles of training presented in this text.

Exercise During Pregnancy

A review of the research indicates that women may safely participate in physical fitness programs during pregnancy. The type of exercise and the intensity of the training regimen should be based on the fitness and activity level of the woman before pregnancy. Women who are physically fit can engage in the normal physical activities that they are accustomed to throughout pregnancy. On the other hand, sedentary women should gradually increase their activity level by engaging in such nonstrenuous activities as bending, stretching, and walking; highly active women, such as those who are training for the Olympics, should reduce their training regimen to allow for the increased caloric cost of the pregnancy and to counter the potential adverse effect of exhaustion on uterine blood flow to the fetus.

The normal physiological response of the organism during pregnancy is to increase its cardiovascular and pulmonary activity, both at rest and during exercise. Consequently, it would seem logical that physically fit females entering pregnancy or labor would be better equipped to accommodate the added workload than the less-fit female. Therefore, the recommendation is that women should engage in a program of moderate exercise during pregnancy, providing they have been active during the prepregnancy period. The caution in recommending vigorous activity for all pregnant women is the paucity of evidence about fetal response to exercise. Of particular concern are the effects of increased body temperature and oxygen deprivation to the fetus.[4]

Specific activities to be engaged in by the pregnant woman should be those she is accustomed to. Swimming, jogging (at a moderate pace), tennis, squash, paddleball, and racquetball are generally safe activities. Regardless of the activity, core body temperature must be checked continually. One authority recommends that a pregnant woman should limit her temperature rise to 1.5°F. to 2°F until research shows what is safe.[5]

Here are some concrete guidelines for pregnant women who want to begin an exercise program.[6] All women are urged to see their physician for professional guidance before starting an exercise program.

1. The exercise prescription should be based on the person's medical and exercise history and complications encountered in the pregnancy.
2. A submaximal exercise stress test should be administered to provide information regarding the exercise prescription for trained women who wish to remain active during the later stages of pregnancy.
3. Women contemplating pregnancy should begin their conditioning program before conception.
4. A sedentary, healthy woman with an absence of pregnancy-related problems should be able to exercise 20 to 40 minutes on alternate days at an intensity less than 85 percent of her age-predicted maximum heart rate.
5. It might be more beneficial for some women who have been sedentary before conception to join an exercise class for pregnant women. (Check with the local YMCA or a reputable health and fitness establishment to determine if such programs are available.)
6. Proper support should be provided for the larger breasts of the pregnant woman to protect the heavier and more glandular breast tissue from becoming stretched and injured. It might be wise to check with manufacturers of the "athletic bras" that are now on the market.
7. Avoid exercising in extreme heat and at high altitudes.
8. Coordinate caloric intake and physical activity to permit a gradual weight gain of approximately 25 pounds during pregnancy.
9. Following an uncomplicated pregnancy in which no episiotomy* is needed, a woman can resume physical training without delay. When an episiotomy is needed, a woman can resume physical conditioning when her incision has healed. (The ability to exercise without pain is an indication that healing has occurred.)
10. After a cesarean section, a woman may safely resume physical training when she can participate without pain.
11. Swimming should be postponed until the cervix has closed (normally about three weeks after delivery), to avoid endometritis.†
12. Be aware of the reduction in joint flexibility and changes in ligament structure. Do not overstretch.
13. Listen to your body. When participation in physical activity causes undue pain, lower the level of intensity or discontinue the activity completely and engage in a less strenuous activity.

*An incision of the vulva to allow additional clearance for birth.
†Inflammation of the lining of the uterus.

Physical Activity for Children and Young People

The low level of physical fitness of the youth of America is lamentable in view of the increased interest and participation in fitness activities by adult Americans during the past two decades. According to a two-year study by the U.S. Department of Health and Human Services (HHS), approximately half of American children and adolescents are failing to develop healthy hearts and lungs (cardiorespiratory fitness).

This HHS study surveyed 8000 students in grades 5 through 12 (ages 10 to 17) across the country. There were five important findings:

1. American young people have become fatter since the 1960s, with median skinfold sums 2 to 3 millimeters thicker than in a 1960s sample studied by the Public Health Service (PHS).
2. Only about half the students were achieving the minimum appropriate physical activity to maintain effective functioning cardiorespiratory systems, as measured by exercise and fitness norms that were developed as part of the study.
3. In elementary school, only half the children take physical education class more than twice a week. Programs at the high school level tend to focus on group and team sports rather than on individual and lifetime skills for promoting good health.
4. Only 36.3 percent of students in grades 5 through 12 take physical education classes daily, compared with the 1990 goal of 90 percent.
5. More than 80 percent of the physical activity of students was performed outside school physical education classes.[7]

Physicial activities for children should be structured so that a majority participate rather than watch.

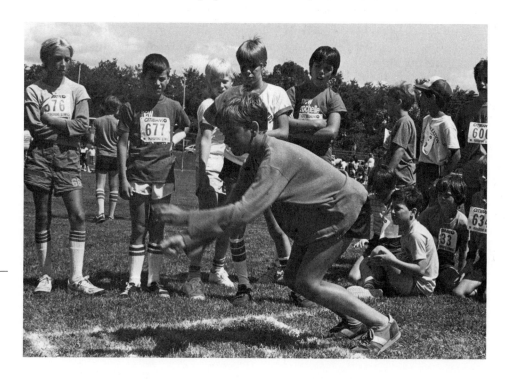

There are no simple solutions to this complex problem. However, apparently school programs of physical education must concentrate on teaching for and achieving the objective of physical fitness, particularly cardiorespiratory fitness. The secretary of the U.S. Department of Health and Human Services indicated that in addition to improved fitness programs in schools, community programs should be coordinated as an integral part of overall physical development of children and youth.

The United States Public Health Service has also expressed concern about the fitness of American youth. In a 1980 publication this group listed among its objectives that by 1990 more than 90 percent of children and adolescents ages 10 to 17 will participate regularly in appropriate physical activities, particularly cardiorespiratory fitness programs.[8]

Recognizing the gravity of the problem, the President's Council on Physical Fitness and Sports (PCPFS) established the area of youth fitness as its top priority for 1985 and 1986. The council conducted public hearings on the physical fitness needs of American youth and received hundreds of written statements from a wide variety of organizations and individuals representing all segments of government, educational institutions, recreation and sports groups, youth agencies, and parents.

A preliminary summary of the testimony gathered during the hearings was presented at the National Conference on Youth Fitness held in Washington, D.C., on June 8 and 9, 1984. Both the importance of physical fitness for children and youth and the low level of fitness in many school-aged populations were emphasized. Among other conclusions was the recognition that the major responsibility for physical fitness for children and youth rests with educational institutions, with youth-serving agencies in public and private sectors having supporting roles. It was acknowledged that there are some exemplary school physical education programs, but many physical educators experience low morale due to lack of administrative support and a host of other negative factors.

What Are the Solutions?

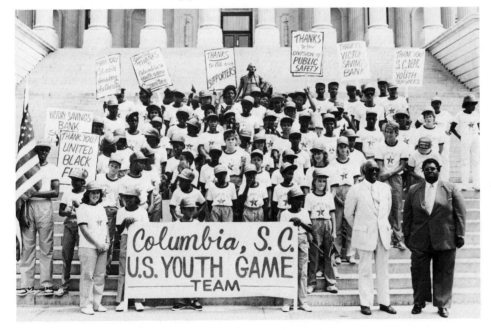

Columbia, South Carolina, is helping to foster fitness in its youth through the Youth Game Team.

Representative Mario Biaggi of New York indicated what must be done by schools to achieve the fitness objective for children and youth when he stated:

> Given the importance of physical fitness for America's youth, I feel that all schools should incorporate physical fitness education into their daily curriculum, and they should also stress participation in intramural and varsity sports programs. By working towards these goals and providing leadership at the state and local level, youth physical fitness programs can become an integral part of every school's curriculum.[9]

The testimony of Representative Biaggi and countless others prompted the council to issue many recommendations for policy and programs for the future. Specifically regarding school programs of physical education, the council made the following recommendations:

1. All schoolchildren in grades kindergarten through 12 should be required to participate in daily programs of physical education that emphasize the development of physical fitness and skills for growth and development and encourage a lifetime of vigor and health.
2. Every pupil should have an understanding of the basic principles of exercise science and how to apply them.
3. Every pupil should have posture checks, body composition assessments, and routine health screenings with appropriate follow up.[10]

Fundamental reform will be needed to achieve the President's Council's objective. This will include massive additional funding from state departments of education and local school boards to provide a daily program of physical education for grades K through 12 in schools where this is not the present practice. (It has already been noted that only 36.3 percent of students in grades 5 through 12 have

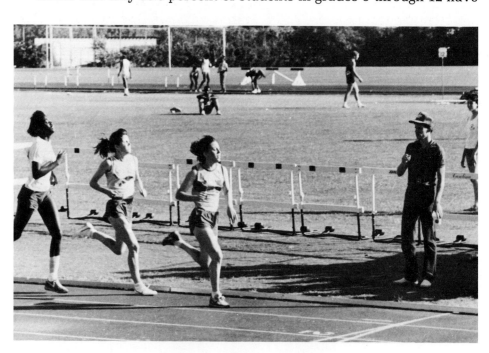

Track and field is excellent exercise for physical fitness, for girls as well as boys.

daily physical education classes, and only half of the children in elementary schools take physical education more than twice a week.) Teachers who are knowledgeable in the area of exercise science and committed to the teaching of fitness at the elementary and high school level will be needed. In many schools this will require hiring additional physical education teachers and/or retraining many of those presently on the staff. Positive attitudes toward fitness must be fostered in students to have them participate enthusiastically in the program. Finally, a positive and effective public relations program must be undertaken to convince the various publics of the importance of and necessity for fitness programs for children and youth.

I believe that the elementary school level is the place to begin refocusing physical activity programs to include greater emphasis on health-related fitness. Vern Seedfeldt offers the following four-step process for forging new directions for physical activity programs:

1. Communicate to parents and administrators what we currently know about the benefits inherent in well-conceived activity programs.
2. Ensure that children have ample opportunity to participate in the activity programs.
3. Employ strategies to encourage teachers and supervisors to concentrate on changing present levels of motor behavior and fitness.
4. Determine which procedures and activities produce the expected outcomes.[11]

One new national program developed to measure and improve the fitness of children and youth is the Fitnessgram, a computerized report card based on a student's performance on the Youth Fitness Test or the Health Related Physical Fitness Test of the American Alliance for Health, Physical Education, Recreation and Dance (AAHPERD). Besides reporting the test results, the Fitnessgram provides the following information: a student's rank against a national norm for each test; an overall fitness score and its rank against the norm; the student's height and weight; and where appropriate, recommended activities for improving fitness.

The Fitnessgram program was developed by the Institute for Aerobic Research in Dallas and is presented by the President's Council on Physical Fitness and Sports and the AAHPERD. Teachers interested in the Fitnessgram program should contact Ms. Marilu Meredith, Project Director of Fitnessgram, Institute for Aerobics Research, 12200 Preston Road, Dallas, TX 75230.

It will take the conscientious effort of all physical educators working as a collective force to create the atmosphere and provide the programs that will help to improve the fitness levels of the children and youth of America. It can be accomplished. By beginning exemplary fitness programs at the elementary school level, we will create a positive attitude toward fitness and provide students with the knowledge and understanding of fitness they need to practice healthful habits throughout a lifetime.

Special Considerations for the Elderly

Much of the information in this book applies to everyone. Do the elderly really need special considerations? The answer is yes—because many older adults who have not been active in the past few years might be unable to perform some of the activities presented in this text without adaptation to their present condition and health status. Of particular concern are senior citizens with arthritis and/or osteoporosis. Some of these elderly people are chairbound and need specially modified exercises to enable them to become more active.

Principles and Considerations of Fitness Programs for the Elderly

Information regarding principles, procedures, and guidelines applicable to the elderly has been presented in various parts of this book. The recommendations by the Council on Scientific Affairs of the American Medical Association regarding physical activity by the older adult are included here as a summary statement. This AMA council recommends that physicians and fitness leaders do the following:

1. Stress the importance of exercise for older patients, explaining in detail its physiological and psychological benefits.
2. Obtain a complete and reliable medical history and perform a physical examination, employing exercise testing for quantification of cardiovascular and physical fitness as appropriate, before the specific exercise prescription.
3. Maintain an active interest in patients' exercise practices through appropriate follow-up.
4. Encourage all patients to establish an exercise program as a lifetime commitment in preparation for their later years.[12]

Exercise for the Chairbound Elderly

The exercises presented in this section were developed by Lawrence J. Frankel and Betty B. Richard and are included with their permission.[13] The exercises may be modified according to each person's strength, and they should be performed at least three days a week (persons who are institutionalized should perform the exercise five days a week).

Some of the exercises included elsewhere in this text are adapted here for use with chairbound persons. The exercises are designed to improve muscle function and flexibility of the major joints of the body.

1.   Head Back and Forward (Figure 14.1)

Instructions: a. Start by sitting erect, back in the chair.
                       b. Slowly move the head back as far as possible.
                       c. Slowly bend the head forward, dropping chin to chest.

Repetitions: 5 times in each direction.

Count: 1 (head back) and (head forward), 2 (head back) and (head forward), and so on.

Neck Exercises

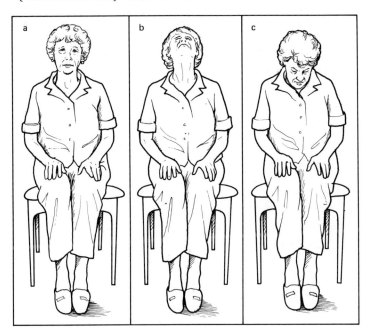

Figure 14.1
Head back and forward.

Source: Lawrence J. Frankel and Betty Byrd Richard, Be Alive as Long as You Live *(Charleston, W.V.: Lawrence Frankel Foundation), 1977. Used by permission of the authors.*

2.   Ear Toward Shoulder (Figure 14.2)

Instructions: Sitting back in the chair, alternately move right ear toward right shoulder, then left ear toward left shoulder, keeping shoulders perfectly still.

Repetitions: 5 times in each direction

Count: 1 (move to right) and (move to left), 2 (move to right) and (move to left), and so on.

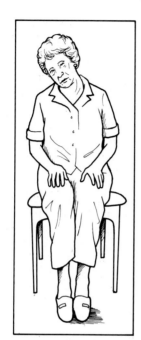

Figure 14.2
Ear toward shoulder.

Source: Lawrence J. Frankel and Betty Byrd Richard, Be Alive as Long as You Live (Charleston, W.V.: Lawrence Frankel Foundation), 1977. Used by permission of the authors.

3.   Head Turns (Figure 14.3)

Instructions: Sitting erect, turn head first to look over right shoulder, then to look over left shoulder.

Repetitions: 5 times in each direction

Count: 1 (turn right) and (turn left), and so on.

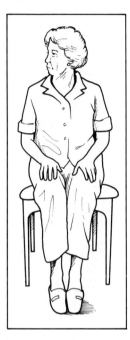

Figure 14.3
Head turns.

Source: Lawrence J. Frankel and Betty Byrd Richard, Be Alive as Long as You Live *(Charleston, W.V.: Lawrence Frankel Foundation), 1977. Used by permission of the authors.*

4.   Shoulder Shrugs (Figure 14.4)

Instructions: Sit back in the chair with hands on thighs. Shrug shoulders up toward ears and back down.

Repetitions: 5 times in each direction

Count: 1 (up) and (down), 2 (up) and (down), and so on.

Shoulder and Arm Exercises

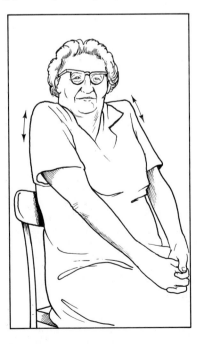

Figure 14.4
Shoulder shrugs.

Source: Lawrence J. Frankel and Betty Byrd Richard, Be Alive as Long as You Live *(Charleston, W.V.: Lawrence Frankel Foundation), 1977. Used by permission of the authors.*

5. Shoulder Rotations (Figure 14.5)

Instructions:	Sitting erect, shrug the shoulders and slowly rotate them forward, making 5 complete rotations. Then rotate shoulders backward, making 5 complete rotations.
Repetitions:	5 forward and backward
Count:	1 and (complete rotation), 2 and (complete rotation), and so on.

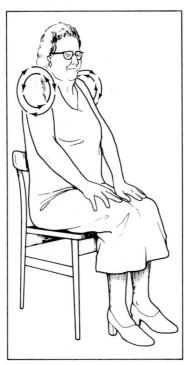

Figure 14.5
Shoulder rotations.

Source: Lawrence J. Frankel and Betty Byrd Richard, Be Alive as Long as You Live (Charleston, W.V.: Lawrence Frankel Foundation), 1977. Used by permission of the authors.

6. Arm Circles (Figure 14.6)

Instructions:	Sitting back in the chair, extend arms horizontally at shoulder level, palms down. Stretch arms outward without bending elbows, holding head up. Rotate arms slowly from the shoulders, making very small circles.
Repetitions:	10 complete circles forward, then 10 backward
Count:	1 and (complete rotation), 2 and (complete rotation), and so on.

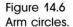

Figure 14.6
Arm circles.

Source: Lawrence J. Frankel and Betty Byrd Richard, Be Alive as Long as You Live (Charleston, W.V.: Lawrence Frankel Foundation), 1977. Used by permission of the authors.

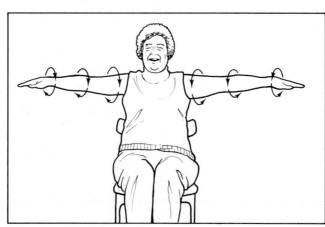

7. Hand Rotations (Figure 14.7)

Instructions: Grasp right wrist with left hand and slowly rotate the right hand, making large complete circles. Keep palm facing down. Exercise both hands.

Repetitions: 10 times clockwise, and 10 times counterclockwise with right and left hands

Count: 1 and (complete rotation), and so on.

Hand, Wrist, and Finger Exercises

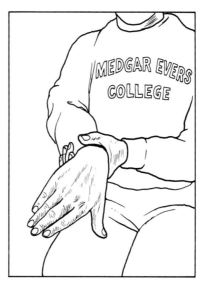

Figure 14.7
Hand rotations.

Source: Lawrence J. Frankel and Betty Byrd Richard, Be Alive as Long as You Live *(Charleston, W.V.: Lawrence Frankel Foundation), 1977. Used by permission of the authors.*

8. Finger Stretching (Figure 14.8)

Instructions: a. Hold right hand with palm facing down. Gently force fingers back toward forearm with left hand.

b. Place left hand on top of right hand and gently force fingers down

Repetitions: 5 times in each direction, then repeat with opposite hand

Count: 1 (pull fingers back) and (push fingers down), 2 (pull fingers back) and (push fingers down), and so on.

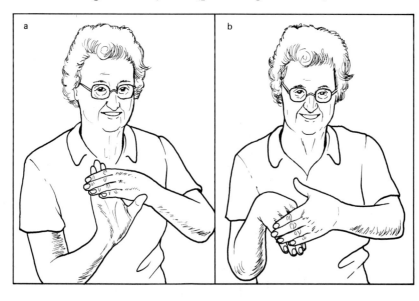

Figure 14.8
Finger stretching.

Source: Lawrence J. Frankel and Betty Byrd Richard, Be Alive as Long as You Live *(Charleston, W.V.: Lawrence Frankel Foundation), 1977. Used by permission of the authors.*

9. Finger Flexion and Extension (Figure 14.9)

Instructions: a. Extend arms forward at shoulder height and close fists tightly.

b. Extend fingers.

Repetitions: 10

Count: 1 (close fists) and (extend fingers), 2 (close fists) and (extend fingers), and so on.

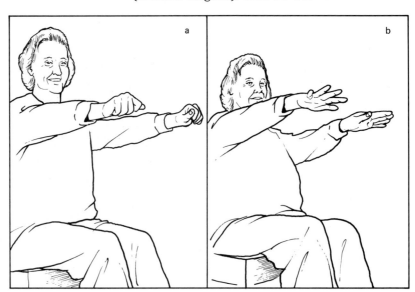

Figure 14.9
Finger flexion and extension.

Source: Lawrence J. Frankel and Betty Byrd Richard, Be Alive as Long as You Live *(Charleston, W.V.: Lawrence Frankel Foundation), 1977. Used by permission of the authors.*

10.   Finger Abduction and Adduction (Figure 14.10)

Instructions: a. Extend arms forward, palms facing down. Spread
                       fingers wide apart.
                       b. Bring fingers back together.

Repetitions: 5

Count: 1 (fingers apart) and (fingers together), 2 (fingers
                       apart) and (fingers together), and so on.

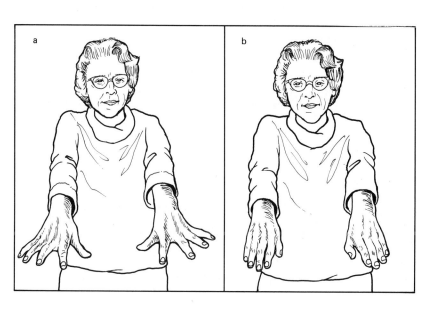

Figure 14.10
Finger abduction and
adduction.

*Source: Lawrence J.
Frankel and Betty Byrd
Richard, Be Alive as
Long as You Live
(Charleston, W.V.:
Lawrence Frankel
Foundation), 1977.
Used by permission of
the authors.*

11.   Thumb Rotations (Figure 14.11)

Instructions: Extend arms forward, palms down, with fingers
                       closed. Rotate both thumbs, making a complete cir-
                       cle forward, then backward.

Repetitions: 5 times in each direction

Count: 1 and (complete rotation), and so on.

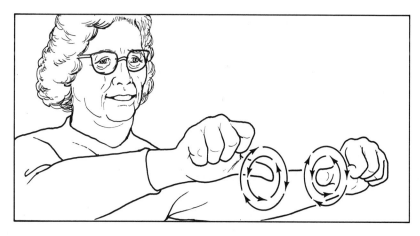

Figure 14.11
Thumb rotations.

*Source: Lawrence J.
Frankel and Betty Byrd
Richard, Be Alive as
Long as You Live
(Charleston, W.V.:
Lawrence Frankel
Foundation), 1977.
Used by permission of
the authors.*

Foot and Ankle Exercises

12.   Foot and Ankle Rotations (Figure 14.12)

Instructions:	Sitting back in the chair, cross right leg over left knee. Rotate right foot slowly, making large complete circles.
Repetitions:	10 to the right and 10 to the left.
Count:	1 and (complete rotation), 2 and (complete rotation), and so on.

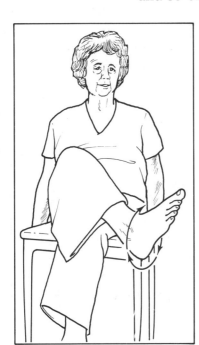

Figure 14.12
Foot and ankle
rotations.

Source: Lawrence J. Frankel and Betty Byrd Richard, Be Alive as Long as You Live (Charleston, W.V.: Lawrence Frankel Foundation), 1977. Used by permission of the authors.

13. Ankle Eversion and Inversion (Figure 14.13.)

Instructions: a. Sitting back in the chair, extend legs forward. Evert ankles so that soles of feet approximate each other. Hold for one or two seconds.

b. Invert ankles as far as possible. Hold for one or two seconds.

Repetitions: 5 times in each direction

Count: 1 (evert) and (invert), 2 (evert) and (invert), and so on.

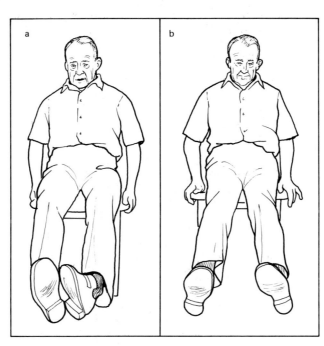

Figure 14.13
Ankle eversion and inversion.

Source: Lawrence J. Frankel and Betty Byrd Richard, Be Alive as Long as You Live *(Charleston, W.V.: Lawrence Frankel Foundation), 1977. Used by permission of the authors.*

14. Ankle Flexion and Extension (Figure 14.14)

Instructions: a. Sitting back in the chair with legs extended, flex ankles toward body.

b. Extend away from body.

Repetitions: 5 flexions and extensions in each direction

Count: 1 (flex) and (extend), 2 (flex) and (extend), and so on.

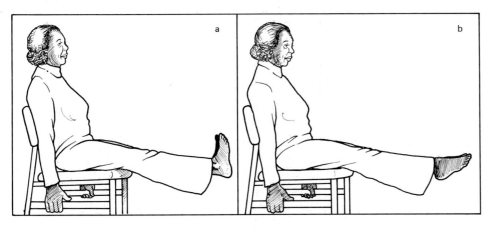

Figure 14.14
Ankle flexion and extension.

Source: Lawrence J. Frankel and Betty Byrd Richard, Be Alive as Long as You Live *(Charleston, W.V.: Lawrence Frankel Foundation), 1977. Used by permission of the authors.*

Combination Abdominal and Cardiorespiratory Exercises

15.   Bicycling (Figure 14.15)

Instructions:	Sitting near the front of the chair, raise both knees toward chest and make pedaling movements, as if riding a bicycle.
Repetitions:	10 times forward and 10 times backward
Count:	1 (Pedal forward with right leg), 2 (Pedal forward with left leg), and so on.

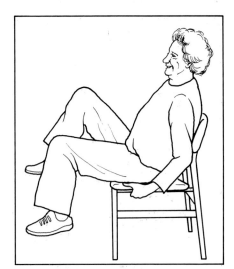

Figure 14.15
Bicycling.

Source: Lawrence J. Frankel and Betty Byrd Richard, Be Alive as Long as You Live *(Charleston, W.V.: Lawrence Frankel Foundation), 1977. Used by permission of the authors.*

16.   Scissors Kick (Figure 14.16)

Instructions:	Sitting near the front of the chair, extend both legs forward. Vigorously kick up and down, alternately, in a "scissors" motion.
Repetitions:	10
Count:	1 (Kick up with right leg), 2 (Kick up with left leg), and so on.

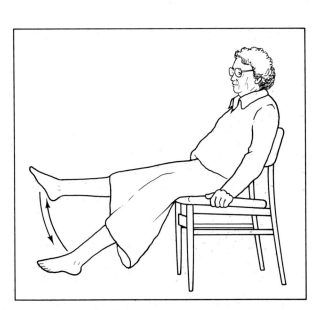

Figure 14.16
Scissors kick.

Source: Lawrence J. Frankel and Betty Byrd Richard, Be Alive as Long as You Live *(Charleston, W.V.: Lawrence Frankel Foundation), 1977. Used by permission of the authors.*

17.   Crossover (Figure 14.17)

Instructions: Sitting near the front of the chair, extend legs forward. Vigorously cross right leg over left, then left leg over right, in fast cadence (rhythmic movements).

Repetitions: 10

Count: 1 (Cross right leg over left), 2 (Cross left leg over right), and so on.

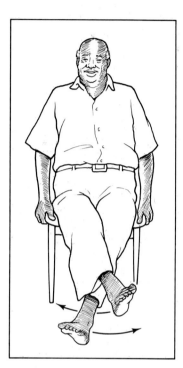

Figure 14.17
Crossover.

Source: Lawrence J. Frankel and Betty Byrd Richard, Be Alive as Long as You Live *(Charleston, W.V.: Lawrence Frankel Foundation), 1977. Used by permission of the authors.*

Some of you might have to begin by performing fewer repetitions of some of the exercises than indicated. As you gain in strength and flexibility, however, you should increase both the duration and intensity of the exercises. For example, you might wish to perform exercises 14, 16, and 17 with one-pound weights added. (Fill a bag with rice or sand to make the weights.) Once you can perform these exercises with ease, you might wish to try some of the other exercises in this book.

Recommendations

Make every effort to progress from sitting exercises to those that you can perform while standing. Do no let your age become a hindrance to joyful and exciting movement. Get up and about. Make physical activity a meaningful part of every day.

Exercising in Urban Environments

People who exercise in urban environments should be aware of the increased exposure to air pollutants and the effects that such exposure can have on them. The major environmental pollutants (also identified

Hazards of Air Pollutants

as primary pollutants) are carbon monoxide, sulfur dioxide, and particulates (solid and liquid substances from heating, power generation, incineration, industrial, and automotive sources). These pollutants, along with a secondary pollutant, ozone (also called an oxidant), should be of great concern to all, especially to those who exercise in environments where the concentration of these pollutants renders the air quality below standard.

Research studies have linked air pollutants to various disease states (bronchitis and bronchial asthma, for example), and these conditions have reduced the capacity of such individuals to engage in physical activity. The capacity of otherwise healthy individuals is also reduced in heavily polluted environments. Steven Horvath, of the Institute of Environmental Stress at the University of California at Santa Barbara, indicates that the most precise information on the human capacity to perform work as modified by ambient pollutents has been gathered from experimental studies conducted on carbon monoxide, oxidants, and particulates.[14] For example, regular exposure to sulfur dioxide can cause chronic bronchitis. Carbon monoxide, probably the greatest environmental pollutant in urban areas because of the many automobiles with internal combustion engines, decreases the oxygen-carrying capacity of blood. Inhaling high levels of carbon monoxide can cause headaches, nausea, convulsions, coma, and respiratory failure, sometimes resulting in death.

Although the respiratory apparatus is equipped to filter out many of the pollutants in the air, some do get into the lungs and eventually into the bloodstream. Exercising in environments of high pollutant concentrations significantly increases the effect of such pollutants due to increased lung ventilation. Therefore, precautions must be taken when exercising in polluted urban environments. Here are some suggestions for persons who exercise in highly polluted environments:

1. Exercise away from areas congested with automobiles and factories. Use parks, grassy areas, and exercise areas such as jogging trails in open spaces.
2. Exercise early in the morning or late in the evening rather than during the day (10:00 A.M. to 7:00 P.M.), when air pollution is greatest.
3. Exercise indoors if the air quality is rated low. (The air quality index may be secured by calling the local air quality control agency in your area.)
4. Reduce the intensity and duration of the physical activity if you must exercise in an environment of less than satisfactory air quality.
5. Do not exercise outdoors when a smog alert is in effect.
6. Avoid exercising in highly polluted areas if you have respiratory infections such as asthma, a cold, or bronchitis.
7. Be especially careful when exercising in hot climates where the air quality is poor. It was reported in one study that the combination of ambient heat (35° C) and 0.30 parts per million (of) ozone caused such pulmonary impairment and respiratory discomfort that three of the ten aerobically trained subjects had to stop exercise prematurely.[15]

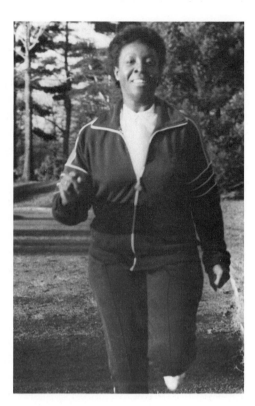

This woman is jogging on a cinder track surrounded by trees— much more desirable than a paved city street, where many joggers run.

Running on Hard Surfaces

Another problem encountered by individuals who exercise in urban environments is the increased risk of injuries to the joints caused by the added shock of the body when it comes in contact with the hard concrete surfaces. Tendonitis, shin splints, and blisters are common injuries that occur with increased frequency among people who exercise on concrete, asphalt, and other hard surfaces. The prevention and care of common sports injuries are discussed later in this chapter; it is sufficient to state here that proper footwear when exercising, especially when jogging, will help to reduce injuries to the feet and the joints of the legs. Also, run on soft surfaces such as grass, cinder tracks, and gravel. Finally, undertake a conditioning program, following the principles of training, before participating in competitive racing events.

Exercising Under Extreme Environmental Conditions

Exercising under extremely hot or cold weather conditions is of concern because of the deleterious effects such participation can cause if proper precautions are not taken.

Exercising in Hot Weather

The temperature of the body should be between 36° and 38° C (96.8° and 100.4° F) to maintain optimal functioning. The body is better equipped to maintain this temperature by a process called acclimatization. Specifically, the heat dissipation from the body is regulated to equal that of the heat generated in the body plus external heat. However, a malfunction in the homeostatic mechanisms regulating temperature control can occur, resulting in extreme body heat. Body temperatures exceeding 42° C (107.6° F) may cause heat stroke, a medical emergency that can lead to death.[16]

Heat must be dissipated from the body in hot climates in order for individuals to maintain normal body temperatures. The body loses heat through the basic processes of radiation, conduction, convection, and evaporation. *Radiation* is the transfer of heat as infrared heat rays from one object to another without physical contact. In order for the body to lose heat through radiation, the other objects, such as walls, ceilings, and floors, must have a temperature that is lower than the body's temperature. *Conduction* is the transfer of heat away from the skin by direct contact with cooler objects or substances, such as clothing, chairs, cool air, or water. *Convection* involves the forced transfer of heat induced by movement of air past the body. For instance, when cool air comes in contact with the body, it becomes warmed and is carried away by convection currents.

These mechanisms are incapable of cooling the body when the environmental heat or heat from the other object is higher than the skin temperature. Under extreme heat and humidity conditions, the only way to dissipate heat is by the *evaporation* of sweat, whereby water vaporizes from the skin, causing a great cooling effect. Evaporation of a liter of sweat from the skin surface can rid the body of about 600 kilocalories of accumulated heat.[17] However, as the humidity increases, the percentage of sweat that is evaporated from the skin decreases. It is prudent, therefore, not to engage in strenuous aerobic exercises of long durations in extremely hot and humid weather.

Besides the reduced evaporation of heat from the skin during hot and humid weather conditions, there is also a significant loss of tissue fluid because of the increased sweating. This substantial decrease in body fluid can lead to dehydration unless adequate fluids are taken in during prolonged physical activity in hot and humid weather. The fluid loss is accompanied by a diminishment of blood volume. Consequently, blood pressure falls, and the body labors harder to supply oxygen to the working muscles. This places greater stress on the heart and blood vessels as well as the respiratory organs.

Health Hazards Related to Physical Activity in Hot Climates

The basic health hazards associated with hyperthermia are muscle cramps, heat exhaustion, and heat stroke. (see details in Table 14.1). All persons who exercise in hot climates should become familiar with these hazards. Although each of the heat stress conditions requires first aid treatment, heat stroke is the most life-threatening and requires immediate attention. The most immediate problem is to cool the person suffering from heat stroke to lower the body temperature below 40° C (104° F). The prognosis is described as poor if diagnosis and treatment are delayed for as little as two hours.

Preventive Measures.   It may sound axiomatic, but the best cure for the health hazards associated with exercising in extremely hot and humid climates is prevention. Two of the first preventive measures are to establish an adequate training base and slowly to acclimatize yourself to hot weather. Acclimatization to hot weather (often called "acclimation") is usually complete within 10 to 14 days of exposure.[18]

To help reduce the possibility of heat stress during distance running, the American College of Sports Medicine has issued the following recommendations:

1. A medical director knowledgeable in exercise physiology and sports medicine should coordinate the preventive and therapeutic aspect of the running event and work closely with the race director.
2. Races should be organized to avoid the hottest summer months and the hottest part of the day. Organizers should be cautious of unseasonably hot days in early spring as entrants will almost certainly not be heat-acclimatized.
3. The environmental heat stress prediction for the day should be obtained from the meteorological service. It can be measured as wet bulb globe temperature (WBGT), which is a temperature/humidity/radiation index. If WBGT is above 28° C (82° F), consideration should be given to rescheduling or delaying the race until safer conditions prevail. If below 28° C, participants may be alerted to the degree of heat stress by using color-coded flags at the start of the race and at key points along the course.

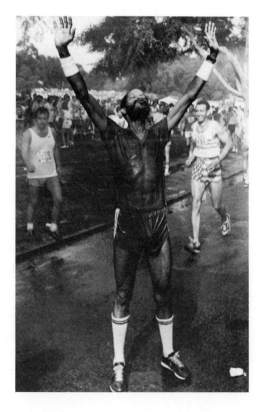

A cool sprinkler of water is a welcome part of a cool-down after a hard run road race.

TABLE 14.1   **Health Hazards Associated with Hyperthermia**

Health Hazard	Symptoms	First Aid
Muscle Cramps		
An involuntary contraction of the affected muscles due to an inadequate replacement of salt lost in sweat.	Constriction of muscle(s) Pain in muscle area Reduced flexibility	Discontinue the activity. Replace body fluids. Increase salt intake in meals; do not take salt tablets.
Heat Exhaustion		
A condition characterized by inability to continue muscular work. Occurs when excessive sweating and fluid loss lead to dehydration.	Headache Nausea Cool, sweaty skin Disorientation Dizziness	Discontinue activity. Go to a shady area. Take a cool shower or bath. Ingest fluids.
Heat Stroke		
A condition characterized by a profound increase in body temperature resulting from a breakdown of the heat regulatory mechanisms. A serious medical emergency that can lead to death.	High body temperature and fever (up to 41°C) Disorientation Dry, hot skin Rapid, faint pulse Shock Coma	Discontinue the activity at once. Reduce the body temperature immediately by immersing the patient in a bath of cold tap water and fanning with cool air. Request medical assistance.

4. All summer events should be scheduled for the early morning, ideally before 8:00 A.M., or in the evening after 6:00 P.M., to minimize exposure to solar radiation.

5. An adequate supply of water should be available before the race and every 2 to 3 kilometers during the race. Runners should be encouraged to consume 100 to 200 milliliters at each station.

6. Race officials should be educated to recognize the warning signs of an impending collapse. Each official should wear an identifiable arm band or badge and should warn runners to stop if they appear to be in difficulty.

7. Medical support staff and facilities should be available at the race site, staffed with personnel capable of instituting immediate and

appropriate resuscitation measures when necessary. Apart from the routine resuscitation equipment, ice packs and fans for cooling are required.

8. Persons trained in first aid, appropriately identified with an arm band, badge, and so forth, should be stationed along the course to warn runners to stop if runners exhibit signs of impending heat injury.

9. All runners should wear proper clothing.[19]

Are Women More Prone to Heat Stress than Men?   The answer to this question is yes and no. Based on the results of many studies at the Laboratory for Human Performance Research at the Pennsylvania State University and on reviews of more than 35 other studies on the topic, Larry Kenney states that women, as a population, are less tolerant to a given imposed heat stress; however, if they are matched for cardiovascular fitness level, body size, and acclimatization state, the differences tend to disappear. He further indicates that "women have a lower sweat rate than men of equal fitness, size, and acclimation, which is disadvantageous in hot-dry environments, but advantageous in hot-wet environments; and menstrual cycle effects are minimal." Kenny concluded that "aerobic capacity, surface-to-mass ratio, and state of acclimation are more important than sex in determining physiological responses to heat stress."[20]

Exercising in Cold Weather

Exercising in the outdoors during extremely cold weather conditions, including a high wind-chill factor* and precipitation, is permissible, provided certain precautions are taken. In fact, it is advantageous to exercise during slightly cold weather because it helps to maintain a constant core temperature. A constant core temperature can be maintained by exercise energy in air temperature as low as $-30°$ C $(-22°$ F) without the need for heavy, restrictive clothing.[21]

While you may engage in outdoor physical activities (such as jogging, skiing, ice skating, and snowmobiling), prolonged exposure to the cold and wind without proper protection can lead to hypothermia (abnormally low body temperature), a potentially fatal condition. Another possible health hazard resulting from exposure to the elements during cold weather is frostbite (freezing of a body part, usually the fingers, toes, ears, cheeks, or nose, sometimes destroying the underlying tissue of the affected body part).

Cold weather hazards, symptoms, and first aid procedures are presented in Table 14.2. Although knowledge of the information in the table is important, people who engage in physical activities in the outdoors during cold weather should try to prevent these health hazards.

---

*The temperature equivalent of the combined absolute temperature and wind velocity.

TABLE 14.2   **Health Hazards Associated with Exposure to Cold Weather**

HYPOTHERMIA

An abnormally low core body temperature due to prolonged exposure to cold weather. Other factors contributing to hypothermia include fatigue, hunger, improper or inadequate amount or type of clothing, thin build, inadequate protection from the elements.

Symptoms

Shivering, numbness
Poor coordination
Fatigue, apathy
Dilation of pupils
Very slow pulse and respiratory rates
Slurring of speech
Low body temperature
Reduced shivering and generalized rigidity of muscles
Blueness of skin
Disorientation, amnesia

First Aid

Administer artificial respiration if necessary.
Take the victim to a warm area.
Remove wet or frozen clothing and constricting clothing.
Rewarm victim by wrapping in warm blankets or by placing in a tub of warm water (not hot to hands or feet). Use your own body heat if other procedures are not possible.
Give hot liquids to a victim who is still conscious.
Dry victim thoroughly if water is used for rewarming. Get victim to a medical facility as soon as possible, especially if victim loses consciousness.

FROSTBITE

A condition in which a body part (usually fingers, toes, ears, cheeks, or nose) becomes frozen due to prolonged exposure to subfreezing temperatures, especially when combined with wind. In some cases the underlying tissue is damaged.

Symptoms

White or grayish yellow discoloration of the skin
Feeling of pain, which subsides as frostbite progresses
Blisters
Cold and numbness of body parts
Pale, glossy skin
Disorientation, mental instability, hallucinations
Unconsciousness, shock
Cessation of breathing
Death, which sometimes occurs, is usually due to heart failure.

First Aid

Protect the frozen area from cold and dampness by:
    Covering the frozen part
    Providing extra dry clothes and blankets
    Taking the victim indoors as soon as possible
Do not rub any affected part.

TABLE 14.2 (*Continued*)

Do not apply heat lamps or hot water bottles.

Do not break blisters.

Give the victim a warm drink (not alcohol).

Rewarm the frozen part quickly by placing it in warm water (not hot to the inner surface of the forearm). Water temperature should be between 39° and 41°C (102° and 105°F).

Have the victim exercise the rewarmed body part.

Do not let the victim bring the affected part near a hot stove.

If the feet are involved, do not allow the victim to walk even after the affected part thaws.

Place dry, sterile gauze between fingers and toes that have been frostbitten to keep them separated.

Do not apply other dressings unless the victim is to be transported for medical help.

If travel is necessary, cover the affected parts with sterile or clean clothes and keep the injured parts elevated.

Elevate the frostbitten parts and protect them from contact with bedclothes.

Get medical help as soon as possible.

Source: Adapted from the American National Red Cross, Standard First Aid and Personal Safety *(New York: Doubleday, 1973), pp. 160–165.*

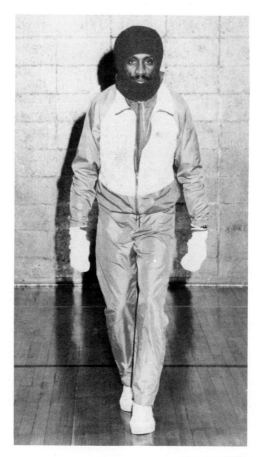

This person is properly dressed for physical activity during cold weather.

The following guidelines and recommendations can help to prevent hypothermia and frostbite when exercising outdoors during extremely cold weather:

1. Dress properly for the activity and weather conditions. Wear several light layers rather than one heavy article of clothing. Remove layers as needed.
2. Increase your intake of food.
3. Don't smoke or drink alcoholic beverages while engaging in outdoor activities during cold weather. Nicotine constricts the blood vessels in the hands and feet and can lower the temperature of these extremities by as much as 5° C (9° F). Alcohol dilates the vascular networks of the hands and feet; although it produces a warming sensation, it also increases radiated and convective heat, cooling the body further.[22]
4. Do not spend long, uninterrupted periods of time exercising in cold weather. Plan your activity program to include brief trips indoors to warm up and dry off. Also, drink some hot liquids while indoors.
5. Get yourself in good condition before engaging in strenuous outdoor activities during cold weather conditions.
6. Consider the wind-chill factor, remembering that it makes the absolute temperature (actual thermometer reading) feel even colder. For example, a wind speed of 20 miles per hour at an absolute temperature of 5° F will create a wind-chill equivalent temperature of −32° F, a temperature cold enough to cause considerable danger of freezing exposed flesh within a few minutes.
7. Work out with at least one other person. Another person is more apt to notice signs of hypothermia than the affected person.
8. If you are not accustomed to exercising in cold climates, give your body time to become acclimated to the elements. Increase the time spent warming up, and start at a lower intensity level than you would under normal environmental conditions.
9. Become acquainted with the signs and symptoms of hypothermia and frostbite, and take appropriate first aid measures if you notice any of them.

Exercising at Altitude

The problems of exercising at altitude depend on the distance above sea level: The higher the elevation, the lower the total barometric pressure and the partial pressure of oxygen. This lowered oxygen pressure results in a decrease in the oxygen content of arterial blood and thus diminishes the oxygen supply to the working muscles. Sometimes there is a lack of adequate oxygen (hypoxia), which places greater stress on the cardiovascular and respiratory systems when exercising at elevations well above sea level.

High elevations are categorized as moderate altitude (8,000–14,000 ft), high altitude (14,000–18,000 ft), and very high altitude (18,000–29,000 ft). The health hazards or medical problems associated with ascending to these altitudes range from acute mountain sickness (AMS) at altitudes above 9,000 or 10,000 feet to acute hypoxia and high-altitude deterioration at altitudes above 18,000 to 19,000 feet. The symptoms of acute mountain sickness are headache, nausea, vomiting, insomnia, and dyspnea. Insomnia, fatigue, weight loss, and general deterioration are symptoms of high-altitude deterioration. With acute hypoxia, mental impairment and collapse usually occur after rapid exposure above 18,000 feet. Altitude illness of any type is rare at elevations below 8,000 feet, and permanent residence is not possible above 17,000 feet. Prolonged stay above 18,000 feet results in progressive deterioration rather than further acclimatization.[23]

Certain precautions are advised for those who engage in physical activities at high altitudes. One important caveat is not to engage in strenuous exercise at altitudes above 18,000 feet. Other recommendations are to get in good physical conditions before going to high altitudes, make slow ascents to increased altitudes, and give yourself time to become acclimatized to higher altitudes.

The need for physical fitness (especially cardiorespiratory fitness) when engaging in physical activities at high altitudes is obvious. A strong heart and lungs will enable more oxygen to be transported to the working muscles, reducing the stress to these organs caused by the decreased availability of oxygen at high altitude.

Exercise prudence, and adapt to changes in altitude slowly. Mountain climbers and others who ascend to higher altitudes must be alert to the symptoms of altitude sickness to determine whether they are ascending too rapidly. Make changes in the speed of ascent accordingly.

Although the rate at which acclimatization occurs depends on the altitude level, at moderate altitudes one can expect major adjustments to take place in two or three weeks. In general, a minimal time of one week should be allowed for acclimatizing to every increase in altitude of about 3000 feet.[24] People who plan to remain at a high altitude for some time and participate in physical activities should reduce the distance and intensity of the exercise by about one-fourth of their sea-level performance.

Persons with cardiovascular and respiratory diseases, the obese, and those in poor physical condition should be especially careful when engaging in physical activity at high altitudes. You are advised to check with your physician to get medical clearance for such activity. If permission to exercise is granted and you do participate in a physical activity, pay attention to your body. If you feel uncomfortable or out of breath, reduce the intensity level of the activity or discontinue the activity entirely.

Dressing for Physical Activity

Proper attire for participation in physical activity includes certain basic items, such as a good pair of athletic shoes, socks, undergarments, and outerwear, and special clothing for certain activities (ski suit for skiing, for example) and weather conditions (such as a windproof, water-repellent outer garment during cold and rainy weather). Supportive and protective equipment such as athletic supporters (jocks) for males and brassieres (bras) for females are required. The clothing should be loose-fitting and comfortable to allow for complete freedom of movement.

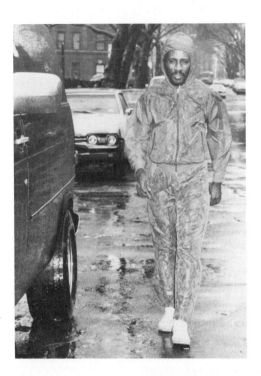

Proper attire for activity during rainy weather.

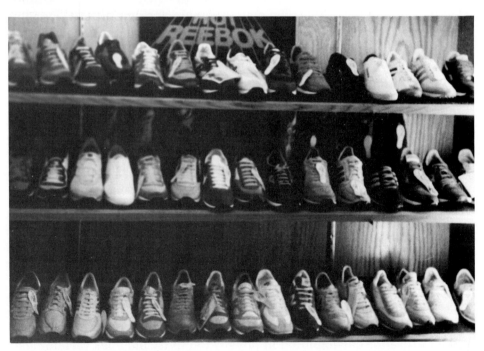

There is a wide variety of running shoes from which to choose.

Proper footwear is a must for anyone participating in physical activity. Although there are specialized shoes for different sports activities (tennis shoes, basketball sneakers, dance pumps, bowling shoes, ski boots), all footwear should possess three essential features: adequate gripping action (traction), shock absorption, and proper support. (Refer to Table 14.3 and Figure 14.18 as needed during this discussion.)

Athletic Shoes

In activities such as distance running, where great stress is placed on the feet and weight-bearing joints, proper shoes can help to protect against injuries to the feet and joints. A good running shoe is one that has the following features: a heel counter that is firm enough to stabilize the hindfoot and padded enough to prevent irritation or inflammation of the heel area (Achilles tendon); a heel that is flared and beveled to provide stability; a sole that is thick and sturdy enough under the heel (between the outsole and insole) to adequately absorb the shock of running; a high arch support; and a round toe with a toe box that is high enough to prevent crowding of the toes or blisters.

Additional features to note are outsole and last of shoes. Shoes with studded outsoles, called "waffle soles," provide added cushioning and better traction. As for shoe lasts, almost all shoes are designed with a slight inflare. However, experiments with runners for more than two years have led one group of researchers to conclude that the shoe last should be straight. They assert that the normal foot does not have an adducted (curved toward the midline of the body) forefoot, and thus there is no logical reason for an inflare last.[25]

Always try on shoes before you purchase them. Try both shoes because one foot is usually larger than the other. Check the fit of the shoes while standing, preferably near the end of the day, when the feet are their largest. Also consider the possibility of wearing two pairs of socks during the winter months. To allow for the extra pair of socks, some runners buy shoes that are one size larger than their normal shoe size. For those planning to run 20 to 30 miles a week, two pairs of shoes might be purchased—one pair for hot weather and the other for cold weather.

TABLE 14.3   Glossary of Shoe Terms

Heel counter: The back portion of the shoe that supports the heel to prevent rotation of the foot during the striking motion of the foot.

Insole: The inner portion of the sole of the shoe that absorbs the force of the foot strike under the heel.

Midsole: The portion of the sole of the shoe that cushions the midfoot and toes.

Outsole: The bottom part of the sole of the shoe that comes in contact with the surface being run on. "Waffle sole" outsoles, resembling the pattern of a waffle iron, provide very good cushion and traction.

Toe box: The front part of the shoe in which the toes are encased.

Shoe last: The shape of the length of the shoe, using the sole as the reference point.

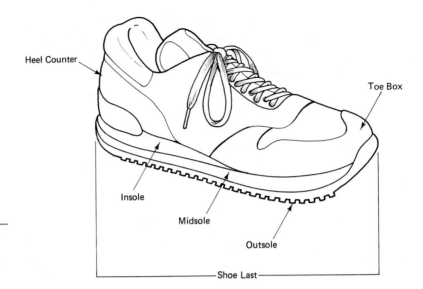

Figure 14.18
The parts of a running shoe.

Purchase training shoes rather than racing shoes. Racing shoes are for people involved in competitive racing.

Once purchased, break in running shoes gradually. Do not wear new shoes on long runs; wear them around the house and on short runs to get used to them. Keep your running shoes in good repair. The wear of the shoes should be on the outer back side of the heel, with an even distribution over the forefoot. An uneven wearing down of the outer edge of the heel portends foot problems. Replace the heel when it wears down a quarter inch or more. Check with a podiatrist or orthopedist if you have problems with your feet.

Dressing for Hot Weather

In hot, humid weather, anyone engaging in physical activity should wear loose-fitting and light-colored clothing. The basic outfit should include undergarments (brassieres and underpants for females, briefs for males*), shorts, a T-shirt, and proper footwear. Ankle-length socks might also be worn. An athletic supporter (jockstrap) should be worn by some males, and a special athletic bra may be necessary for females with large or pendulous breasts. A lightweight warm-up suit might be needed, especially for those who exercise in areas where the weather can turn cool before the end of the workout.

Shorts.   There are many types and brands of shorts from which to choose. A basic guideline when selecting a pair of shorts is to select those made from a material that is nonabrasive and nonirritating and that absorbs water quickly. Cottons and linens absorb water readily and thus meet this last criterion. Also, choose a light color because it reflects heat rays away from the body. A salesperson in a reputable sporting goods store will be able to recommend shorts made of specific material for hot weather.

Proper fit and quality construction are also important considerations

---

*Briefs are not necessary if shorts have an inner lining.

when purchasing shorts. Examine the shorts to make sure they are sewn smoothly and are bar-tacked (stitched more heavily) at the crotch and other stress points. A durable waistband is needed in shorts; tug at the waistband to see if the stitches hold firmly.

Shirts.   The T-shirt should be one that dissipates heat from the body and minimizes chafing. Cotton blends are excellent for summer athletic wear since they provide the absorbency needed and are inexpensive and durable. Nylon is not recommended for T-shirt material because it traps too much water, reducing the cooling process.

Dressing for Cold Weather

The primary objective when dressing for cold weather activity is to provide insulation from the cold elements by trapping in body heat and slowing the heat loss from the body. To achieve this objective, people who exercise outdoors in the cold weather should wear several layers of loose-fitting clothing that is not constricting around the ankles and wrists. Remove layers as necessary as the body warms up.

The layers of clothing should be arranged so that the layer next to the skin will pull the warm moisture away from the skin to the surface of the material, where it will evaporate. A synthetic material such as Gore-tex* is ideal as a first layer of clothing. The outer layer should be a material that is porous enough to trap the air. Wool fits the bill since it dries from the inside out and has a porous density that allows air to be trapped and warmed. A middle layer should be a light material that is lined with animal fur, feathers, or down. Depending on the activity level and weather, additional layers of clothing might be necessary. Check with the salesperson at a reputable sporting goods store for help in selecting winter clothing for physical activity.

The head, hands, and feet must also be protected from the elements during outdoor activity in cold weather. Since almost 50 percent of the body's heat can escape through the surface of the head, it is important to wear a good hat. A hat or cap made of synthetic material that keeps the head both dry and warm is recommended. A wool stocking cap may also be worn.

Mittens are recommended for the hands; wool socks can also be used effectively to keep the fingers warm. Gloves are not recommended because they keep the fingers isolated from each other, preventing the conservation of body heat that results from the fingers' being in contact with each other.

The feet should be well protected since they are among the first body parts to be affected by cold weather. Knee-length socks of a synthetic material should be worn next to the skin. Two pairs of socks are suggested if you spend long periods of time exercising outdoors. Individuals who have problems with poor circulation might consider wearing wool socks next to the skin and a second pair made of synthetic material on top of them.

*This material has many very small holes that prohibit water from passing through. So besides being porous enough to permit body sweat to pass through the material to prevent condensation and being rainproof, it is also windproof.

In extreme cold and windy conditions, a face mask and scarf (a cotton towel is good, since it doesn't chafe much) will provide much needed protection. Cross-country skiers should also protect their eyes by wearing goggles (ski goggles provide protection of the upper face and forehead). Thermal underwear* and turtleneck pullovers might also be needed. It is wise to experiment with different combinations of clothing for winter activity until you discover the proper mix to keep you warm and dry.

Injuries Resulting from Physical Activity

The reasons for participating in an organized physical fitness program were presented in Section One and reinforced in other parts of the text. Important values that can be derived from engaging in a fitness program have also been discussed (see Chapter 7). Unfortunately, individuals who participate in various forms of physical activity are also susceptible to injuries.

Preventing Injuries

Following the principles and procedures for program development presented in Chapter 9 should enable anyone to become physically fit with a minimum of injuries. Preventive measures include the following:

1. Get a medical examination and evaluate your present fitness status before engaging in a vigorous program of physical activity.
2. Begin your fitness program at an appropriate intensity level (based on the results of the medical examination and your present fitness level), and progress toward your optimal level of fitness (observe the principles of progression and overload).
3. Adhere to the principle of specificity (refer to Chapter 9).
4. Choose an exercise program consisting of activities that you enjoy.
5. Be sure to warm up before beginning the conditioning bout of your exercise program and to cool down at the end of the conditioning bout.
6. Be sensible about the duration and frequency of your fitness program (see Chapter 9). In other words, do not overtrain.
7. Become familiar with the human body and how it is affected by varying intensities, frequencies, and durations of physical activity. Review Chapter 3 as needed.

*Specially designed bodywear made of polypropylene fabric is now available. It does not absorb moisture, and thus it keeps the body dry when you sweat. A catalog can be ordered from Moss Brown, a firm that specializes in exercise clothing, by calling (800) 424-2772.

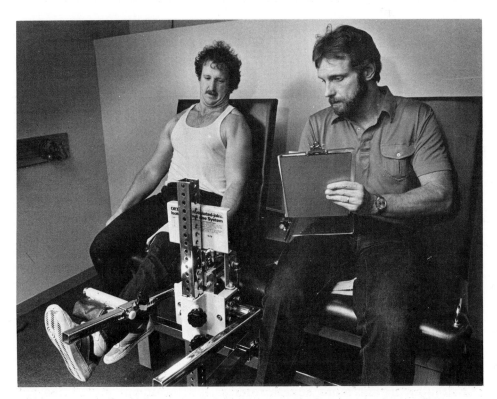

Stretching the various muscle groups through progressive resistance exercises is a preventive measure for injury. This person is working out on an isokinetic weight machine.

Exercise Injuries: Classification, Description, and Emergency Treatment

Space and time limitations dictate the need for a selective discussion of activity-related injuries. This discussion includes a classification of injuries in general; a description of and the emergency treatment for strains and sprains; the description, treatment, and preventive measures for five injuries commonly sustained by runners; and the description, treatment, and preventive measures for other selected injuries or problems that are related to exercise.

Of the many possible classification schemes, two broad classes—exposed and unexposed—are used to identify injuries. *Exposed* injuries are external, resulting in the exposure of the superficial and underlying tissue. An *unexposed* injury is one that does not break the skin and is therefore entirely internal. Injuries are also classified according to the predisposing condition and may be either acute (caused by overstress) or chronic (caused by overuse).

Classification of Injuries

Strains and Sprains.   Two of the most common unexposed injuries sustained by participants in various physical activities are strains and sprains. A *strain,* commonly called a muscle pull, is a stretch or tear of a muscle or tendon (fibrous tissue that connects muscles to bones). The injury might result from either overuse or overstress of some part of the muscle-tendon unit and is caused by an improper or abnormal muscular contraction. A strain is graded as first degree (mild), second degree (moderate), or third degree (severe), according to the severity of the injury (see Table 14.4). Strains most commonly occur to the hamstrings, gastrocnemius, quadriceps, spinalis of the back, deltoid, and rotator cuff muscles of the shoulder.

A *sprain* is a stretch or tear of a ligament (tough connective tissue that attaches bones together at the joints). Sprains, like strains, are also graded as first, second, and third degree, depending on the extent of the injury (see Table 14.4). The joints that are most vulnerable to sprains are the ankles, knees, and shoulders. Participation in a particular physical activity may increase the incidence of sprains in some other body joint. For example, sprains of the elbow occur in tennis players.

Treatment of Strains and Sprains.   The treatment of both strains and sprains, as well as other unexposed injuries in which there is tissue disruption, consists of five procedures: cold application, compression, elevation, immobilization, and rest. Ice applications, compression bandages, and elevation of the injured body part during the first 24 to 48 hours following the injury constitute the standard first aid procedure for mild (first-degree) strains and sprains. This procedure is sometimes called the ICE treatment. For more severe injuries, all treatment modalities are required. Surgery may be necessitated by some third-degree strains and sprains.

Although it has traditionally been the practice to alternate cold and heat treatments after the first 48 hours, the heat modality is not emphasized in the ICE procedure. Cold application is stressed, particularly during the early stages of treatment. One reason heat application is not emphasized by some physical therapists and athletic trainers is the knowledge that a reversion of vasoconstriction (reduction of blood vessel size) to vasodilatation occurs after 20 to 30 minutes of cold application. This "rebound" phenomenon lasts about 15 minutes. Vasodilatation, the enlargement of a blood vessel, results in an increase in the blood and lymph in the injured area. Therefore, cold applications serve the purposes of controlling the bleeding and minimizing swelling.

Despite the vasoconstriction-vasodilatation reversal phenomenon, heat might be warranted during the later stages of injury management. Direct heat, whether penetrating or superficial, causes an immediate dilatation of blood vessels. Thus heat facilitates the pickup and elimination of waste products and debris in the area and accelerates the normal healing process. Consequently, serious strains and sprains should be treated with alternating cold and heat applications. The heat should not be administered until the cold application has stopped the hemorrhage and has begun to heal the injured tissue. There is a wide variation in the time required for cold applications, ranging from 1 to 2 hours to 72 hours, depending on the extent of the injury. A first-degree strain, for instance, in which there is a slightly pulled muscle and little hemorrhage, may

TABLE 14.4   Characteristics of the Three Degrees of Strains and Sprains

First Degree	Second Degree	Third Degree
Strains		
Symptoms: Local pain, aggravated by movement or tension of muscle; minor disability	Local pain, aggravated by movement or tension of muscle; moderate disability	Severe pain; disability
Physical Signs: Mild spasm, swelling, ecchymosis; local tenderness; minor loss of function and strength	Moderate spasm, swelling, ecchymosis; local tenderness; impaired muscle function	Severe spasm, swelling, ecchymosis; hematoma; tenderness, loss of muscle function; defect usually palpable
Complications: Tendency to recurrence, aggravation; tendonitis; periostitis at attachment	Tendency to recurrence, aggravation	Prolonged disability
Pathology: No appreciable hemorrhage, being confined to low-grade inflammation and some disruption of muscle-tendon tissue	Stretching and tearing of fibers without complete disruption	Muscle or tendon ruptured, separating muscle from muscle, muscle from tendon, or avulsion of tendon from bone
Sprains		
Symptoms: Pain; mild disability	Pain; moderate disability	Pain; disability
Physical Signs: Mild point tenderness; no abnormal motion; little or no swelling; minimal functional loss	Point tenderness; moderate loss of function; slight to moderate abnormal motion; swelling; localized hemorrhage	Loss of function; marked abnormal motion; possible deformity; tenderness; swelling; hemorrhage
Complications: Tendency to recurrence, aggravation	Tendency to recurrence, aggravation; persistent instability; traumatic arthritis	Persistent instability; traumatic arthritis
Pathology: Minor tearing of ligament fibers	Partial tear of ligament	Complete tear of ligament

Source: Adapted from American Medical Association, Standard Nomenclature of Athletic Injuries *(Chicago: 1976), pp. 99–101. Reprinted by permission.*

require cold application for only one hour. On the other hand, a third-degree sprain with considerable hemorrhage would require cold application for 72 hours or more. The primary objective is to prevent recurrence of the hemorrhage.

The application of pressure to the injured area should be continued until the internal bleeding is under control. An elastic bandage should be used if the injured area is large; for a small area with a superficial hematoma, a sponge-rubber pressure pad will suffice.

The next stage of the treatment process involves elevation and immobilization of the injured body part. These treatment modalities are designed to help decrease hemorrhage and the escape of fluids at the injury site. Immobilization might be accomplished with tape, elastic tape, or a plaster cast, depending on the extent of the injury. Care should be taken when immobilizing an injured part so that there is no tissue disruption (further injury).

Resting the injured body part is the final phase of the immediate management of strains and sprains. Although rest is listed last, it is by no means unimportant. In fact, rest should be of vital concern throughout the initial treatment process. Along with immobilization, rest allows the body time to organize its natural healing processes and lessens the chances of further injury to tissues in the injured area.

Progressive resistance exercise of the injured body part should begin during follow-up treatment and rehabilitation. The objective is to prevent atrophy and weakness of the muscles surrounding the injured body part. The amount and intensity of the exercise therapy should be dictated by the degree of tenderness and pain indicated by palpating the injured part. Participation in controlled all-body exercises to maintain flexibility, muscular endurance, and cardiorespiratory endurance is also important during the convalescent period.

Injuries Commonly Incurred by Runners

Of all the physical activities in which Americans participate, the most injuries are sustained during running. Injuries sustained by runners are usually chronic injuries caused by overuse. Different runners who log an average of approximately 100 miles per week complain of the same injuries. For example, a survey of over 4000 runners by *Runner's World* magazine and a more controlled study of 180 runners by Stanley James and colleagues revealed that the majority of the runners sustained the following injuries: knee pain (mostly condromalacia of the knee), shin splints, tendonitis (primarily of the Achilles tendon and iliotibial tract*), plantar fasciitis, and stress fractures.[26]

What can be done to prevent these injuries, and what treatment measures are recommended if they occur? Obviously, since they are overuse injuries, rest is a general treatment modality. However, individual runners react differently to the stress of running; therefore, individualized treatment is warranted. Several treatment modalities might be

---

*The iliotibial tract is a wide, strong band of longitudinal fibers of the deep connective tissue (fascia) attached above the iliac crest and below to the lateral condyle of the tibia and capsule of the knee joint.

necessary. In the study by James and colleagues, seven treatment modalities were used (see Table 14.5). You will note in the table that 5 percent of the runners required surgery. Rest was the most widely used treatment modality (47 percent). Note that reduced mileage was the treatment used for 26 percent of the runners. This is understandable because it is known that dedicated runners are loath to abstain from training. If you are in this category, temper your desire to continue your running schedule with the knowledge that rest or a reduction in the intensity, frequency, and/or duration of the exercise can help to prevent recurrent chronic injuries.

TABLE 14.5 **Prevalence of Treatment Methods for Runners' Injuries**

1. Rest	47%[a]
2. Orthotics	46
3. Reduced mileage	26
4. Shoe change or modification	19
5. Steriod injection	17
6. Anti-inflammatory drugs	14
7. Surgery	5

[a]The percentages do not add to 100 because more than one treatment method was used for some individuals.

Source: Stanley L. James, Barry T. Bates, and Louis R. Ostering, "Injuries to Runners," American Journal of Sports Medicine 6 (1978): 45.

Table 14.6 identifies and describes the five most common injuries sustained by runners and their probable causes and suggests preventive and treatment measures. Some of these injuries, although related specifically to runners in this instance, are also sustained by individuals who participate in other types of physical activity. For example, shin splints and stress fractures are common injuries for persons who play basketball and tennis. Some injuries, like tendonitis, also occur in various joints, depending on where the stress is placed. Runners and basketball players suffer tendonitis of the Achilles tendon, for instance, whereas people who engage in swimming and baseball (which involve constant movement of the upper arms) develop tendonitis in the shoulder tendon and tennis and paddleball players, whose sports require snapping or rotation of the elbow, experience tendonitis of the elbow.

Rest is one recommended treatment for all injuries. Rest does not mean total inactivity. You should exercise areas of the body other than the injured part while you are recuperating from a specific injury. You can achieve this objective by switching to other activities. For instance, runners who develop stress fractures of the feet or legs might try swimming or riding a stationary bicycle for exercise. The idea is to reduce the stress placed on the injured body part. However, an attempt should be made to prevent atrophy and weakness in major muscle groups and to maintain cardiorespiratory fitness.

TABLE 14.6 Common Injuries to Runners: Description, Probable Causes, Prevention, and Treatment

Injury and Description	Probable Causes	Preventive Measures	Treatment
Chondromalacia patellae			
A degenerative process that results in a softening of the undersurface of the kneecap. The condition is characterized by swelling, pain when the knee is moved, a catching or locking of the knee, and stiffness when it is held in one position.	Overuse stress Irritation of the bones at the knee joint Faulty running mechanics Improper running shoes Anatomically unbalanced foot or knee joint	Use heel and arch supports. Engage in strength and flexibility exercises of hamstrings, quadriceps, and Achilles tendon. Reduce mileage. Wear proper running shoes. Use proper running mechanics.	Rest. Exercise the hamstrings, quadriceps, and Achilles tendon. See an orthopedist if the condition persists for more than a week.
Plantar fasciitis			
A strain or tear of the plantar fascia, a band of dense connective tissue that runs the length of the sole of the foot.	Overuse stress Faulty running mechanics Improper running shoe (inadequate padding at heel and stiff soles) Excessive pronation of feet	Reduce mileage. Wear properly constructed running shoes. Use correct running mechanics. Use heel cup.	Rest. Perform strength and flexibility exercises for the gastrocnemius and soleus muscles. See an orthopedist or podiatrist if the condition persists for more than a week.
Shin splints			
An inflammation of the front and back tendons of the large bone (tibia) of the lower leg. A shin splint is characterized by pain and irritation in the shin area.	Overuse stress Running on hard surfaces Falling arches Fatigue of foot and leg muscles Doing too much Improper running shoes Faulty postural alignment	Reduce mileage. Run on soft surfaces. Engage in exercises that stretch the calf muscles and strengthen the weaker shin muscles. Wear properly constructed running shoes. Use orthotic shoe inserts.	Rest. Use the ICE procedure. See an orthopedist if the condition persists for more than two weeks.

Injury and Description	Probable Causes	Preventive Measures	Treatment
Tendonitis (Achilles)			
Irritation and inflammation of the Achilles tendon (heel cord). Achilles tendonitis is characterized by pain, swelling, and restricted flexibility of the ankle joint.	Overuse stress Overstretching of the Achilles tendon Slight tear of Achilles tendon or muscle sheath Improper running mechanics Improper running shoes	Wear properly constructed running shoes. Engage in exercises that stretch the calf muscle and heel cord. Run on soft surfaces. Reduce mileage.	Rest. Use the ICE procedure. Perform stretching exercises for calf and heel cord. See an orthopedist or podiatrist if the condition persists for more than two weeks.
Stress fracture			
A small crack in a bone's surface (the foot and leg are the usual bones runners fracture). It is characterized by pain, swelling, and tenderness in the injured area. A callus (scar tissue) forms as the bone heals.	Abnormal foot conditions such as hallux valgus, flatfeet, Morton's foot, and Haglund's disease Overuse stress Improper running mechanics Improperly constructed running shoes Running on hard surfaces	Reduce mileage. Wear properly constructed running shoes. Run on soft surfaces.	Rest. See an orthopedist if pain persists for more than two weeks.

Sources: Isao Hiratha, Jr., The Doctor and the Athlete (Philadelphia: Lippincott, 1974); Stanley L. James, Barry T. Bates, and Louis R. Ostering, "Injury to Runners," American Journal of Sports Medicine 6 (1978): 40–45; Carl E. Klafs and Daniel D. Arnheim, Modern Principles of Athletic Training, 5th ed. (St. Louis: Mosby, 1981); Gabe Mirkin and Marshall Hoffman, The Sportsmedicine Book (Boston: Little, Brown, 1978); Don H. O'Donoghue, Treatment of Athletic Injuries, 3d ed. (Philadelphia: Saunders, 1976); George Sheehan, "Foot Faults: The Symptoms," Physician and Sportsmedicine 6 (April 1978): 41.

TABLE 14.7 Exercise-related Injuries

Injury and Description	Probable Causes	Preventive Measures	Treatment
Athlete's foot			
A fungus infection of the foot, characterized by extreme itching on the soles of the feet and between the toes. There also are usually small pimples or blisters that break and emit pus.	Growth of a fungus in the moist, dark environment of shoes in which the toes are close together Exercise and hot weather conditions	Wash the feet and dry thoroughly on a daily basis (be careful to dry between the toes). Use a talcum powder to help keep the feet dry. Wear clean socks. Keep the shoes dry by dusting them with powder on a daily basis.	Use a fungicide such as Desenex or Tinactin. If the condition persists for more than two weeks, see a dermatologist.
Blisters			
Localized collections of fluid in the outer part of the skin (usually on the toes, feet, heel, hands, and fingers), characterized by swelling and the formation of clear or yellowish fluid under the top layer of skin.	Friction of some object against a body part, causing the top skin layer (epidermis) to separate from the second layer (dermis). For example, tennis players get blisters in the hand and on the fingers because of the friction between the racquet and the skin.	Wear comfortable, snug-fitting shoes. Wear snug-fitting socks and keep them clean. Use petroleum jelly on the blister site to reduce friction. Wear gloves for golf and other sports where blisters are common on the hands.	Cleanse the blister site with alcohol and puncture the blister at its edge with a sterilized needle (heated over an open flame until it is red, then allowed to cool). Tape lightly with plain adhesive tape (no gauze). Consult a dermatologist if the blister becomes painful, emits pus, or develops red streaks that remain for a week.
Bursitis			
An inflammation of the bursa within a joint (commonly the knee, shoulder, and elbow are affected), characterized by point tenderness, pain, and reduced flexibility at the affected joint and fluid accumulation at the injured site.	Overuse stress An injury such as a blow to the joint.	Avoid overuse of the joint. Engage in stretching exercises before beginning activity in which vigorous movement of the joint is necessary.	Use the ICE treatment procedure. Perform stretching exercises once the soreness is gone. Consult an orthopedist if pain persists.

Injury and Description	Probable Causes	Preventive Measures	Treatment
Low back pain			
A chronic condition characterized by pain in the lower back area, abnormal curvature of the spine, and a sagging midsection. Sciatica (an inflammation of the sciatic nerve), and lumbosacral strain are two specific low-back-pain conditions. May require traction or, in severe cases, surgery.	Sprains of muscles and ligaments Postural abnormalities (mainly in the spinal column) Weak muscles in the lower back and abdominal area Slipped disk Arthritic condition	Engage in stretching exercises focusing on the abdominal area and the lower back (bent-knee sit-ups are good). Engage in aerobic exercises for weight control. Be careful to lift heavy objects properly.	Rest. Recondition the muscles of the spine, lower back, and abdominal area. Consult an orthopedist or chiropractor if pain persists.
Muscle cramp			
Tightness in a muscle resulting from sustained contractions of the muscle fibers in that muscle, characterized by pain and stiffness in the cramped area. The gastrocnemius, hamstrings, and quadriceps are the muscles that commonly cramp.	Salt deficiency Deficiency of minerals such as potassium and magnesium An injury or strain of the muscle Overuse fatigue of the muscle Disruption of blood supply to the muscle	Stretch thoroughly before engaging in physical activities. Increase intake of fruits and vegetables. Ingest adequate amounts of fluids. Ensure that mineral deficiency is corrected.	Rest. Stretch and squeeze the cramped muscle. Increase intake of minerals. Consult a physician if the cramp persists.

TABLE 14.7 (*Continued*)

Injury and Description	Probable Causes	Preventive Measures	Treatment
Muscle soreness			
A discomforting condition of the muscle or muscles that can be general or localized. General soreness appears immediately after exercise and lasts for three to four hours. Localized soreness usually does not appear until 8 to 24 hours after the exercise bout. If the discomfort is localized in a specific muscle group, the muscle may be injured (pulled, torn, or the like). Muscle soreness is common at the start of a conditioning program or after use of muscles that have not been used for some time.	Insufficient warm-up Overuse stress Poor flexibility Mineral deficiency Structural abnormality of the body	Warm up thoroughly before engaging in strenuous physical activity. Ingest adequate amounts of minerals. Avoid overtraining. Pay attention to the principle of progression (start with low levels of exercise dosage—intensity, duration, and frequency—and increase gradually).	Use the ICE procedure. Strengthen and stretch the muscles involved. Consult a physician if pain and discomfort persist in a localized area or muscle.

Sources: Carl E. Clafs and Daniel D. Arnheim, Modern Principles of Athletic Training, *5th ed. (St. Louis: Mosby, 1981); Gabe Mirkin and Marshall Hoffman,* The Sportsmedicine Book *(Boston: Little, Brown, 1978).*

354

A few of the other exercise-related injuries and problems are presented in Table 14.7. For discussion of injuries or problems that are not covered, refer to the sources of Tables 14.6 and 14.7. Also refer to other parts of this chapter for information on exercising under extreme environmental conditions and at high altitude for a discussion of injuries commonly associated with exercising under those conditions.

Other Exercise-related Injuries and Problems

Notes

1. Rose E. Frisch, Grace Wyshak, and Larry Vincent, "Delayed Menarche and Amenorrhea in Ballet Dancers," *New England Journal of Medicine* 303 (1980):18.
2. Ibid., 17.
3. Mona M. Shangold, "The Pain of Dysmenorrhea," *Journal of the American Medical Women's Association* 38 (1983):12–17.
4. Terry Jopke, "Pregnancy: A Time to Exercise Judgment," *Physician and Sportsmedicine* 11 (July 1983):139.
5. Ibid., 143.
6. Ibid., 143–144; Mona M. Shangold, "Pregnancy," in Christine E. Haycock, ed., *Sports Medicine for the Athletic Female* (Oradell, N.J.: Medical Economics Co., 1980), pp. 332–338.
7. "Study Shows Students Fatter, Less Fit," *Journal of Physical Education, Recreation and Dance* 55 (1984):12.
8. U.S. Department of Health and Human Services, *Promoting Health/Preventing Disease: Objectives for the Nation* (Washington, D.C.: U.S. Government Printing Office, 1980).
9. Ash Hayes, "Youth Physical Fitness Hearings," *Journal of Physical Education, Recreation and Dance* 55 (1984):30–31.
10. Ibid., 32, 40.
11. Vern Seedfeldt, "Physical Fitness in Preschool and Elementary School-aged Children," *Journal of Physical Education, Recreation and Dance* 55 (1984):36–37.
12. Council on Scientific Affairs, American Medical Association, "Exercise Programs for the Elderly," *Journal of the American Medical Association* 25 (1984):546.
13. Lawrence J. Frankel and Betty B. Richard, *Be Alive As Long As You Live* (Charleston, W.Va.: Preventicare Publications, 1977).
14. Steven M. Horvath, "Impact of Air Quality on Exercise Performance," in Doris I. Miller, ed., *Exercise and Sport Sciences Reviews* 9 (1981):267.
15. Suzanne I. Gibbons and William C. Adams, "Combined Effects of Ozone Exposure and Ambient Heat on Exercising Females," *Journal of Applied Physiology* 57 (1984):450–456.
16. G. Keren, Y. Shonfeld, and E. Sohar, "Prevention of Damage by Sport Activity in Hot Climates," *Journal of Sports Medicine* 20 (1980):452.
17. Ibid.
18. Abdel Halim, "Fluid and Electrolyte Balance and Physical Training in Hot Climates," *Journal of Sports Medicine* 20 (1980):350.
19. American College of Sports Medicine, "Prevention of Thermal Injuries During Distance Running," *Medicine and Science in Sports* 16 (October 1984):ix–xiv.
20. W. Larry Kenney, "A Review of Comparative Responses of Men and Women to Heat Stress," in *Environmental Research* (New York: Academic Press, 1985), p. 1.

21. Alan D. Claremont, "Taking Winter in Stride Requires Proper Attire," *Physician and Sportsmedicine* 4 (December 1976):65–68.

22. Charles S. Houston, "Oxygen Lack at High Altitude: A Mountaineer's Problem," in John R. Sutton et al., *Hypoxia: Man at Altitude* (New York: Thieme-Stratton, Inc., 1982), pp. 156–157.

23. Herbert N. Hultgren, "High Altitude Medical Problems," in John R. Sutton, et al., p. 161.

24. Bruno Balke, "Work Capacity at Altitude," in Warren R. Johnson, ed., *Science and Medicine of Exercise and Sports* (New York: Harper & Row, 1960), p. 339.

25. Stanley L. James, Barry T. Bates, and Louis R. Ostering, "Injuries to Runners," *American Journal of Sports Medicine* 6 (1978):40–46.

26. J. Henderson, "First Aid for the Injured," *Runner's World,* July 1977, p. 37; James et al., 45.

APPENDIXES

Appendix

Appendix A
Units of Measurement

The Metric System   Increasingly, the metric system is being used as the worldwide standard system of measurement. In fact, the metric system is now used by all major countries except the United States. Scientific notations in the fields of science (including nutrition and dietetics) and mathematics are almost universally expressed in metric units. In the metric system the multiples and submultiples of any given unit are always related by powers of 10. For example, there are 10 millimeters in one centimeter, 100 centimeters in one meter, and 1000 meters in one kilometer. Also, one meter is 10 decimeters or 100 centimeters or 1000 millimeters. This system allows easy conversions from one unit to another.

Metric Prefixes

Prefix	Means	Prefix	Means
kilo- (10^3)	one thousand times	deci- (10^{-1})	one-tenth of
hecto- (10^2)	one hundred times	centi- (10^{-2})	one-hundredth of
deka- (10^1)	ten times	milli- (10^{-3})	one-thousandth of

TABLE A-1   Household Measures of Volume and Weight

	Volume	
Household Measure	Fluid Ounces (fl oz)	Metric Equivalent[a] (ml)
1 quart (qt)	32	946
1 pint (pt)	16	473
1 cup (c)	8	237
2 tablespoons (tbsp)	1	30
1 tablespoon (tbsp)	1/2	15
1 teaspoon (tsp)	1/6	5

Weight	
	Metric Equivalent (g)
1 pound (lb) = 16 ounces =	453.6
1 ounce	28.35
3½ ounces	100.00

[a]In some cases the equivalent is an approximation rather than the exact figure.

TABLE A-2 Units of Length, Mass, and Volume

Metric Unit	Metric Equivalent	English Equivalent
Length		
1 kilometer (km)	1000 m	3280 ft = 0.62 mi
1 meter (m)	100 cm	39.37 in. = 3.28 ft
	1000 mm	= 1.09 yd
1 centimeter (cm)	0.01 m	0.394 in.
1 millimeter (mm)	0.001 m	0.0394 in.
	0.1 cm	

To convert inches to centimeters, multiply inches by 2.5.
To convert centimeters to inches, multiply centimeters by 0.4 or divide centimeters by 2.5.
To convert miles to kilometers, multiply miles by 1.6.
To convert kilometers to miles, multiply kilometers by 0.6.

Metric Unit	Metric Equivalent	English Equivalent
Mass		
1 kilogram (kg)	1000 g	2.205 lb = 35.3 oz
1 gram (g)	0.001 kg	0.04 oz
	1000 mg	
1 milligram (mg)	0.001 g	0.00004 oz.
	0.000001 kg	

To convert pounds to kilograms, divide pounds by 2.2 or multiply pounds by 0.45.
To convert kilograms to pounds, multiply kilograms by 2.2.

Metric Unit	Metric Equivalent	English Equivalent
Volume		
1 liter (l)	1000 ml	33.81 fl oz = 1.057 qt
		946 ml = 1 qt
1 milliliter (ml)	0.001 liter	0.0338 fl oz
		30 ml = 1 fl oz
1 cubic centimeter (cm^3)	0.999972 ml[a]	0.0338 fl oz

To convert ounces to milliliters, multiply ounces by 30.
To convert milliliters to ounces, multiply milliliters by 0.034.
To convert quarts to liters, multiply liters by 0.95.
To convert liters to quarts, multiply quarts by 1.06.

[a]For computational purposes, this number can be rounded off to one (1) so that 1 cm^3 = 1 ml.

TABLE A-3   **Temperature and Energy Conversions**

Temperature

To convert a Fahrenheit (F) temperature to Celsius (C), subtract 32 from °F and then multiply by 5/9.

To convert Celsius to Fahrenheit, multiply °C by 9/5 and then add 32.

Energy

KILOCALORIES (KCAL) (CALORIES)

1 kcal = 1000 calories = 4.2 kilojoules (kj)
1 kcal = 3086 ft-lb of work
1 kcal = 426.8 kg

METABOLIC ENERGY[a]

1 MET = 3.5 millimeters of oxygen per kilogram of body weight per minute during basal metabolism (at rest)
1 MET = 1 kilocalorie per kilogram of body weight per hour
1 liter of oxygen consumed equals 5 Calories of energy expenditure

[a]These are approximate equivalent figures.

Appendix B
Recommended Daily Dietary Allowances

These Recommended Daily Dietary Allowances (RDA) are designed for the maintenance of good nutrition of practically all healthy persons in the United States. The Recommended Daily Dietary Allowances (RDA) should not be confused with the U.S. Recommended Daily Dietary Allowances (U.S. RDA). The RDA are amounts of nutrients recommended by the Food and Nutrition Board of the National Research Council and are considered adequate for maintenance of good nutrition in healthy persons in the United States. The allowances are revised from time to time in accordance with newer knowledge of nutritional needs.

The U.S. RDA are the amounts of proteins, vitamins, and minerals established by the Food and Drug Administration as standards for nutrition labeling. These allowances were derived from the RDA set by the Food and Nutrition Board. The U.S. RDA for most nutrients approximates the highest RDA of the sex-age categories in this table, excluding the allowances for pregnant and lactating females. Therefore, a diet that furnishes the U.S. RDA for a nutrient will furnish the RDA for most people and more than the RDA for many. U.S. RDA are protein, 45 grams (eggs, fish, meat, milk, poultry), 65 grams (other foods); vitamin A, 5000 International Units; thiamin, 1.5 milligrams; riboflavin, 1.7 milligrams; niacin, 20 milligrams; ascorbic acid, 60 milligrams; calcium, 1 gram; phosphorus, 1 gram; iron, 18 milligrams. For additional information on U.S. RDA, see the *Federal Register*, vol. 38, no. 49 (March 14, 1973), pp. 6959–6960, and Agriculture Information Bulletin 382, *Nutritional Labeling: Tools for Its Use.*

Sex-age category	Age (years)	Weight (kg)	Weight (lb)	Height (cm)	Height (in.)	Food energy (Cal.)	Protein (g)	Minerals Calcium (mg)	Phosphorus (mg)	Iron (mg)	Vitamin A (I.U.)	Thiamin (mg)	Riboflavin (mg)	Niacin (mg)	Ascorbic acid (mg)
Infants	0–0.5	6	13	60	24	kg × 115 / lb × 52.3	kg × 2.2 / lb × 1.0	360	240	10	1400	0.3	0.4	6	35
	0.5–1	9	20	71	28	kg × 105 / lb × 47.7	kg × 2.0 / lb × 0.9	540	360	15	2000	.5	.6	8	35
Children	1–3	13	29	90	35	1300	23	800	800	15	2000	.7	.8	9	45
	4–6	20	44	112	44	1700	30	800	800	10	2500	.9	1.0	11	45
	7–10	28	62	132	52	2400	34	800	800	10	3300	1.2	1.4	16	45
Males	11–14	45	99	157	62	2700	45	1200	1200	18	5000	1.4	1.6	18	50
	15–18	66	145	176	69	2800	56	1200	1200	18	5000	1.4	1.7	18	60
	19–22	70	154	177	70	2900	56	800	800	10	5000	1.5	1.7	19	60
	23–50	70	154	178	70	2700	56	800	800	10	5000	1.4	1.6	18	60
	51+	70	154	178	70	2400[a]	56	800	800	10	5000	1.2	1.4	16	60
Females	11–14	46	101	157	62	2200	46	1200	1200	18	4000	1.1	1.3	15	50
	15–18	55	120	163	64	2100	46	1200	1200	18	4000	1.1	1.3	14	60
	19–22	55	120	163	64	2100	44	800	800	18	4000	1.1	1.3	14	60
	23–50	55	120	163	64	2000	44	800	800	18	4000	1.0	1.2	13	60
	51+	55	120	163	64	1800[a]	44	800	800	10	4000	1.0	1.2	13	60
Pregnant						+300	+30	+400	+400	18+[b]	+1000	+.4	+.3	+2	+20
Lactating						+500	+20	+400	+400	18	+2000	+.5	+.5	+5	+40

[a]After age 75 years, energy requirement is 2050 calories for males and 1600 calories for females.

[b]The increased requirement cannot be met by ordinary diets; therefore, the use of supplemental iron is recommended.

Source: Adapted from National Academy of Sciences, National Research Council. Recommended Dietary Allowances, 9th ed. (Washington, D.C.: 1980), 185 pp. This publication tabulates the RDA for selected nutrients, discusses the basis for all the RDA, and reviews current knowledge of the dietary needs for other nutrients. Used by permission.

Appendix C
Mean Heights and Weights and Recommended Energy Intake

Sex-age Category	Age (years)	Weight		Height		Energy Needs (range)[a]	
		(kg)	(lb)	(cm)	(in.)	(kcal)	
Infants	0–0.5	6	13	60	24	kg × 115	(95–145)
	0.5–1	9	20	71	28	kg × 105	(80–135)
Children	1–3	13	29	90	35	1300	(900–1800)
	4–6	20	44	112	44	1700	(1300–2300)
	7–10	28	62	132	52	2400	(1650–3300)
Males	11–14	45	99	157	62	2700	(2000–3700)
	15–18	66	145	176	69	2800	(2100–3900)
	19–22	70	154	177	70	2900	(2500–3300)
	23–50	70	154	178	70	2700	(2300–3100)
	51–75	70	154	178	70	2400	(2000–2800)
	76+	70	154	178	70	2050	(1650–2450)
Females	11–14	46	101	157	62	2200	(1500–3000)
	15–18	55	120	163	64	2100	(1200–3000)
	19–22	55	120	163	64	2100	(1700–2500)
	23–50	55	120	163	64	2000	(1600–2400)
	51–75	55	120	163	64	1800	(1400–2200)
	76+	55	120	163	64	1600	(1200–2000)
Pregnant						+300	
Lactating						+500	

[a]The energy allowances for the young adults are for men and women doing light work. The allowances for the two older age groups represent mean energy needs over these age spans, allowing for a 2 percent decrease in basal (resting) metabolic rate per decade and a reduction in activity of 200 kcal/day for men and women between 51 and 75 years, 500 kcal for men over 75 years, and 400 kcal for women over 75 years.

Energy allowances for children through age 18 are based on median energy intakes of children of these ages followed in longitudinal growth studies. The values in parentheses are 10th and 90th percentiles of energy intake, to indicate the range of energy consumption among children of these ages.

Source: Adapted from National Academy of Sciences, National Research Council, Recommended Daily Allowances, 9th ed. (Washington, D.C.: 1980), 185 pp. Used by permission.

Appendix D
Nutritive Values of the Edible Part of Foods

Item No.	Foods, approximate measures, units, and weight (edible part unless footnotes indicate otherwise)	Serving	Weight (g)	Water (%)	Food Energy (Cal.)	Protein (g)	Fat (g)	Saturated (total) (g)	Oleic (g)	Linoleic (g)	Carbohydrate (g)	Calcium (mg)	Phosphorus (mg)	Iron (mg)	Potassium (mg)	Vitamin A value (I.U.)	Thiamin (mg)	Riboflavin (mg)	Niacin (mg)	Ascorbic acid (mg)
	Dairy products (cheese, cream, imitation cream, milk; related products)																			
	Butter. See Fats, oils; related products, items 103–108.																			
	Cheese:																			
	Natural:																			
1	Blue	1 oz	28	42	100	6	8	5.3	1.9	.2	1	150	110	.1	73	200	.01	.11	.3	0
2	Camembert (3 wedges per 4-oz container)	1 wedge	38	52	115	8	9	5.8	2.2	.2	*	147	132	.1	71	350	.01	.19	.2	0
	Cheddar:																			
3	Cut pieces	1 oz	28	37	115	7	9	6.1	2.1	.2	*	204	145	.2	28	300	.01	.11	*	0
4		1 cu in.	17.2	37	70	4	6	3.7	1.3	.1	*	124	88	.1	17	180	*	.06	*	0
5	Shredded	1 cup	113	37	455	28	37	24.2	8.5	.7	1	815	579	.8	111	1,200	.03	.42	.1	0
	Cottage (curd not pressed down):																			
	Creamed (cottage cheese, 4% fat):																			
6	Large curd	1 cup	225	79	235	28	10	6.4	2.4	.2	6	135	297	.3	190	370	.05	.37	.3	*
7	Small curd	1 cup	210	79	220	26	9	6.0	2.2	.2	6	126	277	.3	177	340	.04	.34	.3	*
8	Low fat (2%)	1 cup	226	79	205	31	4	2.8	1.0	.1	8	155	340	.4	217	160	.05	.42	.3	*
9	Low fat (1%)	1 cup	226	82	165	28	2	1.5	.5	.1	6	138	302	.3	193	80	.05	.37	.3	*
10	Uncreamed (cottage cheese, dry curd, less than ½% fat)	1 cup	145	80	125	25	1	.4	.1	*	3	46	151	.3	47	40	.04	.21	.2	0
11	Cream	1 oz	28	54	100	2	10	6.2	2.4	.2	1	23	30	.3	34	400	*	.06	*	0
	Mozzarella, made with:																			
12	Whole milk	1 oz	28	48	90	6	7	4.4	1.7	.2	1	163	117	.1	21	260	*	.08	*	0
13	Part skim milk	1 oz	28	49	80	8	5	3.1	1.2	.1	1	207	149	.1	27	180	.01	.10	*	0
	Parmesan, grated:																			
14	Cup, not pressed down	1 cup	100	18	455	42	30	19.1	7.7	.3	4	1376	807	1.0	107	700	.05	.39	.3	0
15	Tablespoon	1 tbsp	5	18	25	2	2	1.0	.4	*	*	69	40	*	5	40	*	.02	*	0
16	Ounce	1 oz	28	18	130	12	9	5.4	2.2	.1	1	390	229	.3	30	200	.01	.11	.1	0
17	Provolone	1 oz	28	41	100	7	8	4.8	1.7	.1	1	214	141	.1	39	230	.01	.09	*	0
	Ricotta, made with:																			
18	Whole milk	1 cup	246	72	430	28	32	20.4	7.1	.7	7	509	389	.9	257	1210	.03	.48	.3	0
19	Part skim milk	1 cup	246	74	340	28	19	12.1	4.7	.5	13	669	449	1.1	308	1060	.05	.46	.2	0
20	Romano	1 oz	28	31	110	9	8	—	—	—	1	302	215	—	—	160	—	.11	*	0
21	Swiss	1 oz	28	37	105	8	8	5.0	1.7	.2	1	272	171	*	31	240	.01	.10	*	0
	Pasteurized process cheese:																			
22	American	1 oz	28	39	105	6	9	5.6	2.1	.2	*	174	211	.1	46	340	.01	.10	*	0
23	Swiss	1 oz	28	42	95	7	7	4.5	1.7	.1	1	219	216	.2	61	230	*	.08	*	0
24	Pasteurized process cheese food, American	1 oz	28	43	95	6	7	4.4	1.7	.1	2	163	130	.2	79	260	.01	.13	*	0
25	Pasteurized process cheese spread, American	1 oz	28	48	80	5	6	3.8	1.5	.1	2	159	202	.1	69	220	.01	.12	*	0
	Cream, sweet:																			
26	Half-and-half (cream and milk)	1 cup	242	81	315	7	28	17.3	7.0	.6	10	254	230	.2	314	260	.08	.36	.2	2
27		1 tbsp	15	81	20	*	2	1.1	.4	*	1	16	14	*	19	20	.01	.02	*	*

Nutrients in Indicated Quantity / Fatty Acids / Unsaturated (column group headers)

Appendix D
Nutritive Values of the Edible Part of Foods (Continued)

| | | | | | | | | Fatty Acids | | | | | | | | | | | | |
| | | | | | | | | | Unsaturated | | | | | | | | | | | |
Item No.	Foods, approximate measures, units, and weight (edible part unless footnotes indicate otherwise)	Serving	Weight (g)	Water (%)	Food Energy (Cal.)	Protein (g)	Fat (g)	Saturated (total) (g)	Oleic (g)	Linoleic (g)	Carbohydrate (g)	Calcium (mg)	Phosphorus (mg)	Iron (mg)	Potassium (mg)	Vitamin A value (I.U.)	Thiamin (mg)	Riboflavin (mg)	Niacin (mg)	Ascorbic acid (mg)
28	Light, coffee, or table	1 cup	240	74	470	6	46	28.8	11.7	1.0	9	231	192	.1	292	1730	.08	.36	.1	2
29		1 tbsp	15	74	30	*	3	1.8	.7	.1	1	14	12	*	18	110	*	.02	*	*
	Whipping, unwhipped (volume about double when whipped):																			
30	Light	1 cup	239	64	700	5	74	46.2	18.3	1.5	7	166	146	.1	231	2690	.06	.30	.1	1
31		1 tbsp	15	64	45	*	5	2.9	1.1	.1	*	10	9	*	15	170	*	.02	*	*
32	Heavy	1 cup	238	58	820	5	88	54.8	22.2	2.0	7	154	149	.1	179	3500	.05	.26	.1	1
33		1 tbsp	15	58	80	*	6	3.5	1.4	.1	*	10	9	*	11	220	*	.02	*	*
34	Whipped topping, (pressurized)	1 cup	60	61	155	2	13	8.3	3.4	.3	7	61	54	*	88	550	.02	.04	*	0
35		1 tbsp	3	61	10	*	1	.4	.2	*	*	3	3	*	4	30	*	*	*	0
36	Cream, sour	1 cup	230	71	495	7	48	30.0	12.1	1.1	10	268	195	.1	331	1820	.08	.34	.2	2
37		1 tbsp	12	71	25	*	3	1.6	.6	.1	1	14	10	*	17	90	*	.02	*	*
	Cream products, imitation (made with vegetable fat): Sweet: Creamers:																			
38	Liquid (frozen)	1 cup	245	77	335	2	24	22.8	.3	*	28	23	157	.1	467	220[a]	0	0	0	0
39		1 tbsp	15	77	20	*	1	1.4	*	0	2	1	10	*	29	10[a]	0	0	0	0
40	Powdered	1 cup	94	2	515	5	33	30.6	.9	*	52	21	397	.1	763	190[a]	0	.16[a]	0	0
41		1 tsp	2	2	10	*	1	.7	*	0	1	*	8	*	16	*[a]	0	*[a]	0	0
	Whipped topping:																			
42	Frozen	1 cup	75	50	240	1	19	16.3	1.0	.2	17	5	6	.1	14	650[a]	0	0	0	0
43		1 tbsp	4	50	15	*	1	.9	.1	*	1	*	*	*	1	30[a]	0	0	0	0
44	Powdered, made with whole milk	1 cup	80	67	150	3	10	8.5	.6	.1	13	72	69	*	121	290[a]	.02	.09	*	1
45		1 tbsp	4	67	10	*	*	.4	*	*	1	4	3	*	6	10[a]	*	*	*	*
46	Pressurized	1 cup	70	60	185	1	16	13.2	1.4	.2	11	4	13	*	13	330[a]	0	0	0	0
47		1 tbsp	4	60	10	*	1	.8	.1	*	1	*	1	*	1	20[a]	0	0	0	0
48	Sour dressing (imitation sour cream) made with nonfat dry milk	1 cup	235	75	415	8	39	31.2	4.4	1.1	11	266	205	.1	380	20[a]	.09	.38	.2	2
49		1 tbsp	12	75	20	*	2	1.6	.2	.1	1	14	10	*	19	*[a]	.01	.02	*	*
	Ice cream. See Milk desserts, frozen (items 75–80). Ice milk. See Milk desserts, frozen (items 81–83). Milk: Fluid:																			
50	Whole (3.3% fat)	1 cup	244	88	150	8	8	5.1	2.1	.2	11	291	228	.1	370	310[b]	.09	.40	.2	2
	Lowfat (2%):																			
51	No milk solids added Milk solids added:	1 cup	244	89	120	8	5	2.9	1.2	.1	12	297	232	.1	377	500	.10	.40	.2	2
52	Label claim less than 10 g of protein per cup	1 cup	245	89	125	9	5	2.9	1.2	.1	12	313	245	.1	397	500	.10	.42	.2	2
53	Label claim 10 or more grams of protein per cup (protein fortified)	1 cup	246	88	135	10	5	3.0	1.2	.1	14	352	276	.1	447	500	.11	.48	.2	3

Nutrients in Indicated Quantity

No.	Food	Measure	Grams	Water (%)	Food energy	Protein (g)	Fat (g)	Saturated fat (g)	Oleic (g)	Linoleic (g)	Carbohydrate (g)	Calcium (mg)	Phosphorus (mg)	Iron (mg)	Potassium (mg)	Vitamin A (IU)	Thiamin (mg)	Riboflavin (mg)	Niacin (mg)	Ascorbic acid (mg)
	Lowfat (1%):																			
54	No milk solids added	1 cup	244	90	100	8	3	1.6	.7	.1	12	300	235	.1	381	500	.10	.41	.2	2
	Milk solids added:																			
55	Label claim less than 10 g of protein per cup	1 cup	245	90	105	9	2	1.5	.6	.1	12	313	245	.1	397	500	.10	.42	.2	2
56	Label claim 10 or more grams of protein per cup (protein fortified)	1 cup	246	89	120	10	3	1.8	.7	.1	14	349	273	.1	444	500	.11	.47	.2	3
	Nonfat (skim):																			
57	No milk solids added	1 cup	245	91	85	8	*	.3	.1	*	12	302	247	.1	406	500	.09	.34	.2	2
	Milk solids added:																			
58	Label claim less than 10 g of protein per cup	1 cup	245	90	90	9	1	.4	.1	*	12	316	255	.1	418	500	.10	.43	.2	2
59	Label claim 10 or more grams of protein per cup (protein fortified)	1 cup	246	89	100	10	1	.4	.1	*	14	352	275	.1	446	500	.11	.48	.2	3
60	Buttermilk	1 cup	245	90	100	8	2	1.3	.5	*	12	285	219	.1	371	80[c]	.08	.38	.1	2
	Canned:																			
	Evaporated, unsweetened:																			
61	Whole milk	1 cup	252	74	340	17	19	11.6	5.3	0.4	25	657	510	.5	764	610[c]	.12	.80	.5	5
62	Skim milk	1 cup	255	79	200	19	1	.3	.1	*	29	738	497	.7	845	1,000[d]	.11	.79	.4	3
63	Sweetened, condensed	1 cup	306	27	980	24	27	16.8	6.7	.7	166	868	775	.6	1,136	1,000[c]	.28	1.27	.6	8
	Dried:																			
64	Buttermilk	1 cup	120	3	465	41	7	4.3	1.7	.2	59	1,421	1,119	.4	1,910	260[c]	.47	1.90	1.1	7
	Nonfat instant:																			
65	Envelope, net wt., 3.2 oz	1 envelope	91	4	325	32	1	.4	.1	*	47	1,120	896	.3	1,552	2,160[f]	.38	1.59	.8	5
66	Cup[g]	1 cup	68	4	245	24	*	.3	.1	*	35	837	670	.2	1,160	1,610[f]	.28	1.19	.6	4
	Milk beverages:																			
	Chocolate milk (commercial):																			
67	Regular	1 cup	250	82	210	8	8	5.3	2.2	.2	26	280	251	.6	417	300[c]	.09	.41	.3	2
68	Lowfat (2%)	1 cup	250	84	180	8	5	3.1	1.3	.1	26	284	254	.6	422	500	.10	.42	.3	2
69	Lowfat (1%)	1 cup	250	85	160	8	3	1.5	.7	.1	26	287	257	.6	426	500	.10	.40	.2	2
70	Eggnog (commercial)	1 cup	254	74	340	10	19	11.3	5.0	.6	34	330	278	.5	420	890	.09	.48	.3	4
	Malted milk, home-prepared with 1 cup of whole milk and 2 to 3 heaping tsp of malted milk powder (about 3/4 oz):																			
71	Chocolate	1 cup of milk plus 3/4 oz of powder	265	81	235	9	9	5.5	—	—	29	304	265	.5	500	330	.14	.43	.7	2
72	Natural	1 cup of milk plus 3/4 oz of powder	265	81	235	11	10	6.0	—	—	27	347	307	.3	529	380	.20	.54	1.3	2
	Shakes, thick:[h]																			
73	Chocolate, container, net wt., 10.6 oz	1 container	300	72	355	9	8	5.0	2.0	.2	63	396	378	.9	672	260	.14	.67	.4	0
74	Vanilla, container, net wt., 11 oz	1 container	313	74	350	12	9	5.9	2.4	.2	56	457	361	.3	572	360	.09	.61	.5	0
	Milk desserts, frozen:																			
	Ice cream:																			
	Regular (about 11% fat):																			
75	Hardened	1/2 gal	1064	61	2155	38	115	71.3	28.8	2.6	254	1,406	1,075	1.0	2,052	4,340	.42	2.63	1.1	6
76		1 cup	133	61	270	5	14	8.9	3.6	.3	32	176	134	.1	257	540	.05	.33	.1	1
77		3-fl-oz container	50	61	100	2	5	3.4	1.4	.1	12	66	51	*	96	200	.02	.12	.1	*
78	Soft serve (frozen custard)	1 cup	173	60	375	7	23	13.5	5.9	.6	38	236	199	.4	338	790	.08	.45	.2	1
79	Rich (about 16% fat), hardened	1/2 gal	1188	59	2805	33	190	118.3	47.8	4.3	256	1,213	927	.8	1,771	7,200	.36	2.27	.9	5
80		1 cup	148	59	350	4	24	14.7	6.0	.5	32	151	115	.1	221	900	.04	.28	.1	1
	Ice milk:																			
81	Hardened (about 4.3% fat)	1/2 gal	1048	69	1470	41	45	28.1	11.3	1.0	232	1,409	1,035	1.5	2,117	1,710	.61	2.78	.9	6
82		1 cup	131	69	185	5	6	3.5	1.4	.1	29	176	129	.1	265	210	.08	.35	.1	1
83	Soft serve (about 2.6% fat)	1 cup	175	70	225	8	5	2.9	1.2	.1	38	274	202	.3	412	180	.12	.54	.2	1
84	Sherbet (about 2% fat)	1/2 gal	1542	66	2160	17	31	19.0	7.7	.7	469	827	594	2.5	1,585	1,480	.26	.71	1.0	31
85		1 cup	193	66	270	2	4	2.4	1.0	.1	59	103	74	.3	198	190	.03	.09	.1	4

Appendix D
Nutritive Values of the Edible Part of Foods (*Continued*)

| | | | | | | | | Fatty Acids | | | | | | | | | | | | |
| | | | | | | | | | Unsaturated | | | | | | | | | | | |
Item No.	Foods, approximate measures, units, and weight (edible part unless footnotes indicate otherwise) / Serving	Weight (g)	Water (%)	Food Energy (Cal.)	Pro-tein (g)	Fat (g)	Satu-rated (total) (g)	Oleic (g)	Lino-leic (g)	Carbo-hydrate (g)	Cal-cium (mg)	Phos-phorus (mg)	Iron (mg)	Potas-sium (mg)	Vitamin A value (I.U.)	Thiamin (mg)	Ribo-flavin (mg)	Niacin (mg)	Ascor-bic acid (mg)
	Milk desserts, other:																		
86	Custard, baked — 1 cup	265	77	305	14	15	6.8	5.4	.7	29	297	310	1.1	387	930	.11	.50	.3	1
	Puddings:																		
	From home recipe:																		
	Starch base:																		
87	Chocolate — 1 cup	260	66	385	8	12	7.6	3.3	.3	67	250	255	1.3	445	390	.05	.36	.3	1
88	Vanilla (blancmange) — 1 cup	255	76	285	9	10	6.2	2.5	.2	41	298	232	*	352	410	.08	.41	.3	2
89	Tapioca cream — 1 cup	165	72	220	8	8	4.1	2.5	.5	28	173	180	.7	223	480	.07	.30	.2	2
	From mix (chocolate) and milk:																		
90	Regular (cooked) — 1 cup	260	70	320	9	8	4.3	2.6	.2	59	265	247	.8	354	340	.05	.39	.3	2
91	Instant — 1 cup	260	69	325	8	7	3.6	2.2	.3	63	374	237	1.3	335	340	.08	.39	.3	2
	Yogurt:																		
	With added milk solids:																		
	Made with lowfat milk:																		
92	Fruit-flavored[j] — 1 container, net wt., 8 oz	227	75	230	10	3	1.8	.6	.1	42	343	269	.2	439	120[j]	.08	.40	.2	1
93	Plain — 1 container, net wt., 8 oz	227	85	145	12	4	2.3	.8	.1	16	415	326	.2	531	150[j]	.10	.49	.3	2
94	Made with nonfat milk — 1 container, net wt., 8 oz	227	85	125	13	*	.3	.1	*	17	452	355	.2	579	20[j]	.11	.53	.3	1
	Without added milk solids:																		
95	Made with whole milk — 1 container, net wt., 8 oz	227	88	140	8	7	4.8	1.7	.1	11	274	215	.1	351	280	.07	.32	.2	1
	Eggs																		
	Eggs, large (24 oz per dozen):																		
	Raw:																		
96	Whole, without shell — 1 egg	50	75	80	6	6	1.7	2.0	.6	1	28	90	1.0	65	260	.04	.15	*	0
97	White — 1 white	33	88	15	3	*	0	0	0	*	4	4	*	45	0	*	.09	*	0
98	Yolk — 1 yolk	17	49	65	3	6	1.7	2.1	.6	*	26	86	.9	15	310	.04	.07	*	0
	Cooked:																		
99	Fried in butter — 1 egg	46	72	85	5	6	2.4	2.2	.6	1	26	80	.9	58	290	.03	.13	*	0
100	Hard-cooked, shell removed — 1 egg	50	75	80	6	6	1.7	2.0	.6	1	28	90	1.0	65	260	.04	.14	*	0
101	Poached — 1 egg	50	74	80	6	6	1.7	2.0	.6	1	28	90	1.0	65	260	.04	.13	*	0
102	Scrambled (milk added) in butter. Also omelet. — 1 egg	64	76	95	6	7	2.8	2.3	.6	1	47	97	.9	85	310	.04	.16	*	0
	Fats, Oils; Related Products																		
	Butter:																		
	Regular (1 brick or 4 sticks per lb):																		
103	Stick (½ cup) — 1 stick	113	16	815	1	92	57.3	23.1	2.1	*	27	26	.2	29	3470[b]	.01	.04	*	0
104	Tablespoon (about ⅛ stick) — 1 tbsp	14	16	100	*	12	7.2	2.9	.3	*	3	3	*	4	430[b]	*	*	*	0
105	Pat (1 in. square, ⅓ in. high; 90 per lb) — 1 pat	5	16	35	*	4	2.5	1.0	.1	*	1	1	*	1	150[b]	*	*	*	0
	Whipped (6 sticks or two 8-oz containers per lb):																		

No.	Food, approximate measure	Measure	Grams	Water (%)	Food energy (Cal)	Protein (g)	Fat (g)	Saturated (g)	Oleic (g)	Linoleic (g)	Carbohydrate (g)	Calcium (mg)	Phosphorus (mg)	Iron (mg)	Potassium (mg)	Vitamin A (IU)	Thiamin (mg)	Riboflavin (mg)	Niacin (mg)	Ascorbic acid (mg)
106	Stick (½ cup)	1 stick	76	16	540	1	61	38.2	15.4	1.4	*	18	17	.1	20	2310[k]	*	.03	*	0
107	Tablespoon (about ⅛ stick)	1 tbsp	9	16	65	*	8	4.7	1.9	.2	*	2	2	*	2	290[k]	*	*	*	0
108	Pat (1¼ in. square, ⅓ in. high; 120 per lb)	1 pat	4	16	25	*	3	1.9	.8	.1	*	1	1	*	1	120[k]	*	*	*	0
109	Fats, cooking (vegetable shortenings)	1 cup	200	0	1770	0	200	48.8	88.2	48.4	0	0	0	0	0	—	0	0	0	0
110		1 tbsp	13	0	110	0	13	3.2	5.7	3.1	0	0	0	0	0	—	0	0	0	0
111	Lard	1 cup	205	0	1850	0	205	81.0	83.8	20.5	0	0	0	0	0	0	0	0	0	0
112		1 tbsp	13	0	115	0	13	5.1	5.3	1.3	0	0	0	0	0	0	0	0	0	0
	Margarine:																			
	Regular (1 brick or 4 sticks per lb):																			
113	Stick (½ cup)	1 stick	113	16	815	1	92	16.7	42.9	24.9	*	27	26	.2	29	3750[l]	.01	.04	*	0
114	Tablespoon (about ⅛ stick)	1 tbsp	14	16	100	*	12	2.1	5.3	3.1	*	3	3	*	4	470[l]	*	*	*	0
115	Pat (1 in. square, ⅓ in. high; 90 per lb)	1 pat	5	16	35	*	4	.7	1.9	1.1	*	1	1	*	1	170[l]	*	*	.1	0
116	Soft, two 8-oz containers per lb	1 container	227	16	1635	1	184	32.5	71.5	65.4	*	53	52	.4	59	7500[l]	.01	.08	*	0
117		1 tbsp	14	16	100	*	12	2.0	4.5	4.1	*	3	3	*	4	470[l]	*	*	*	0
	Whipped (6 sticks per lb):																			
118	Stick (½ cup)	1 stick	76	16	545	*	61	11.2	28.7	16.7	.1	18	17	.1	20	2500[l]	*	.03	*	0
119	Tablespoon (about ⅛ stick)	1 tbsp	9	16	70	*	8	1.4	3.6	2.1	*	2	2	*	2	310[l]	*	*	*	0
	Oils, salad or cooking:																			
120	Corn	1 cup	218	0	1925	0	218	27.7	53.6	125.1	0	0	0	0	0	—	0	0	0	0
121		1 tbsp	14	0	120	0	14	1.7	3.3	7.8	0	0	0	0	0	—	0	0	0	0
122	Olive	1 cup	216	0	1910	0	216	30.7	154.4	17.7	0	0	0	0	0	—	0	0	0	0
123		1 tbsp	14	0	120	0	14	1.9	9.7	1.1	0	0	0	0	0	—	0	0	0	0
124	Peanut	1 cup	216	0	1910	0	216	37.4	98.5	67.0	0	0	0	0	0	—	0	0	0	0
125		1 tbsp	14	0	120	0	14	2.3	6.2	4.2	0	0	0	0	0	—	0	0	0	0
126	Safflower	1 cup	218	0	1925	0	218	20.5	25.9	159.8	0	0	0	0	0	—	0	0	0	0
127		1 tbsp	14	0	120	0	14	1.3	1.6	10.0	0	0	0	0	0	—	0	0	0	0
128	Soybean oil, hydrogenated (partially hardened)	1 cup	218	0	1925	0	218	31.8	93.1	75.6	0	0	0	0	0	—	0	0	0	0
129		1 tbsp	14	0	120	0	14	2.0	5.8	4.7	0	0	0	0	0	—	0	0	0	0
130	Soybean-cottonseed oil blend, hydrogenated	1 cup	218	0	1925	0	218	38.2	63.0	99.6	0	0	0	0	0	—	0	0	0	0
131		1 tbsp	14	0	120	0	14	2.4	3.9	6.2	0	0	0	0	0	—	0	0	0	0
	Salad dressings:																			
	Commercial:																			
	Blue cheese:																			
132	Regular	1 tbsp	15	32	75	1	8	1.6	1.7	3.8	1	12	11	*	6	30	*	.02	*	*
133	Low calorie (5 Cal per tsp)	1 tbsp	16	84	10	*	1	.5	.3	*	1	10	8	*	5	30	*	.01	*	*
	French:																			
134	Regular	1 tbsp	16	39	65	*	6	1.1	1.3	3.2	3	2	2	.1	13	—	—	—	—	—
135	Low calorie (5 Cal per tsp)	1 tbsp	16	77	15	*	1	.1	.4	.2	2	2	.1	13	—	—	—	—	—	—
	Italian:																			
136	Regular	1 tbsp	15	28	85	*	9	1.6	1.9	4.7	1	2	1	*	2	*	*	*	*	—
137	Low calorie (2 Cal per tsp)	1 tbsp	15	90	10	*	1	.1	.1	.4	*	*	1	*	2	*	*	*	*	—
138	Mayonnaise	1 tbsp	14	15	100	*	11	2.0	2.4	5.6	*	3	4	.1	5	40	*	.01	*	—
	Mayonnaise type:																			
139	Regular	1 tbsp	15	41	65	*	6	1.1	1.4	3.2	2	2	4	*	1	30	*	*	*	—
140	Low calorie (8 Cal per tsp)	1 tbsp	16	81	20	*	2	.4	.4	1.0	2	3	4	*	1	40	*	*	*	—
141	Tartar sauce, regular	1 tbsp	14	34	75	*	8	1.5	1.8	4.1	1	3	4	.1	11	30	*	*	*	*
	Thousand Island:																			
142	Regular	1 tbsp	16	32	80	*	8	1.4	1.7	4.0	2	2	3	.1	18	50	*	*	*	*
143	Low calorie (10 Cal per tsp)	1 tbsp	15	68	25	*	2	.4	.4	1.0	2	2	3	.1	17	50	*	*	*	*
	From home recipe:																			
144	Cooked type[m]	1 tbsp	16	68	25	1	2	.5	.6	.3	2	14	15	.1	19	80	.01	.03	*	*

Appendix D
Nutritive Values of the Edible Part of Foods (Continued)

Nutrients in Indicated Quantity

Item No.	Foods, approximate measures, units, and weight (edible part unless footnotes indicate otherwise) — Serving	Weight (g)	Water (%)	Food Energy (Cal.)	Protein (g)	Fat (g)	Fatty Acids Saturated (total) (g)	Unsaturated Oleic (g)	Unsaturated Linoleic (g)	Carbohydrate (g)	Calcium (mg)	Phosphorus (mg)	Iron (mg)	Potassium (mg)	Vitamin A value (I.U.)	Thiamin (mg)	Riboflavin (mg)	Niacin (mg)	Ascorbic acid (mg)
	Fish, shellfish, meat, poultry; related products																		
	Fish and shellfish:																		
145	Bluefish, baked with butter or margarine — 3 oz	85	68	135	22	4	—	—	—	0	25	244	.6	—	40	.09	.08	1.6	—
	Clams:																		
146	Raw, meat only — 3 oz	85	82	65	11	1	—	—	—	2	59	138	5.2	154	90	.08	.15	1.1	8
147	Canned, solids and liquid — 3 oz	85	86	45	7	1	0.2	*	*	2	47	116	3.5	119	—	.01	.09	.9	—
148	Crabmeat (white or king), canned, not pressed down — 1 cup	135	77	135	24	3	.6	0.4	0.1	1	61	246	1.1	149	—	.11	.11	2.6	—
149	Fish sticks, breaded, cooked, frozen (stick, 4 by 1 by ½ in.) — 1 fish stick or 1 oz	28	66	50	5	3	—	—	—	2	3	47	.1	—	0	.01	.02	.5	—
150	Haddock, breaded, fried[a] — 3 oz	85	66	140	17	5	1.4	2.2	1.2	5	34	210	1.0	296	—	.03	.06	2.7	2
151	Ocean perch, breaded, fried[a] — 1 fillet	85	59	195	16	11	2.7	4.4	2.3	6	28	192	1.1	242	—	.10	.10	1.6	—
152	Oysters, raw, meat only (13–19 medium Selects) — 1 cup	240	85	160	20	4	1.3	.2	.1	8	226	343	13.2	290	740	.34	.43	6.0	—
153	Salmon, pink, canned, solids and liquid — 3 oz	85	71	120	17	5	.9	.8	.1	0	167[a]	243	.7	307	60	.03	.16	6.8	—
154	Sardines, Atlantic, canned in oil, drained solids — 3 oz	85	62	175	20	9	3.0	2.5	.5	0	372	424	2.5	502	190	.02	.17	4.6	—
155	Scallops, frozen, breaded, fried, reheated — 6 scallops	90	60	175	16	8	—	—	—	9	—	—	—	—	—	—	—	—	—
156	Shad, baked with butter or margarine, bacon — 3 oz	85	64	170	20	10	—	—	—	0	20	266	.5	320	30	.11	.22	7.3	—
	Shrimp:																		
157	Canned meat — 3 oz	85	70	100	21	1	.1	.1	*	1	98	224	2.6	104	50	.01	.03	1.5	—
158	French fried[p] — 3 oz	85	57	190	17	9	2.3	3.7	2.0	9	61	162	1.7	195	—	.03	.07	2.3	—
159	Tuna, canned in oil, drained solids — 3 oz	85	61	170	24	7	1.7	1.7	.7	0	7	199	1.6	—	70	.04	.10	10.1	—
160	Tuna salad[q] — 1 cup	205	70	350	30	22	4.3	6.3	6.7	7	41	291	2.7	—	590	.08	.23	10.3	2
	Meat and meat products:																		
161	Bacon (20 slices per lb, raw), broiled or fried, crisp — 2 slices	15	8	85	4	8	2.5	3.7	.7	*	2	34	.5	35	0	.08	.05	.8	—
	Beef,[r] cooked:																		
	Cuts braised, simmered or pot roasted:																		
162	Lean and fat (piece, 2½ by 2½ by ¾ in.) — 3 oz	85	53	245	23	16	6.8	6.5	.4	0	10	114	2.9	184	30	.04	.18	3.6	—
163	Lean only from item 162 — 2.5 oz	72	62	140	22	5	2.1	1.8	.2	0	10	108	2.7	176	10	.04	.17	3.3	—
	Ground beef, broiled:																		
164	Lean with 10% fat — 3 oz or patty 3 by 5/8 in.	85	60	185	23	10	4.0	3.9	.3	0	10	196	3.0	261	20	.08	.20	5.1	—
165	Lean with 21% fat — 2.9 oz or patty 3 by 5/8 in.	82	54	235	20	17	7.0	6.7	.4	0	9	159	2.6	221	30	.07	.17	4.4	—
	Roast, oven cooked, no liquid added: Relatively fat, such as rib:																		

No.	Food, approximate measure, and weight		(g)	Water (%)	Food energy (cal)	Protein (g)	Fat (g)	Sat. fat (g)	Oleic (g)	Linoleic (g)	Carbo. (g)	Calcium (mg)	Phos. (mg)	Iron (mg)	Potas. (mg)	Vit. A (IU)	Thiamin (mg)	Ribo. (mg)	Niacin (mg)	Asc. acid (mg)
166	Lean and fat (2 pieces, 4⅛ by 2¼ by ¼ in.)	3 oz	85	40	375	17	33	14.0	13.6	.8	0	8	158	2.2	189	70	.05	.13	3.1	—
167	Lean only from item 166	1.8 oz	51	57	125	14	7	3.0	2.5	.3	0	6	131	1.8	161	10	.04	.11	2.6	—
	Relatively lean, such as heel of round:																			
168	Lean and fat (2 pieces, 4⅛ by 2¼ by ¼ in.)	3 oz	85	62	165	25	7	2.8	2.7	.2	0	11	208	3.2	279	10	.06	.19	4.5	—
169	Lean only from item 168	2.8 oz	78	65	125	24	3	1.2	1.0	.1	0	10	199	3.0	268	*	.06	.18	4.3	—
	Steak:																			
	Relatively fat—sirloin, broiled:																			
170	Lean and fat (piece, 2½ by 2½ by ¾ in.)	3 oz	85	44	330	20	27	11.3	11.1	.6	0	9	162	2.5	220	50	.05	.15	4.0	—
171	Lean only from item 170	2.0 oz	56	59	115	18	4	1.8	1.6	.2	0	7	146	2.2	202	10	.05	.14	3.6	—
	Relatively lean—round, braised:																			
172	Lean and fat (piece, 4⅛ by 2¼ by ½ in.)	3 oz	85	55	220	24	13	5.5	5.2	.4	0	10	213	3.0	272	20	.07	.19	4.8	—
173	Lean only from item 172	2.4 oz	68	61	130	21	4	1.7	1.5	.2	0	9	182	2.5	238	10	.05	.16	4.1	—
	Beef, canned:																			
174	Corned beef	3 oz	85	59	185	22	10	4.9	4.5	.2	0	17	90	3.7	—	—	.01	.20	2.9	0
175	Corned beef hash	1 cup	220	67	400	19	25	11.9	10.9	.5	24	29	147	4.4	440	—	.02	.20	4.6	0
176	Beef, dried, chipped	2½-oz jar	71	48	145	24	4	2.1	2.0	.1	0	14	287	3.6	142	—	.05	.23	2.7	0
177	Beef and vegetable stew	1 cup	245	82	220	16	11	4.9	4.5	.2	15	29	184	2.9	613	2400	.15	.17	4.7	17
178	Beef potpie (home recipe), baked (piece, ⅓ of 9-in.-diam. pie)	1 piece	210	55	515	21	30	7.9	12.8	6.7	39	29	149	3.8	334	1720	.30	.30	5.5	6
179	Chili con carne with beans, canned	1 cup	255	72	340	19	16	7.5	6.8	.3	31	82	321	4.3	594	150	.08	.18	3.3	—
180	Chop suey with beef and pork (home recipe)	1 cup	250	75	300	26	17	8.5	6.2	.7	13	60	248	4.8	425	600	.28	.38	5.0	33
181	Heart, beef, lean, braised	3 oz	85	61	160	27	5	1.5	1.1	.6	1	5	154	5.0	197	20	.21	1.04	6.5	1
	Lamb, cooked:																			
	Chop, rib (cut 3 per lb with bone), broiled:																			
182	Lean and fat	3.1 oz	89	43	360	18	32	14.8	12.1	1.2	0	8	139	1.0	200	—	.11	.19	4.1	—
183	Lean only from item 182	2 oz	57	60	120	16	6	2.5	2.1	.2	0	6	121	1.1	174	—	.09	.18	3.4	—
	Leg, roasted:																			
184	Lean and fat (2 pieces, 4⅛ by 2¼ by ¼ in.)	3 oz	85	54	235	22	16	7.3	6.0	.6	0	9	177	1.4	241	—	.13	.23	4.7	—
185	Lean only from item 184	2.5 oz	71	62	130	20	5	2.1	1.8	.2	0	9	169	1.4	227	—	.12	.21	4.4	—
	Shoulder, roasted:																			
186	Lean and fat (3 pieces, 2½ by 2½ by ¼ in.)	3 oz	85	50	285	18	23	10.8	8.8	.9	0	9	146	1.0	206	—	.11	.20	4.0	—
187	Lean only from item 186	2.3 oz	64	61	130	17	6	3.6	2.3	.2	0	8	140	1.0	193	—	.10	.18	3.7	—
188	Liver, beef, fried (slice, 6½ by 2⅜ by ⅜ in.)	3 oz	85	56	195	22	9	2.5	3.5	.9	5	9	405	7.5	323	45,390[d]	.22	3.56	14.0	23
	Pork, cured, cooked:																			
189	Ham, light cure, lean and fat, roasted (2 pieces, 4⅛ by 2¼ by ¼ in.)	3 oz	85	54	245	18	19	6.8	7.9	1.7	0	8	146	2.2	199	0	.40	.15	3.1	—
	Luncheon meat:																			
190	Boiled ham, slice (8 per 8-oz pkg.)	1 oz	28	59	65	5	5	1.7	2.0	.4	0	3	47	.8	—	0	.12	.04	.7	—
191	Canned, spiced or unspiced: Slice, approx. 3 by 2 by ½ in.	1 slice	60	55	175	9	15	5.4	6.7	1.0	1	5	65	1.3	133	0	.19	.13	1.8	—
	Pork, fresh, cooked:																			
	Chops, loin (cut 3 per lb with bone), broiled:																			
192	Lean and fat	2.7 oz	78	42	305	19	25	8.9	10.4	2.2	0	9	209	2.7	216	0	.75	.22	4.5	—
193	Lean only from item 192	2 oz	56	53	150	17	9	3.1	3.6	.8	0	7	181	2.2	192	0	.63	.18	3.8	—
	Roast, oven cooked, no liquid added:																			

Appendix D
Nutritive Values of the Edible Part of Foods (*Continued*)

Item No.	Foods, approximate measures, units, and weight (edible part unless footnotes indicate otherwise) / Serving	Weight (g)	Water (%)	Food Energy (Cal.)	Protein (g)	Fat (g)	Saturated (total) (g)	Oleic (g)	Linoleic (g)	Carbohydrate (g)	Calcium (mg)	Phosphorus (mg)	Iron (mg)	Potassium (mg)	Vitamin A value (I.U.)	Thiamin (mg)	Riboflavin (mg)	Niacin (mg)	Ascorbic acid (mg)
194	Lean and fat (piece, 2½ by 2½ by ¾ in.) / 3 oz	85	46	310	21	24	8.7	10.2	2.2	0	9	218	2.7	233	0	.78	.22	4.8	—
195	Lean only from item 194 / 2.4 oz	68	55	175	20	10	3.5	4.1	.8	0	9	211	2.6	224	0	.73	.21	4.4	—
	Shoulder cut, simmered:																		
196	Lean and fat (3 pieces, 2½ by 2½ by ¼ in.) / 3 oz	85	46	320	20	26	9.3	10.9	2.3	0	9	118	2.6	158	0	.46	.21	4.1	—
197	Lean only from item 196 / 2.2 oz	63	60	135	18	6	2.2	2.6	.6	0	8	111	2.3	146	0	.42	.19	3.7	—
	Sausages (see also Luncheon meat, items 190–191):																		
198	Bologna, slice (8 per 8-oz pkg.) / 1 slice	28	56	85	3	8	3.0	3.4	.5	*	2	36	.5	65	—	.05	.06	.7	—
199	Braunschweiger, slice (6 per 6-oz pkg.) / 1 slice	28	53	90	4	8	2.6	3.4	.8	1	3	69	1.7	—	1850	.05	.41	2.3	—
200	Brown and serve (10–11 per 8-oz pkg.), browned / 1 link	17	40	70	3	6	2.3	2.8	.7	*	—	—	—	—	—	—	—	—	—
201	Deviled ham, canned / 1 tbsp	13	51	45	2	4	1.5	1.8	.4	0	1	12	.3	—	0	.02	.01	.2	—
202	Frankfurter (8 per 1-lb pkg.), cooked (reheated) / 1 frankfurter	56	57	170	7	15	5.6	6.5	1.2	1	3	57	.8	—	—	.08	.11	1.4	—
203	Meat, potted (beef, chicken, turkey), canned / 1 tbsp	13	61	30	2	2	—	—	—	0	—	—	—	—	—	*	.03	.2	—
204	Pork link (16 per 1-lb pkg.), cooked / 1 link	13	35	60	2	6	2.1	2.4	.5	*	1	21	.3	35	0	.10	.04	.5	—
	Salami:																		
205	Dry type, slice (12 per 4-oz pkg.) / 1 slice	10	30	45	2	4	1.6	1.6	.1	*	1	28	.4	—	—	.04	.03	.5	—
206	Cooked type, slice (8 per 8-oz pkg.) / 1 slice	28	51	90	5	7	3.1	3.0	.2	*	3	57	.7	—	—	.07	.07	1.2	—
207	Vienna sausage (7 per 4-oz can) / 1 sausage	16	63	40	2	3	1.2	1.4	.2	*	1	24	.3	—	—	.01	.02	.4	—
	Veal, medium fat, cooked, bone removed:																		
208	Cutlet (4⅛ by 2¼ by ½ in.), braised or broiled / 3 oz	85	60	185	23	9	4.0	3.4	.4	0	9	196	2.7	258	—	.06	.21	4.6	—
209	Rib (2 pieces, 4⅛ by 2¼ by ¼ in.), roasted / 3 oz	85	55	230	23	14	6.1	5.1	.6	0	10	211	2.9	259	—	.11	.26	6.6	—
	Poultry and poultry products: Chicken, cooked:																		
210	Breast, fried," bones removed, ½ breast (3.3 oz with bones) / 2.8 oz	79	58	160	26	5	1.4	1.8	1.1	1	9	218	1.3	—	70	.04	.17	11.6	—
211	Drumstick, fried," bones removed (2 oz with bones) / 1.3 oz	38	55	90	12	4	1.1	1.3	.9	*	6	89	.9	—	50	.03	.15	2.7	—
212	Half broiler, broiled, bones removed (10.4 oz with bones) / 6.2 oz	176	71	240	42	7	2.2	2.5	1.3	0	16	355	3.0	483	160	.09	.34	15.5	—
213	Chicken, canned, boneless / 3 oz	85	65	170	18	10	3.2	3.8	2.0	0	18	210	1.3	117	200	.03	.11	3.7	3
214	Chicken à la king, cooked (home recipe) / 1 cup	245	68	470	27	34	2.7	14.3	3.3	12	127	358	2.5	404	1130	.10	.42	5.4	12

No.	Food	Measure	Grams	Water (%)	Food energy (cal)	Protein (g)	Fat (g)	Saturated fat (g)	Oleic (g)	Linoleic (g)	Carbohydrate (g)	Calcium (mg)	Phosphorus (mg)	Iron (mg)	Potassium (mg)	Vitamin A (IU)	Thiamin (mg)	Riboflavin (mg)	Niacin (mg)	Ascorbic acid (mg)
215	Chicken and noodles, cooked (home recipe)	1 cup	240	71	365	22	18	5.9	7.1	3.5	26	26	247	2.2	149	430	.05	.17	4.3	*
	Chicken chow mein:																			
216	Canned	1 cup	250	89	95	7	*	—	—	—	18	45	85	1.3	418	150	.05	.10	1.0	13
217	From home recipe	1 cup	250	78	255	31	10	2.4	3.4	3.1	10	58	293	2.5	473	280	.08	.23	4.3	10
218	Chicken potpie (home recipe), baked,[s] piece (1/3 or 9-in.-diam. pie)	1 piece	232	57	545	23	31	11.3	10.9	5.6	42	70	232	3.0	343	3090	.34	.31	5.5	5
	Turkey, roasted, flesh without skin:																			
219	Dark meat, piece, 2½ by ⅝ by ¼ in.	4 pieces	85	61	175	26	7	2.1	1.5	1.5	0	—	—	2.0	338	—	.03	.20	3.6	—
220	Light meat, piece, 4 by 2 by ¼ in.	2 pieces	85	62	150	28	3	.9	.6	.7	0	—	—	1.0	349	—	.04	.12	9.4	—
	Light and dark meat:																			
221	Chopped or diced	1 cup	140	61	265	44	9	2.5	1.7	1.8	0	11	351	2.5	514	—	.07	.25	10.8	—
222	Pieces (1 slice white meat, 4 by 2 by ¼ in., with 2 slices dark meat, 2½ by 1⅝ by ¼ in.)	3 pieces	85	61	160	27	5	1.5	1.0	1.1	0	7	213	1.5	312	—	.04	.15	6.5	—

Fruits and fruit products

No.	Food	Measure	Grams	Water (%)	Food energy (cal)	Protein (g)	Fat (g)	Saturated fat (g)	Oleic (g)	Linoleic (g)	Carbohydrate (g)	Calcium (mg)	Phosphorus (mg)	Iron (mg)	Potassium (mg)	Vitamin A (IU)	Thiamin (mg)	Riboflavin (mg)	Niacin (mg)	Ascorbic acid (mg)
	Apples, raw, unpeeled, without cores:																			
223	2¾-in. diam. (about 3 per lb with cores)	1 apple	138	84	80	*	1	—	—	—	20	10	14	.4	152	120	.04	.03	.1	6
224	3¼-in. diam. (about 2 per lb with cores)	1 apple	212	84	125	*	1	—	—	—	31	15	21	.6	233	190	.06	.04	.2	8
225	Applejuice, bottled or canned[v]	1 cup	248	88	120	*	*	—	—	—	30	15	22	1.5	250	—	.02	.05	.2	2[v]
	Applesauce, canned:																			
226	Sweetened	1 cup	255	76	230	1	*	—	—	—	61	10	13	1.3	166	100	.05	.03	.1	3[y]
227	Unsweetened	1 cup	244	89	100	*	*	—	—	—	26	10	12	1.2	190	100	.05	.02	.1	2[y]
	Apricots:																			
228	Raw, without pits (about 12 per lb with pits)	3 apricots	107	85	55	1	*	—	—	—	14	18	25	.5	301	2890	.03	.04	.6	11
229	Canned in heavy sirup (halves and sirup)	1 cup	258	77	220	2	*	—	—	—	57	28	39	.8	604	4490	.05	.05	1.0	10
	Dried:																			
230	Uncooked (28 large or 37 medium halves per cup)	1 cup	130	25	340	7	1	—	—	—	86	87	140	7.2	1273	14,170	.01	.21	4.3	16
231	Cooked, unsweetened, fruit and liquid	1 cup	250	76	215	4	1	—	—	—	54	55	88	4.5	795	7500	.01	.13	2.5	8
232	Apricot nectar, canned	1 cup	251	85	145	1	*	—	—	—	37	23	30	.5	379	2380	.03	.03	.5	36[z]
	Avocados, raw, whole, without skins and seeds:																			
233	California, mid- and late-winter (with skin and seed, 3⅛-in. diam.; wt., 10 oz)	1 avocado	216	74	370	5	37	5.5	22.0	3.7	13	22	91	1.3	1303	630	.24	.43	3.5	30
234	Florida, late summer and fall (with skin and seed, 3⅝-in. diam.; wt., 1 lb)	1 avocado	304	78	390	4	33	6.7	15.7	5.3	27	30	128	1.8	1836	880	.33	.61	4.9	43
235	Banana without peel (about 2.6 per lb with peel)	1 banana	119	76	100	1	*	—	—	—	26	10	31	.8	440	230	.06	.07	.8	12
236	Banana flakes	1 tbsp	6	3	20	*	*	—	—	—	5	2	6	.2	92	50	.01	.01	.2	*
237	Blackberries, raw	1 cup	144	85	85	2	1	—	—	—	19	46	27	1.3	245	290	.04	.06	.6	30
238	Blueberries, raw	1 cup	145	83	90	1	1	—	—	—	22	22	19	1.5	117	150	.04	.09	.7	20
	Cantaloupe. See Muskmelons (item 271).																			
	Cherries:																			
239	Sour (tart), red, pitted, canned, water pack	1 cup	244	88	105	2	*	—	—	—	26	37	32	.7	317	1,660	.07	.05	.5	12
240	Sweet, raw, without pits and stems	10 cherries	68	80	45	1	*	—	—	—	12	15	13	.3	129	70	.03	.04	.3	7
241	Cranberry juice cocktail, bottled, sweetened	1 cup	253	83	165	*	*	—	—	—	42	13	8	.8	25	*	.03	.03	.1	81[aa]
242	Cranberry sauce, sweetened, canned, strained	1 cup	277	62	405	*	*	—	—	—	104	17	11	.6	83	60	.03	.03	.1	6
	Dates:																			
243	Whole, without pits	10 dates	80	23	220	2	*	—	—	—	58	47	50	2.4	518	40	.07	.08	1.8	0
244	Chopped	1 cup	178	23	490	4	1	—	—	—	130	105	112	5.3	1,153	90	.16	.18	3.9	0

Appendix D
Nutritive Values of the Edible Part of Foods (Continued)

| | | | | | | | | | Fatty Acids | | | | | | | | | | | | |
| | | | | | | | | | Saturated | Unsaturated | | | | | | | | | | | | |
Item No.	Foods, approximate measures, units, and weight (edible part unless footnotes indicate otherwise)	Serving	Weight (g)	Water (%)	Food Energy (Cal.)	Protein (g)	Fat (g)	Saturated (total) (g)	Oleic (g)	Linoleic (g)	Carbohydrate (g)	Calcium (mg)	Phosphorus (mg)	Iron (mg)	Potassium (mg)	Vitamin A value (I.U.)	Thiamin (mg)	Riboflavin (mg)	Niacin (mg)	Ascorbic acid (mg)
245	Fruit cocktail, canned, in heavy sirup	1 cup	255	80	195	1	*	—	—	—	50	23	31	1.0	411	360	.05	.03	1.0	5
	Grapefruit:																			
	Raw, medium, 3¾-in. diam. (about 1 lb 1 oz):																			
246	Pink or red	½ grapefruit with peel	241^bb	89	50	1	*	—	—	—	13	20	20	.5	166	540	.05	.02	.2	44
247	White	½ grapefruit with peel	241^bb	89	45	1	*	—	—	—	12	19	19	.5	159	10	.05	.02	.2	44
248	Canned, sections with sirup	1 cup	254	81	180	2	*	—	—	—	45	33	36	.8	343	30	.08	.05	.5	76
	Grapefruit juice:																			
249	Raw, pink, red, or white	1 cup	246	90	95	1	*	—	—	—	23	22	37	.5	399	(cc)	.10	.05	.5	93
	Canned, white:																			
250	Unsweetened	1 cup	247	89	100	1	*	—	—	—	24	20	35	1.0	400	20	.07	.05	.5	84
251	Sweetened	1 cup	250	86	135	1	*	—	—	—	32	20	35	1.0	405	30	.08	.05	.5	78
	Frozen, concentrate, unsweetened:																			
252	Undiluted, 6-fl-oz can	1 can	207	62	300	4	1	—	—	—	72	70	124	.8	1,250	60	.29	.12	1.4	286
253	Diluted with 3 parts water by volume	1 cup	247	89	100	1	*	—	—	—	24	25	42	.2	420	20	.10	.04	.5	96
254	Dehydrated crystals, prepared with water (1 lb yields about 1 gal)	1 cup	247	90	100	1	*	—	—	—	24	22	40	.2	412	20	.10	.05	.5	91
	Grapes, European type (adherent skin), raw:																			
255	Thompson Seedless	10 grapes	50	81	35	*	*	—	—	—	9	6	10	.2	87	50	.03	.02	.2	2
256	Tokay and Emperor, seeded types	10 grapes	60^dd	81	40	*	*	—	—	—	10	7	11	.2	99	60	.03	.02	.2	2
	Grapejuice:																			
257	Canned or bottled	1 cup	253	83	165	1	*	—	—	—	42	28	30	.8	293	—	.10	.05	.5	*^y
	Frozen concentrate, sweetened:																			
258	Undiluted, 6-fl-oz can	1 can	216	53	395	1	*	—	—	—	100	22	32	.9	255	40	.13	.22	1.5	32^ee
259	Diluted with 3 parts water by volume	1 cup	250	86	135	1	*	—	—	—	33	8	10	.3	85	10	.05	.08	.5	10^ee
260	Grape drink, canned	1 cup	250	86	135	*	*	—	—	—	35	8	10	.3	88	—	.03^ff	.03^ff	.3	(f)
261	Lemon, raw, size 165, without peel and seeds (about 4 per lb with peels and seeds)	1 lemon	74	90	20	1	*	—	—	—	6	19	12	.4	102	10	.03	.01	.1	39
	Lemon juice:																			
262	Raw	1 cup	244	91	60	1	*	—	—	—	20	17	24	.5	344	50	.07	.02	.2	112
263	Canned, or bottled, unsweetened	1 cup	244	92	55	1	*	—	—	—	19	17	24	.5	344	50	.07	.02	.2	102
264	Frozen, single strength, unsweetened, 6-fl-oz can	1 can	183	92	40	1	*	—	—	—	13	13	16	.5	258	40	.05	.02	.2	81
	Lemonade concentrate, frozen:																			
265	Undiluted, 6-fl-oz can	1 can	219	49	425	*	*	—	—	—	112	9	13	.4	153	40	.05	.06	.7	66
266	Diluted with 4⅓ parts water by volume	1 cup	248	89	105	*	*	—	—	—	28	2	3	.1	40	10	.01	.02	.2	17
	Limeade concentrate, frozen:																			
267	Undiluted, 6-fl-oz can	1 can	218	50	410	*	*	—	—	—	108	11	13	.2	129	*	.02	.02	.2	26
268	Diluted with 4⅓ parts water by volume	1 cup	247	89	100	*	*	—	—	—	27	3	3	*	32	*	*	*	*	6

Nutrients in Indicated Quantity

No.	Food	Measure	Grams	Water (%)	Food energy	Protein (g)	Fat (g)	Saturated (g)	Oleic (g)	Linoleic (g)	Carbohydrate (g)	Calcium (mg)	Phosphorus (mg)	Iron (mg)	Potassium (mg)	Vitamin A (IU)	Thiamin (mg)	Riboflavin (mg)	Niacin (mg)	Ascorbic acid (mg)
	Limejuice:																			
269	Raw	1 cup	246	90	65	1	*	—	—	—	22	22	27	.5	256	20	.05	.02	.2	79
270	Canned, unsweetened	1 cup	246	90	65	1	*	—	—	—	22	22	27	.5	256	20	.05	.02	.2	52
	Muskmelons, raw, with rind, without seed cavity:																			
271	Cantaloupe, orange-fleshed (with rind and seed cavity, 5-in. diam., 2⅓ lb)	½ melon with rind	477[gg]	91	80	2	*	—	—	—	20	38	44	1.1	682	9240	.11	.08	1.6	90
272	Honeydew (with rind and seed cavity, 6½-in. diam., 5¼ lb)	1/10 melon with rind	226[gg]	91	50	1	*	—	—	—	11	21	24	.6	374	60	.06	.04	.9	34
	Oranges, all commercial varieties, raw:																			
273	Whole, 2⅝-in. diam., without peel and seeds (about 2½ per lb with peel and seeds)	1 orange	131	86	65	1	*	—	—	—	16	54	26	.5	263	260	.13	.05	.5	66
274	Sections without membranes	1 cup	180	86	90	2	*	—	—	—	22	74	36	.7	360	360	.18	.07	.7	90
	Orange juice:																			
275	Raw, all varieties	1 cup	248	88	110	2	*	—	—	—	26	27	42	.5	496	500	.22	.07	1.0	124
276	Canned, unsweetened	1 cup	249	87	120	2	*	—	—	—	28	25	45	1.0	496	500	.17	.05	.7	100
	Frozen concentrate:																			
277	Undiluted, 6-fl-oz can	1 can	213	55	360	5	*	—	—	—	87	75	126	.9	1500	1620	.68	.11	2.8	360
278	Diluted with 3 parts water by volume	1 cup	249	87	120	2	*	—	—	—	29	25	42	.2	503	540	.23	.03	.9	120
279	Dehydrated crystals, prepared with water (1 lb yields about 1 gal)	1 cup	248	88	115	1	*	—	—	—	27	25	40	.5	518	500	.20	.07	1.0	109
	Orange and grapefruit juice:																			
	Frozen concentrate:																			
280	Undiluted, 6-fl-oz can	1 can	210	59	330	4	1	—	—	—	78	61	99	.8	1,308	800	.48	.06	2.3	302
281	Diluted with 3 parts water by volume	1 cup	248	88	110	1	*	—	—	—	26	20	32	.2	439	270	.15	.02	.7	102
282	Papayas, raw, ½-in. cubes	1 cup	140	89	55	1	*	—	—	—	14	28	22	.4	328	2450	.06	.06	.4	78
	Peaches:																			
	Raw:																			
283	Whole, 2½-in. diam., peeled, pitted (about 4 per lb with peels and pits)	1 peach	100	89	40	1	*	—	—	—	10	9	19	.5	202	1330[hh]	.02	.05	1.0	7
284	Sliced	1 cup	170	89	65	1	*	—	—	—	16	15	32	.9	343	2260[hh]	.03	.09	1.7	12
	Canned, yellow-fleshed, solids and liquid (halves or slices):																			
285	Sirup pack	1 cup	256	79	200	1	*	—	—	—	51	10	31	.8	333	1100	.03	.05	1.5	8
286	Water pack	1 cup	244	91	75	1	*	—	—	—	20	10	32	.7	334	1100	.02	.07	1.5	7
	Dried:																			
287	Uncooked	1 cup	160	25	420	5	1	—	—	—	109	77	187	9.6	1520	6240	.02	.30	8.5	29
288	Cooked, unsweetened, halves and juice	1 cup	250	77	205	3	1	—	—	—	54	38	93	4.8	743	3050	.01	.15	3.8	5
	Frozen, sliced, sweetened:																			
289	10-oz container	1 container	284	77	250	1	*	—	—	—	64	11	37	1.4	352	1850	.03	.11	2.0	116[ii]
290	Cup	1 cup	250	77	220	1	*	—	—	—	57	10	33	1.3	310	1630	.03	.10	1.8	103[ii]
	Pears:																			
	Raw, with skin, cored:																			
291	Bartlett, 2½-in. diam. (about 2½ per lb with cores and stems)	1 pear	164	83	100	1	1	—	—	—	25	13	18	.5	213	30	.03	.07	.2	7
292	Bosc, 2½-in. diam. (about 3 per lb with cores and stems)	1 pear	141	83	85	1	1	—	—	—	22	11	16	.4	83	30	.03	.06	.1	6
293	D'Anjou, 3-in. diam. (about 2 per lb with cores and stems)	1 pear	200	83	120	1	1	—	—	—	31	16	22	.6	260	40	.04	.08	.2	8
294	Canned, solids and liquid, sirup pack, heavy (halves or slices)	1 cup	255	80	195	1	1	—	—	—	50	13	18	.5	214	10	.03	.05	.3	3
	Pineapple:																			
295	Raw, diced	1 cup	155	85	80	1	*	—	—	—	21	26	12	.8	226	110	.14	.05	.3	26

Item No.	Foods, approximate measures, units, and weight (edible part unless footnotes indicate otherwise) — Serving	Weight (g)	Water (%)	Food Energy (Cal.)	Protein (g)	Fat (g)	Fatty Acids Saturated (total) (g)	Unsaturated Oleic (g)	Linoleic (g)	Carbohydrate (g)	Calcium (mg)	Phosphorus (mg)	Iron (mg)	Potassium (mg)	Vitamin A value (I.U.)	Thiamin (mg)	Riboflavin (mg)	Niacin (mg)	Ascorbic acid (mg)
	Canned, heavy sirup pack, solids and liquid:																		
296	Crushed, chunks, tidbits — 1 cup	255	80	190	1	*	—	—	—	49	28	13	.8	245	130	.20	.05	.5	18
	Slices and liquid:																		
297	Large — 1 slice; 2¼ tbsp liquid.	105	80	80	*	*	—	—	—	20	12	5	.3	101	50	.08	.02	.2	7
298	Medium — 1 slice; 1¼ tbsp liquid.	58	80	45	*	*	—	—	—	11	6	3	.2	56	30	.05	.01	.1	4
299	Pineapple juice, unsweetened, canned — 1 cup	250	86	140	1	*	—	—	—	34	38	23	.8	373	130	.13	.05	.5	80^aa
	Plums: Raw, without pits:																		
300	Japanese and hybrid (2⅛-in. diam., about 6½ per lb with pits) — 1 plum	66	87	30	*	*	—	—	—	8	8	12	.3	112	160	.02	.02	.3	4
301	Prune-type (1½-in. diam., about 15 per lb with pits) — 1 plum	28	79	20	*	*	—	—	—	6	3	5	.1	48	80	.01	.01	.1	1
	Canned, heavy sirup pack (Italian prunes), with pits and liquid:																		
302	Cup — 1 cup	272ʲ	77	215	1	*	—	—	—	56	23	26	2.3	367	3130	.05	.05	1.0	5
303	Portion — 3 plums; 2¾ tbsp liquid	140ʲ	77	110	1	*	—	—	—	29	12	13	1.2	189	1610	.03	.03	.5	3
	Prunes, dried, "softenized," with pits:																		
304	Uncooked — 4 extra large or 5 large prunes	49ʲ	28	110	1	*	—	—	—	29	22	34	1.7	298	690	.04	.07	.7	1
305	Cooked, unsweetened, all sizes, fruit and liquid — 1 cup	250ʲ	66	255	2	1	—	—	—	67	51	79	3.8	695	1590	.07	.15	1.5	2
306	Prune juice, canned or bottled — 1 cup	256	80	195	1	*	—	—	—	49	36	51	1.8	602	—	.03	.03	1.0	5
	Raisins, seedless:																		
307	Cup, not pressed down — 1 cup	145	18	420	4	*	—	—	—	112	90	146	5.1	1106	30	.16	.12	.7	1
308	Packet, ½ oz (1½ tbsp) — 1 packet	14	18	40	*	*	—	—	—	11	9	14	.5	107	*	.02	.01	.1	*
	Raspberries, red:																		
309	Raw, capped, whole — 1 cup	123	84	70	1	1	—	—	—	17	27	27	1.1	207	160	.04	.11	1.1	31
310	Frozen, sweetened, 10-oz container — 1 container	284	74	280	2	1	—	—	—	70	37	48	1.7	284	200	.06	.17	1.7	60
	Rhubarb, cooked, added sugar:																		
311	From raw — 1 cup	270	63	380	1	*	—	—	—	97	211	41	1.6	548	220	.05	.14	.8	16
312	From frozen, sweetened — 1 cup	270	63	385	1	1	—	—	—	98	211	32	1.9	475	190	.05	.11	.5	16
	Strawberries:																		
313	Raw, whole berries, capped — 1 cup	149	90	55	1	1	—	—	—	13	31	31	1.5	244	90	.04	.10	.9	88
	Frozen, sweetened:																		
314	Sliced, 10-oz container — 1 container	284	71	310	1	1	—	—	—	79	40	48	2.0	318	90	.06	.17	1.4	151
315	Whole, 1-lb container (about 1¾ cups) — 1 container	454	76	415	2	1	—	—	—	107	59	73	2.7	472	140	.09	.27	2.3	249
316	Tangerine, raw, 2⅜-in. diam., size 176, without peel (about 4 per lb with peels and seeds) — 1 tangerine	86	87	40	1	*	—	—	—	10	34	15	.3	108	360	.05	.02	.1	27

Item No.	Foods, approximate measures, units	Grams	Water (%)	Food energy (cal)	Protein (g)	Fat (g)	Saturated (g)	Oleic (g)	Linoleic (g)	Carbohydrate (g)	Calcium (mg)	Phosphorus (mg)	Iron (mg)	Potassium (mg)	Vitamin A (IU)	Thiamin (mg)	Riboflavin (mg)	Niacin (mg)	Ascorbic acid (mg)
317	Tangerine juice, canned, sweetened. 1 cup	249	87	125	1	*	—	—	—	30	44	35	.5	440	1040	.15	.05	.2	54
318	Watermelon, raw, 4 by 8 in. wedge with rind and seeds (1/16 of 32 2/3-lb melon, 10 by 16 in.). 1 wedge with rind and seeds	926	93	110	2	1	—	—	—	27	30	43	2.1	426	2510	.13	.13	.9	30

Grain products

Item No.	Foods, approximate measures, units	Grams	Water (%)	Food energy (cal)	Protein (g)	Fat (g)	Saturated (g)	Oleic (g)	Linoleic (g)	Carbohydrate (g)	Calcium (mg)	Phosphorus (mg)	Iron (mg)	Potassium (mg)	Vitamin A (IU)	Thiamin (mg)	Riboflavin (mg)	Niacin (mg)	Ascorbic acid (mg)
	Bagel, 3-in. diam.:																		
319	Egg. 1 bagel	55	32	165	6	2	0.5	0.9	0.8	28	9	43	1.2	41	30	.14	.10	1.2	0
320	Water. 1 bagel	55	29	165	6	1	.2	.4	.6	30	8	41	1.2	42	0	.15	.11	1.4	0
321	Barley, pearled, light, uncooked. 1 cup	200	11	700	16	2	.3	.2	.8	158	32	378	4.0	320	0	.24	.10	6.2	0
	Biscuits, baking powder, 2-in. diam. (enriched flour, vegetable shortening):																		
322	From home recipe. 1 biscuit	28	27	105	2	5	1.2	2.0	1.2	13	34	49	.4	33	*	.08	.08	.7	*
323	From mix. 1 biscuit	28	29	90	2	3	.6	1.1	.7	15	19	65	.6	32	*	.09	.08	.8	*
324	Breadcrumbs (enriched): Dry, grated. 1 cup	100	7	390	13	5	1.0	1.6	1.4	73	122	141	3.6	152	*	.35	.35	4.8	*
	Soft. See White bread (items 349–350).																		
	Breads:																		
325	Boston brown bread, canned, slice, 3 1/4 by 1/2 in. 1 slice	45	45	95	2	1	.1	.2	.2	21	41	72	.9	131	0	.06	.04	.7	0
	Cracked-wheat bread (3/4 enriched wheat flour, 1/4 cracked wheat):																		
326	Loaf, 1 lb. 1 loaf	454	35	1195	39	10	2.2	3.0	3.9	236	399	581	9.5	608	*	1.52	1.13	14.4	*
327	Slice (18 per loaf). 1 slice	25	35	65	2	1	.1	.2	.2	13	22	32	.5	34	*	.08	.06	.8	*
328	French or Vienna bread, enriched: Loaf, 1 lb. 1 loaf	454	31	1315	41	14	3.2	4.7	4.6	251	195	386	10.0	408	*	1.80	1.10	15.0	*
	Slice:																		
329	French (5 by 2 1/2 by 1 in.). 1 slice	35	31	100	3	1	.2	.4	.4	19	15	30	.8	32	*	.14	.08	1.2	*
330	Vienna (4 3/4 by 4 by 1/2 in.). 1 slice	25	31	75	2	1	.2	.3	.3	14	11	21	.6	23	*	.10	.06	.8	*
331	Italian bread, enriched: Loaf, 1 lb. 1 loaf	454	32	1250	41	4	.6	.3	1.5	256	77	349	10.0	336	0	1.80	1.10	15.0	0
332	Slice, 4 1/2 by 3 1/4 by 3/4 in. 1 slice	30	32	85	3	*	*	*	.1	17	5	23	.7	22	0	.12	.07	1.0	0
333	Raisin bread, enriched: Loaf, 1 lb. 1 loaf	454	35	1190	30	13	3.0	4.7	3.9	243	322	395	10.0	1,057	*	1.70	1.07	10.7	*
334	Slice (18 per loaf). 1 slice	25	35	65	2	1	.2	.3	.2	13	18	22	.6	58	*	.09	.06	.6	*
	Rye bread:																		
335	American, light (2/3 enriched wheat flour, 1/3 rye flour): Loaf, 1 lb. 1 loaf	454	36	1100	41	5	.7	.5	2.2	236	340	667	9.1	658	0	1.35	.98	12.9	0
336	Slice (4 3/4 by 3 3/4 by 7/16 in.). 1 slice	25	36	60	2	*	*	*	.1	13	19	37	.5	36	0	.07	.05	.7	0
337	Pumpernickel (2/3 rye flour, 1/3 enriched wheat flour): Loaf, 1 lb. 1 loaf	454	34	1115	41	5	.7	.5	2.4	241	381	1039	11.8	2059	0	1.30	.93	8.5	0
338	Slice (5 by 4 by 3/8 in.). 1 slice	32	34	80	3	*	.1	*	.2	17	27	73	.8	145	0	.09	.07	.6	0
	White bread, enriched: Soft-crumb type:																		
339	Loaf, 1 lb. 1 loaf	454	36	1225	39	15	3.4	5.3	4.6	229	381	440	11.3	476	*	1.80	1.10	15.0	*
340	Slice (18 per loaf). 1 slice	25	36	70	2	2	.2	.3	.3	13	21	24	.6	26	*	.10	.06	.8	*
341	Slice, toasted. 1 slice	22	25	70	2	2	.2	.3	.3	13	21	24	.6	26	*	.08	.06	.8	*
342	Slice (22 per loaf). 1 slice	20	36	55	2	1	.2	.2	.2	10	17	19	.5	21	*	.08	.05	.7	*
343	Slice, toasted. 1-slice	17	25	55	2	1	.2	.2	.2	10	17	19	.5	21	*	.06	.05	.7	*
344	Loaf, 1 1/2 lb. 1 loaf	680	36	1835	59	22	5.2	7.9	6.9	343	571	660	17.0	714	*	2.70	1.65	22.5	*
345	Slice (24 per loaf). 1 slice	28	36	75	2	1	.2	.3	.3	14	24	27	.7	29	*	.11	.07	.9	*
346	Slice, toasted. 1 slice	24	25	75	2	1	.2	.3	.3	14	24	27	.7	29	*	.09	.07	.9	*
347	Slice (28 per loaf). 1 slice	24	36	65	2	1	.2	.3	.2	12	20	23	.6	25	*	.10	.06	.8	*

Appendix D
Nutritive Values of the Edible Part of Foods (Continued)

Item No.	Foods, approximate measures, units, and weight (edible part unless footnotes indicate otherwise) — Serving	Weight (g.)	Water (%)	Food Energy (Cal.)	Protein (g)	Fat (g)	Saturated (total) (g)	Oleic (g)	Linoleic (g)	Carbohydrate (g)	Calcium (mg)	Phosphorus (mg)	Iron (mg)	Potassium (mg)	Vitamin A value (I.U.)	Thiamin (mg)	Riboflavin (mg)	Niacin (mg)	Ascorbic acid (mg)
348	Slice, toasted — 1 slice	21	25	65	2	1	.2	.3	.2	12	20	23	.6	25	*	.08	.06	.8	*
349	Cubes — 1 cup	30	36	80	3	1	.2	.3	.3	15	25	29	.8	32	*	.12	.07	1.0	*
350	Crumbs — 1 cup	45	36	120	4	1	.3	.5	.5	23	38	44	1.1	47	*	.18	.11	1.5	*
	Firm-crumb type:																		
351	Loaf, 1 lb — 1 loaf	454	35	1245	41	17	3.9	5.9	5.2	228	435	463	11.3	549	*	1.80	1.10	15.0	*
352	Slice (20 per loaf) — 1 slice	23	35	65	2	1	.2	.3	.3	12	22	23	.6	28	*	.09	.06	.8	*
353	Slice, toasted — 1 slice	20	24	65	2	1	.2	.3	.3	12	22	23	.6	28	*	.07	.06	.8	*
354	Loaf, 2 lb — 1 loaf	907	35	2495	82	34	7.7	11.8	10.4	455	871	925	22.7	1097	*	3.60	2.20	30.0	*
355	Slice (34 per loaf) — 1 slice	27	35	75	2	1	.2	.3	.3	14	26	28	.7	33	*	.11	.06	.9	*
356	Slice, toasted — 1 slice	23	24	75	2	1	.2	.3	.3	14	26	28	.7	33	*	.09	.06	.9	*
	Whole-wheat bread:																		
	Soft-crumb type:[//]																		
357	Loaf, 1 lb — 1 loaf	454	36	1095	41	12	2.2	2.9	4.2	224	381	1152	13.6	1161	*	1.37	.45	12.7	*
358	Slice (16 per loaf) — 1 slice	28	36	65	3	1	.1	.2	.2	14	24	71	.8	72	*	.09	.03	.8	*
359	Slice, toasted — 1 slice	24	24	65	3	1	.1	.2	.2	14	24	71	.8	72	*	.07	.03	.8	*
	Firm-crumb type:[//]																		
360	Loaf, 1 lb — 1 loaf	454	36	1100	48	14	2.5	3.3	4.9	216	449	1034	13.6	1238	*	1.17	.54	12.7	*
361	Slice (18 per loaf) — 1 slice	25	36	60	3	1	.1	.2	.3	12	25	57	.8	68	*	.06	.03	.7	*
362	Slice, toasted — 1 slice	21	24	60	3	1	.1	.2	.3	12	25	57	.8	68	*	.05	.03	.7	*
	Breakfast cereals:																		
	Hot type, cooked:																		
	Corn (hominy) grits, degermed:																		
363	Enriched — 1 cup	245	87	125	3	*	*	*	.1	27	2	25	.7	27	*[m]	.10	.07	1.0	0
364	Unenriched — 1 cup	245	87	125	3	*	*	*	.1	27	2	25	.2	27	*[m]	.05	.02	.5	0
365	Farina, quick-cooking, enriched — 1 cup	245	89	105	3	*	*	*	.1	22	147	113[oo]	(pp)	25	0	.12	.07	1.0	0
366	Oatmeal or rolled oats — 1 cup	240	87	130	5	2	.4	.8	.9	23	22	137	1.4	146	0	.19	.05	.2	0
367	Wheat, rolled — 1 cup	240	80	180	5	1	—	—	—	41	19	182	1.7	202	0	.17	.07	2.2	0
368	Wheat, whole-meal — 1 cup	245	88	110	4	1	—	—	—	23	17	127	1.2	118	0	.15	.05	1.5	0
	Ready-to-eat:																		
369	Bran flakes (40% bran), added sugar, salt, iron, vitamins — 1 cup	35	3	105	4	1	—	—	—	28	19	125	5.6	137	1540	.46	.52	6.2	0
370	Bran flakes with raisins, added sugar, salt, iron, vitamins — 1 cup	50	7	145	4	1	—	—	—	40+	28	146	7.9	154	2200[qq]	(")	(")	(")	0
	Corn flakes:																		
371	Plain, added sugar, salt, iron, vitamins — 1 cup	25	4	95	2	*	—	—	—	21	(")	9	(")	30	(")	(")	(")	(")	13[qq]
372	Sugar-coated, added salt, iron, vitamins — 1 cup	40	2	155	2	*	—	—	—	37	1	10	(")	27	1760	.53	.50	7.1	21[qq]
373	Corn, oat flour, puffed, added sugar, salt, iron, vitamins — 1 cup	20	4	80	2	1	—	—	—	16	4	18	5.7	—	880	.26	.30	3.5	11
374	Corn, shredded, added sugar, salt, iron, thiamin, niacin — 1 cup	25	3	95	2	*	—	—	—	22	1	10	.6	—	0	.33	.05	4.4	13
375	Oats, puffed, added sugar, salt, minerals, vitamins — 1 cup	25	3	100	3	1	—	—	—	19	44	102	4.0	—	1100	.33	.38	4.4	13

Item No.	Food	Measure	Grams	Water (%)	Food energy (cal)	Protein (g)	Fat (g)	Saturated (g)	Oleic (g)	Linoleic (g)	Carbohydrate (g)	Calcium (mg)	Phosphorus (mg)	Iron (mg)	Potassium (mg)	Vitamin A (IU)	Thiamin (mg)	Riboflavin (mg)	Niacin (mg)	Ascorbic acid (mg)
	Rice, puffed:																			
376	Plain, added iron, thiamin, niacin	1 cup	15	4	60	1	*	—	—	—	13	3	14	.3	15	0	.07	.01	.7	0
377	Presweetened, added salt, iron, vitamins	1 cup	28	3	115	1	0	—	—	—	26	3	14	(")	43	1240[qq]	(")	(")	(")	15[qq]
378	Wheat flakes, added sugar, salt, iron, vitamins	1 cup	30	4	105	3	*	—	—	—	24	12	83	4.8	81	1320	.40	.45	5.3	16
	Wheat, puffed:																			
379	Plain, added iron, thiamin, niacin, vitamins	1 cup	15	3	55	2	*	—	—	—	12	4	48	.6	51	0	.08	.03	1.2	0[qq]
380	Presweetened, added salt, iron, vitamins	1 cup	38	3	140	3	*	—	—	—	33	7	52	(")	63	1680	.50	.57	6.7	20[qq]
381	Wheat, shredded, plain	1 oblong biscuit or 1/2 cup spoon-size biscuits	25	7	90	2	1	—	—	—	20	11	97	.9	87	0	.06	.03	1.1	0
382	Wheat germ, without salt and sugar, toasted	1 tbsp	6	4	25	2	1	—	—	—	3	3	70	.5	57	10	.11	.05	.3	1
383	Buckwheat flour, light, sifted	1 cup	98	12	340	6	1	0.2	0.4	0.4	78	11	86	1.0	314	0	.08	.04	.4	0
384	Bulgur, canned, seasoned	1 cup	135	56	245	8	4	—	—	—	44	27	263	1.9	151	0	.08	.05	4.1	0
	Cake icings. See Sugars and Sweets (items 532–536).																			
	Cakes made from cake mixes with enriched flour:[ss]																			
	Angelfood:																			
385	Whole cake (9 3/4-in.-diam. tube cake)	1 cake	635	34	1645	36	1	—	—	—	377	603	756	2.5	381	0	.37	.95	3.6	0
386	Piece, 1/12 of cake	1 piece	53	34	135	3	*	—	—	—	32	50	63	.2	32	0	.03	.08	.3	0
	Coffeecake:																			
387	Whole cake (7 3/4 by 5 5/8 by 1 1/4 in.)	1 cake	430	30	1385	27	41	11.7	16.3	8.8	225	262	748	6.9	469	690	.82	.91	7.7	1
388	Piece, 1/6 of cake	1 piece	72	30	230	5	7	2.0	2.7	1.5	38	44	125	1.2	78	120	.14	.15	1.3	*
	Cupcakes, made with egg, milk, 2 1/2-in. diam.:																			
389	Without icing	1 cupcake	25	26	90	1	3	.8	1.2	.7	14	40	59	.3	21	40	.05	.05	.4	*
390	With chocolate icing	1 cupcake	36	22	130	2	5	2.0	1.6	.6	21	47	71	.4	42	60	.05	.06	.4	*
	Devil's food with chocolate icing:																			
391	Whole, 2-layer cake (8- or 9-in. diam.)	1 cake	1107	24	3755	49	136	50.0	44.9	17.0	645	653	1162	16.6	1439	1660	1.06	1.65	10.1	1
392	Piece, 1/16 of cake	1 piece	69	24	235	3	8	3.1	2.8	1.1	40	41	72	1.0	90	100	.07	.10	.6	*
393	Cupcake, 2 1/2-in. diam.	1 cupcake	35	24	120	2	4	1.6	1.4	.5	20	21	37	.5	46	50	.03	.05	.3	*
	Gingerbread:																			
394	Whole cake (8-in. square)	1 cake	570	37	1575	18	39	9.7	16.6	10.0	291	513	570	8.6	1562	*	.84	1.00	7.4	*
395	Piece, 1/9 of cake	1 piece	63	37	175	2	4	1.1	1.8	1.1	32	57	63	.9	173	*	.09	.11	.8	*
	White, 2 layer with chocolate icing:																			
396	Whole cake (8- or 9-in. diam.)	1 cake	1140	21	4000	44	122	48.2	46.4	20.0	716	1129	2041	11.4	1322	680	1.50	1.77	12.5	2
397	Piece, 1/16 of cake	1 piece	71	21	250	3	8	3.0	2.9	1.2	45	70	127	.7	82	40	.09	.11	.8	*
	Yellow, 2 layer with chocolate icing:																			

Appendix D
Nutritive Values of the Edible Part of Foods (Continued)

Nutrients in Indicated Quantity

Item No.	Foods, approximate measures, units, and weight (edible part unless footnotes indicate otherwise) / Serving	Weight (g)	Water (%)	Food Energy (Cal)	Protein (g)	Fat (g)	Fatty Acids Saturated (total) (g)	Unsaturated Oleic (g)	Unsaturated Linoleic (g)	Carbohydrate (g)	Calcium (mg)	Phosphorus (mg)	Iron (mg)	Potassium (mg)	Vitamin A value (I.U.)	Thiamin (mg)	Riboflavin (mg)	Niacin (mg)	Ascorbic acid (mg)
398	Whole cake (8- or 9-in. diam.), 1 cake	1108	26	3735	45	125	47.8	47.8	20.3	638	1,008	2017	12.2	1208	1550	1.24	1.67	10.6	2
399	Piece, 1/16 of cake, 1 piece	69	26	235	3	8	3.0	3.0	1.3	40	63	126	.8	75	100	.08	.10	.7	*
	Cakes made from home recipes using enriched flour:[u]																		
	Boston cream pie with custard filling:																			
400	Whole cake (8-in. diam.), 1 cake	825	35	2490	41	78	23.0	30.1	15.2	412	553	833	8.2	734[w]	1730	1.04	1.27	9.6	2
401	Piece, 1/12 of cake, 1 piece	69	35	210	3	6	1.9	2.5	1.3	34	46	70	.7	61[w]	140	.09	.11	.8	*
	Fruitcake, dark:																			
402	Loaf, 1-lb (7½ by 2 by 1½ in.), 1 loaf	454	18	1720	22	69	14.4	33.5	14.8	271	327	513	11.8	2250	540	.72	.73	4.9	2
403	Slice, 1/30 of loaf, 1 slice	15	18	55	1	2	.5	1.1	.5	9	11	17	.4	74	20	.02	.02	.2	*
	Plain, sheet cake:																			
	Without icing:																			
404	Whole cake (9-in. square), 1 cake	777	25	2830	35	108	29.5	44.4	23.9	434	497	793	8.5	614[w]	1320	1.21	1.40	10.2	2
405	Piece, 1/9 of cake, 1 piece	86	25	315	4	12	3.3	4.9	2.6	48	55	88	.9	68[w]	150	.13	.15	1.1	*
	With uncooked white icing:																			
406	Whole cake (9-in. square), 1 cake	1096	21	4020	37	129	42.2	49.5	24.4	694	548	822	8.2	669[w]	2190	1.22	1.47	10.2	2
407	Piece, 1/9 of cake, 1 piece	121	21	445	4	14	4.7	5.5	2.7	77	61	91	.8	74[w]	240	.14	.16	1.1	*
	Pound:[v]																			
408	Loaf, 8½ by 3½ by 3¼ in., 1 loaf	565	16	2725	31	170	42.9	73.1	39.6	273	107	418	7.9	345	1410	.90	.99	7.3	0
409	Slice, 1/17 of loaf, 1 slice	33	16	160	2	10	2.5	4.3	2.3	16	6	24	.5	20	80	.05	.06	.4	0
	Spongecake:																			
410	Whole cake (9¾-in.-diam. tube cake), 1 cake	790	32	2345	60	45	13.1	15.8	5.7	427	237	885	13.4	687	3560	1.10	1.64	7.4	*
411	Piece, 1/12 of cake, 1 piece	66	32	195	5	4	1.1	1.3	.5	36	20	74	1.1	57	300	.09	.14	.6	*
	Cookies made with enriched flour:[ww,xx]																			
	Brownies with nuts:																			
	Home-prepared, 1¾ by 1¾ by ⅞ in.:																			
412	From home recipe, 1 brownie	20	10	95	1	6	1.5	3.0	1.2	10	8	30	.4	38	40	.04	.03	.2	*
413	From commercial recipe, 1 brownie	20	11	85	1	4	.9	1.4	1.3	13	9	27	.4	34	20	.03	.02	.2	*
414	Frozen, with chocolate icing,[yy] 1½ by 1¾ by ⅞ in., 1 brownie	25	13	105	1	5	2.0	2.2	.7	15	10	31	.4	44	50	.03	.03	.2	*
	Chocolate chip:																			
415	Commercial, 2¼-in. diam., ⅜ in. thick, 4 cookies	42	3	200	2	9	2.8	2.9	2.2	29	16	48	1.0	56	50	.10	.17	.9	*
416	From home recipe, 2⅓-in. diam., 4 cookies	40	3	205	2	12	3.5	4.5	2.9	24	14	40	.8	47	40	.06	.06	.5	*
417	Fig bars, square (1⅝ by 1⅝ by ⅜ in.) or rectangular (1½ by 1¾ by ½ in.), 4 cookies	56	14	200	2	3	.8	1.2	.7	42	44	34	1.0	111	60	.04	.14	.9	*
418	Gingersnaps, 2-in. diam., ¼ in. thick, 4 cookies	28	3	90	2	2	.7	1.0	.6	22	20	13	.7	129	20	.08	.06	.7	0
419	Macaroons, 2¾-in. diam., ¼ in. thick, 2 cookies	38	4	180	2	9	—	—	—	25	10	32	.3	176	0	.02	.06	.2	0
420	Oatmeal with raisins, 2⅝-in. diam., ¼ in. thick, 4 cookies	52	3	235	3	8	2.0	3.3	2.0	38	11	53	1.4	192	30	.15	.10	1.0	*
421	Plain, prepared from commercial chilled dough, 2½-in. diam., ¼ in. thick, 4 cookies	48	5	240	2	12	3.0	5.2	2.9	31	17	35	.6	23	30	.10	.08	.9	0

No.	Food, approximate measure, and weight	Measure	Grams	Water (%)	Food energy (Cal)	Protein (g)	Fat (g)	Saturated (g)	Oleic (g)	Linoleic (g)	Carbo-hydrate (g)	Calcium (mg)	Phos-phorus (mg)	Iron (mg)	Potas-sium (mg)	Vitamin A (IU)	Thiamin (mg)	Riboflavin (mg)	Niacin (mg)	Ascorbic acid (mg)
422	Sandwich type (chocolate or vanilla), 1¾-in. diam., ⅜ in. thick	4 cookies	40	2	200	2	9	2.2	3.9	2.2	28	10	96	.7	15	0	.06	.10	.7	0
423	Vanilla wafers, 1¾-in. diam., ¼-in. thick	10 cookies	40	3	185	3	6	—	—	—	30	16	25	.6	29	50	.10	.09	.8	0
	Cornmeal:																			
424	Whole-ground, unbolted, dry form	1 cup	122	12	435	11	5	.5	1.0	2.5	90	24	312	2.9	346	620[zz]	.46	.13	2.4	0
425	Bolted (nearly whole-grain), dry form	1 cup	122	12	440	11	4	.5	.9	2.1	91	21	272	2.2	303	590[zz]	.37	.10	2.3	0
	Degermed, enriched:																			
426	Dry form	1 cup	138	12	500	11	2	.2	.4	.9	108	8	137	4.0	166	610[zz]	.61	.36	4.8	0
427	Cooked	1 cup	240	88	120	3	*	*	.1	.2	26	2	34	1.0	38	140[zz]	.14	.10	1.2	0
	Degermed, unenriched:																			
428	Dry form	1 cup	138	12	500	11	2	.2	.4	.9	108	8	137	1.5	166	610[zz]	.19	.07	1.4	0
429	Cooked	1 cup	240	88	120	3	*	*	.1	.2	26	2	34	.5	38	140[zz]	.05	.02	.2	0
	Crackers:[ll]																			
430	Graham, plain, 2½-in. square	2 crackers	14	6	55	1	1	.3	.5	.3	10	6	21	.5	55	0	.02	.08	.5	0
431	Rye wafers, whole-grain, 1⅞ by 3½ in.	2 wafers	13	6	45	2	*	—	—	—	10	7	50	.5	78	0	.04	.03	.2	0
432	Saltines, made with enriched flour	4 crackers or 1 packet	11	4	50	1	1	.3	.5	.4	8	2	10	.5	13	0	.05	.05	.4	0
	Danish pastry (enriched flour), plain without fruit or nuts:[aaa]																			
433	Packaged ring, 12 oz	1 ring	340	22	1435	25	80	24.3	31.7	16.5	155	170	371	6.1	381	1050	.97	1.01	8.6	*
434	Round piece, about 4¼-in. diam. by 1 in.	1 pastry	65	22	275	5	15	4.7	6.1	3.2	30	33	71	1.2	73	200	.18	.19	1.7	*
435	Ounce	1 oz	28	22	120	2	7	2.0	2.7	1.4	13	14	31	.5	32	90	.08	.08	.7	*
	Doughnuts, made with enriched flour:[ll]																			
436	Cake type, plain, 2½-in. diam., 1 in. high	1 doughnut	25	24	100	1	5	1.2	2.0	1.1	13	10	48	.4	23	20	.05	.05	.4	*
437	Yeast-leavened, glazed, 3¾-in. diam., 1¼ in. high	1 doughnut	50	26	205	3	11	3.3	5.8	3.3	22	16	33	.6	34	25	.10	.10	.8	0
	Macaroni, enriched, cooked (cut lengths, elbows, shells):																			
438	Firm stage (hot)	1 cup	130	64	190	7	1	—	—	—	39	14	85	1.4	103	0	.23	.13	1.8	0
	Tender stage:																			
439	Cold macaroni	1 cup	105	73	115	4	*	—	—	—	24	8	53	.9	64	0	.15	.08	1.2	0
440	Hot macaroni	1 cup	140	73	155	5	1	—	—	—	32	11	70	1.3	85	0	.20	.11	1.5	0
	Macaroni (enriched) and cheese:																			
441	Canned[bbb]	1 cup	240	80	230	9	10	4.2	3.1	1.4	26	199	182	1.0	139	260	.12	.24	1.0	*
442	From home recipe (served hot)[ccc]	1 cup	200	58	430	17	22	8.9	8.8	2.9	40	362	322	1.8	240	860	.20	.40	1.8	*
	Muffins made with enriched flour:[ll]																			
	From home recipe:																			
443	Blueberry, 2⅜-in. diam., 1½ in. high	1 muffin	40	39	110	3	4	1.1	1.4	.7	17	34	53	.6	46	90	.09	.10	.7	*
444	Bran	1 muffin	40	35	105	3	4	1.2	1.4	.8	17	57	162	1.5	172	90	.07	.10	1.7	*
445	Corn (enriched degermed cornmeal and flour), 2⅜-in. diam., 1½ in. high	1 muffin	40	33	125	3	4	1.2	1.6	.9	19	42	68	.7	54	120[ddd]	.10	.10	.7	*
446	Plain, 3-in. diam., 1½ in. high	1 muffin	40	38	120	3	4	1.0	1.7	1.0	17	42	60	.6	50	40	.09	.12	.9	*
	From mix, egg, milk:																			
447	Corn, 2⅜-in. diam., 1½ in. high[eee]	1 muffin	40	30	130	3	4	1.2	1.7	.9	20	96	152	.6	44	100[ddd]	.08	.09	.7	*
448	Noodles (egg noodles), enriched, cooked	1 cup	160	71	200	7	2	—	—	—	37	16	94	1.4	70	110	.22	.13	1.9	0
449	Noodles, chow mein, canned	1 cup	45	1	220	6	11	—	—	—	26	—	—	—	—	—	—	—	—	—
450	Pancakes (4-in. diam.):[ll] Buckwheat, made from mix (with buckwheat and enriched flours), egg and milk added	1 cake	27	58	55	2	2	.8	.9	.4	6	59	91	.4	66	60	.04	.05	.2	*
	Plain:																			
451	Made from home recipe using enriched flour	1 cake	27	50	60	2	2	.5	.8	.5	9	27	38	.4	33	30	.06	.07	.5	*
452	Made from mix with enriched flour, egg and milk added	1 cake	27	51	60	2	2	.7	.7	.3	9	58	70	.3	42	70	.04	.06	.2	*

Appendix D
Nutritive Values of the Edible Part of Foods (Continued)

Item No.	Foods, approximate measures, units, and weight (edible part unless footnotes indicate otherwise)	Serving	Weight (g)	Water (%)	Food Energy (Cal.)	Protein (g)	Fat (g)	Saturated (total) (g)	Unsaturated Oleic (g)	Unsaturated Linoleic (g)	Carbohydrate (g)	Calcium (mg)	Phosphorus (mg)	Iron (mg)	Potassium (mg)	Vitamin A value (I.U.)	Thiamin (mg)	Riboflavin (mg)	Niacin (mg)	Ascorbic acid (mg)
	Pies, piecrust made with enriched flour, vegetable shortening (9-in. diam.):																			
	Apple:																			
453	Whole	1 pie	945	48	2420	21	105	27.0	44.5	25.2	360	76	208	6.6	756	280	1.06	.79	9.3	9
454	Sector, 1/7 of pie	1 sector	135	48	345	3	15	3.9	6.4	3.6	51	11	30	.9	108	40	.15	.11	1.3	2
	Banana cream:																			
455	Whole	1 pie	910	54	2010	41	85	26.7	33.2	16.2	279	601	746	7.3	1847	2280	.77	1.51	7.0	9
456	Sector, 1/7 of pie	1 sector	130	54	285	6	12	3.8	4.7	2.3	40	86	107	1.0	264	330	.11	.22	1.0	1
	Blueberry:																			
457	Whole	1 pie	945	51	2285	23	102	24.8	43.7	25.1	330	104	217	9.5	614	280	1.03	.80	10.0	28
458	Sector, 1/7 of pie	1 sector	135	51	325	3	15	3.5	6.2	3.6	47	15	31	1.4	88	40	.15	.11	1.4	4
	Cherry:																			
459	Whole	1 pie	945	47	2465	25	107	28.2	45.0	25.3	363	132	236	6.6	992	4160	1.09	.84	9.8	*
460	Sector, 1/7 of pie	1 sector	135	47	350	4	15	4.0	6.4	3.6	52	19	34	.9	142	590	.16	.12	1.4	*
	Custard:																			
461	Whole	1 pie	910	58	1985	56	101	33.9	38.5	17.5	213	874	1,028	8.2	1247	2090	.79	1.92	5.6	0
462	Sector, 1/7 of pie	1 sector	130	58	285	8	14	4.8	5.5	2.5	30	125	147	1.2	178	300	.11	.27	.8	0
	Lemon meringue:																			
463	Whole	1 pie	840	47	2140	31	86	26.1	33.8	16.4	317	118	412	6.7	420	1430	.61	.84	5.2	25
464	Sector, 1/7 of pie	1 sector	120	47	305	4	12	3.7	4.8	2.3	45	17	59	1.0	60	200	.09	.12	.7	4
	Mince:																			
465	Whole	1 pie	945	43	2560	24	109	28.0	45.9	25.2	389	265	359	13.3	1682	20	.96	.86	9.8	9
466	Sector, 1/7 of pie	1 sector	135	43	365	3	16	4.0	6.6	3.6	56	38	51	1.9	240	*	.14	.12	1.4	1
	Peach:																			
467	Whole	1 pie	945	48	2410	24	101	24.8	43.7	25.1	361	95	274	8.5	1408	6900	1.04	.97	14.0	28
468	Sector, 1/7 of pie	1 sector	135	48	345	3	14	3.5	6.2	3.6	52	14	39	1.2	201	990	.15	.14	2.0	4
	Pecan:																			
469	Whole	1 pie	825	20	3450	42	189	27.8	101.0	44.2	423	388	850	25.6	1015	1320	1.80	.95	6.9	*
470	Sector, 1/7 of pie	1 sector	118	20	495	6	27	4.0	14.4	6.3	61	55	122	3.7	145	190	.26	.14	1.0	*
	Pumpkin:																			
471	Whole	1 pie	910	59	1920	36	102	37.4	37.5	16.6	223	464	628	7.3	1456	22,480	.78	1.27	7.0	*
472	Sector, 1/7 of pie	1 sector	130	59	275	5	15	5.4	5.4	2.4	32	66	90	1.0	208	3210	.11	.18	1.0	*
473	Piecrust (home recipe) made with enriched flour and vegetable shortening, baked	1 pie shell, 9-in. diam.	180	15	900	11	60	14.8	26.1	14.9	79	25	90	3.1	89	0	.47	.40	5.0	0
474	Piecrust mix with enriched flour and vegetable shortening, 10-oz pkg. prepared and baked	Piecrust for 2-crust pie, 9-in. diam.	320	19	1485	20	93	22.7	39.7	23.4	141	131	272	6.1	179	0	1.07	.79	9.9	0
475	Pizza (cheese) baked, 4³⁄₄-in. sector; ¹⁄₈ of 12-in.-diam. pie⁵	1 sector	60	45	145	6	4	1.7	1.5	.6	22	86	89	1.1	67	230	.16	.18	1.6	4
	Popcorn, popped:																			
476	Plain, large kernel	1 cup	6	4	25	1	*	*	.1	.2	5	1	17	.2	—	—	—	.01	.1	0
477	With oil (coconut) and salt added, large kernel	1 cup	9	3	40	1	2	1.5	.2	.2	5	1	19	.2	—	—	—	.01	.2	0

Item No.	Food, approximate measure	Grams	Water (%)	Food energy (cal)	Protein (g)	Fat (g)	Saturated fatty acids (g)	Oleic (g)	Linoleic (g)	Carbohydrate (g)	Calcium (mg)	Phosphorus (mg)	Iron (mg)	Potassium (mg)	Vitamin A (I.U.)	Thiamin (mg)	Riboflavin (mg)	Niacin (mg)	Ascorbic acid (mg)
478	Sugar-coated	1 cup	35	4	135	2	1	.5	.2	.4	30	2	47	.5	—	—	—	.02	.4	0
	Pretzels, made with enriched flour:																			
479	Dutch, twisted, 2¾ by 2⅝ in.	1 pretzel	16	5	60	2	1	—	—	—	12	4	21	.2	21	0	.05	.04	.7	0
480	Thin, twisted, 3¼ by 2¼ by ¼ in.	10 pretzels	60	5	235	6	3	—	—	—	46	13	79	.9	78	0	.20	.15	2.5	0
481	Stick, 2¼ in. long	10 pretzels	3	5	10	*	*	—	—	—	2	1	4	*	4	0	.01	.01	.1	0
	Rice, white, enriched:																			
	Instant, ready-to-serve, hot:																			
482		1 cup	165	73	180	4	*	*	*	*	40	5	31	1.3	—	0	.21	(ff)	1.7	0
	Long grain:																			
483	Raw	1 cup	185	12	670	12	1	.2	.2	.2	149	44	174	5.4	170	0	.81	.06	6.5	0
484	Cooked, served hot	1 cup	205	73	225	4	*	.1	.1	.1	50	21	57	1.8	57	0	.23	.02	2.1	0
	Parboiled:																			
485	Raw	1 cup	185	10	685	14	1	.2	.1	.2	150	111	370	5.4	278	0	.81	.07	6.5	0
486	Cooked, served hot	1 cup	175	73	185	4	*	.1	.1	.1	41	33	100	1.4	75	0	.19	.02	2.1	0
	Rolls, enriched:																			
	Commercial:																			
487	Brown-and-serve (12 per 12-oz pkg.), browned	1 roll	26	27	85	2	2	.4	.7	.5	14	20	23	.5	25	*	.10	.06	.9	*
488	Cloverleaf or pan, 2½-in. diam., 2 in. high	1 roll	28	31	85	2	2	.4	.6	.4	15	21	24	.5	27	*	.11	.07	.9	*
489	Frankfurter and hamburger (8 per 11½-oz pkg.)	1 roll	40	31	120	3	2	.5	.8	.6	21	30	34	.8	38	*	.16	.10	1.3	*
490	Hard, 3¾-in. diam., 2 in. high	1 roll	50	25	155	5	2	.4	.6	.5	30	24	46	1.2	49	*	.20	.12	1.7	*
491	Hoagie or submarine, 11½ by 3 by 2½ in.	1 roll	135	31	390	12	4	.9	1.4	1.4	75	58	115	3.0	122	*	.54	.32	4.5	*
	From home recipe:																			
492	Cloverleaf, 2½-in. diam., 2 in. high	1 roll	35	26	120	3	3	.8	1.1	.7	20	16	36	.7	41	30	.12	.12	1.2	*
	Spaghetti, enriched, cooked:																			
493	Firm stage, "al dente," served hot	1 cup	130	64	190	7	1	—	—	—	39	14	85	1.4	103	0	.23	.13	1.8	0
494	Tender stage, served hot	1 cup	140	73	155	5	1	—	—	—	32	11	70	1.3	85	0	.20	.11	1.5	0
	Spaghetti (enriched) in tomato sauce with cheese:																			
495	From home recipe	1 cup	250	77	260	9	9	2.0	5.4	.7	37	80	135	2.3	408	1,080	.25	.18	2.3	13
496	Canned	1 cup	250	80	190	6	2	.5	.3	.4	39	40	88	2.8	303	930	.35	.28	4.5	10
	Spaghetti (enriched) with meat balls and tomato sauce:																			
497	From home recipe	1 cup	248	70	330	19	12	3.3	6.3	.9	39	124	236	3.7	665	1,590	.25	.30	4.0	22
498	Canned	1 cup	250	78	260	12	10	2.2	3.3	3.9	29	53	113	3.3	245	1,000	.15	.18	2.3	5
499	Toaster pastries	1 pastry	50	12	200	3	6	—	—	—	36	54''	67''	1.9	74''	500	.16	.17	2.1	('')
	Waffles, made with enriched flour, 7-in. diam.:																			
500	From home recipe	1 waffle	75	41	210	7	7	2.3	2.8	1.4	28	85	130	1.3	109	250	.17	.23	1.4	*
501	From mix, egg and milk added	1 waffle	75	42	205	7	8	2.8	2.9	1.2	27	179	257	1.0	146	170	.14	.22	.9	*
	Wheat flours:																			
	All-purpose or family flour, enriched:																			
502	Sifted, spooned	1 cup	115	12	420	12	1	.2	.1	.5	88	18	100	3.3	109	0	.74	.46	6.1	0
503	Unsifted, spooned	1 cup	125	12	455	13	1	.2	.1	.5	95	20	109	3.6	119	0	.80	.50	6.6	0
504	Cake or pastry flour, enriched, sifted, spooned	1 cup	96	12	350	7	1	.1	.1	.3	76	16	70	2.8	91	0	.61	.38	5.1	0
505	Self-rising, enriched, unsifted, spooned	1 cup	125	12	440	12	1	.2	.1	.5	93	331	583	3.6	—	0	.80	.50	6.6	0
506	Whole-wheat, from hard wheats, stirred	1 cup	120	12	400	16	2	.4	.2	1.0	85	49	446	4.0	444	0	.66	.14	5.2	0

Legumes (dry), nuts, seeds, related products

Item No.	Food, approximate measure	Grams	Water (%)	Food energy (cal)	Protein (g)	Fat (g)	Saturated fatty acids (g)	Oleic (g)	Linoleic (g)	Carbohydrate (g)	Calcium (mg)	Phosphorus (mg)	Iron (mg)	Potassium (mg)	Vitamin A (I.U.)	Thiamin (mg)	Riboflavin (mg)	Niacin (mg)	Ascorbic acid (mg)
	Almonds, shelled:																			
507	Chopped (about 130 almonds)	1 cup	130	5	775	24	70	5.6	47.7	12.8	25	304	655	6.1	1005	0	.31	1.20	4.6	*
508	Slivered, not pressed down (about 115 almonds)	1 cup	115	5	690	21	62	5.0	42.2	11.3	22	269	580	5.4	889	0	.28	1.06	4.0	*

Appendix D
Nutritive Values of the Edible Part of Foods (Continued)

Item No.	Foods, approximate measures, units, and weight (edible part unless footnotes indicate otherwise) — Serving	Water (%)	Food Energy (Cal.)	Protein (g)	Fat (g)	Saturated (total) (g)	Oleic (g)	Linoleic (g)	Carbohydrate (g)	Calcium (mg)	Phosphorus (mg)	Iron (mg)	Potassium (mg)	Vitamin A value (I.U.)	Thiamin (mg)	Riboflavin (mg)	Niacin (mg)	Ascorbic acid (mg)
	Beans, dry:																	
	Common varieties as Great Northern, navy, and others:																	
	Cooked, drained:																	
509	Great Northern, 1 cup	69	210	14	1	—	—	—	38	90	266	4.9	749	0	.25	.13	1.3	0
510	Pea (navy), 1 cup	69	225	15	1	—	—	—	40	95	281	5.1	790	0	.27	.13	1.3	0
	Canned, solids and liquid:																	
	White with—																	
511	Frankfurters (sliced), 1 cup	71	365	19	18	—	—	—	32	94	303	4.8	668	330	.18	.15	3.3	*
512	Pork and tomato sauce, 1 cup	71	310	16	7	2.4	2.8	.6	48	138	235	4.6	536	330	.20	.08	1.5	5
513	Pork and sweet sauce, 1 cup	66	385	16	12	4.3	5.0	1.1	54	161	291	5.9	—	—	.15	.10	1.3	—
514	Red kidney, 1 cup	76	230	15	1	—	—	—	42	74	278	4.6	673	10	.13	.10	1.5	—
515	Lima, cooked, drained, 1 cup	64	260	16	1	—	—	—	49	55	293	5.9	1163	—	.25	.11	1.3	—
516	Blackeye peas, dry, cooked (with residual cooking liquid), 1 cup	80	190	13	1	—	—	—	35	43	238	3.3	573	30	.40	.10	1.0	—
517	Brazil nuts, shelled (6–8 large kernels), 1 oz	5	185	4	19	4.8	6.2	7.1	3	53	196	1.0	203	*	.27	.03	.5	—
518	Cashew nuts, roasted in oil, 1 cup	5	785	24	64	12.9	36.8	10.2	41	53	522	5.3	650	140	.60	.35	2.5	—
	Coconut meat, fresh:																	
519	Piece, about 2 by 2 by ½ in., 1 piece	51	155	2	16	14.0	.9	.3	4	6	43	.8	115	0	.02	.01	.2	1
520	Shredded or grated, not pressed down, 1 cup	51	275	3	28	24.8	1.6	.5	8	10	76	1.4	205	0	.04	.02	.4	2
521	Filberts (hazelnuts), chopped (about 80 kernels), 1 cup	6	730	14	72	5.1	55.2	7.3	19	240	388	3.9	810	—	.53	—	1.0	*
522	Lentils, whole, cooked, 1 cup	72	210	16	*	—	—	—	39	50	238	4.2	498	40	.14	.12	1.2	0
523	Peanuts, roasted in oil, salted (whole, halves, chopped), 1 cup	2	840	37	72	13.7	33.0	20.7	27	107	577	3.0	971	—	.46	.19	24.8	0
524	Peanut butter, 1 tbsp	2	95	4	8	1.5	3.7	2.3	3	9	61	.3	100	—	.02	.02	2.4	0
525	Peas, split, dry, cooked, 1 cup	70	230	16	1	—	—	—	42	22	178	3.4	592	80	.30	.18	1.8	—
526	Pecans, chopped or pieces (about 120 large halves), 1 cup	3	810	11	84	7.2	50.5	20.0	17	86	341	2.8	712	150	1.01	.15	1.1	2
527	Pumpkin and squash kernels, dry, hulled, 1 cup	4	775	41	65	11.8	23.5	27.5	21	71	1,602	15.7	1386	100	.34	.27	3.4	—
528	Sunflower seeds, dry, hulled, 1 cup	5	810	35	69	8.2	13.7	43.2	29	174	1,214	10.3	1334	70	2.84	.33	7.8	—
	Walnuts, Black:																	
529	Chopped or broken kernels, 1 cup	3	785	26	74	6.3	13.3	45.7	19	*	713	7.5	575	380	.28	.14	.9	—
530	Ground (finely), 1 cup	3	500	16	47	4.0	8.5	29.2	12	*	456	4.8	368	240	.18	.09	.6	—
531	Persian or English, chopped (about 60 halves), 1 cup	4	780	18	77	8.4	11.8	42.2	19	119	456	3.7	540	40	.40	.16	1.1	2
	Sugars and sweets																	
	Cake icings:																	
	Boiled, white:																	
532	Plain, 1 cup	18	295	1	0	0	0	0	75	2	2	*	17	0	*	.03	*	0
533	With coconut, 1 cup	15	605	3	13	11.0	.9	*	124	10	50	.8	277	0	.02	.07	.3	0

No.	Food	Measure																		
	Uncooked:																			
534	Chocolate made with milk and butter	1 cup	275	14	1035	9	38	23.4	11.7	1.0	185	165	305	3.3	536	580	.06	.28	.6	1
535	Creamy fudge from mix and water	1 cup	245	15	830	7	16	5.1	6.7	3.1	183	96	218	2.7	238	*	.05	.20	.7	*
536	White	1 cup	319	11	1200	2	21	12.7	5.1	.5	260	48	38	*	57	860	*	.06	*	*
	Candy:																			
537	Caramels, plain or chocolate	1 oz	28	8	115	1	3	1.6	1.1	.1	22	42	35	.4	54	*	.01	.05	.1	*
	Chocolate:																			
538	Milk, plain	1 oz	28	1	145	2	9	5.5	3.0	.3	16	65	65	.3	109	80	.02	.10	.1	*
539	Semisweet, small pieces (60 per oz)	1 cup or 6-oz pkg.	170	1	860	7	61	36.2	19.8	1.7	97	51	255	4.4	553	30	.02	.14	.9	0
540	Chocolate-coated peanuts	1 oz	28	1	160	5	12	4.0	4.7	2.1	11	33	84	.4	143	*	*	.05	2.1	*
541	Fondant, uncoated (mints, candy corn, other)	1 oz	28	8	105	*	1	.1	.3	.1	25	4	2	.3	1	0	.01	*	*	0
542	Fudge, chocolate, plain	1 oz	28	8	115	1	3	1.3	1.4	.6	21	22	24	.3	42	*	.01	.03	.1	*
543	Gum drops	1 oz	28	12	100	*	*	—	—	—	25	2	*	.1	1	0	0	0	0	0
544	Hard	1 oz	28	1	110	0	*	—	—	—	28	6	2	.5	1	0	0	0	0	0
545	Marshmallows	1 oz	28	17	90	1	*	—	—	—	23	5	2	.5	2	0	0	0	*	0
	Chocolate-flavored beverage powders (about 4 heaping tsp per oz):																			
546	With nonfat dry milk	1 oz	28	2	100	5	1	.5	.3	*	20	167	155	.5	227	10	.04	.21	.2	1
547	Without milk	1 oz	28	1	100	1	1	.4	.2	*	25	9	48	.6	142	—	.01	.03	.1	0
548	Honey, strained or extracted	1 tbsp	21	17	65	*	0	0	0	0	17	1	1	.2	11	0	*	.01	.1	*
549	Jams and preserves	1 tbsp	20	29	55	*	*	—	—	—	14	4	2	.2	18	*	*	.01	*	*
550		1 packet	14	29	40	*	*	—	—	—	10	3	1	.1	12	*	*	*	*	*
551	Jellies	1 tbsp	18	29	50	*	*	—	—	—	13	4	1	.3	14	*	*	.01	*	1
552		1 packet	14	29	40	*	*	—	—	—	10	3	1	.2	11	*	0	*	*	*
	Sirups:																			
	Chocolate-flavored sirup or topping:																			
553	Thin type	1 fl oz or 2 tbsp	38	32	90	1	1	.5	.3	*	24	6	35	.6	106	*	.01	.03	.2	0
554	Fudge type	1 fl oz or 2 tbsp	38	25	125	2	5	3.1	1.6	.1	20	48	60	.5	107	60	.02	.08	.2	*
	Molasses, cane:																			
555	Light (first extraction)	1 tbsp	20	24	50	—	—	—	—	—	13	33	9	.9	183	—	.01	.01	*	—
556	Blackstrap (third extraction)	1 tbsp	20	24	45	—	—	—	—	—	11	137	17	3.2	585	—	.02	.04	.4	—
557	Sorghum	1 tbsp	21	23	55	—	—	—	—	—	14	35	5	2.6	—	—	*	.02	*	—
558	Table blends, chiefly corn, light and dark	1 tbsp	21	24	60	0	0	0	0	0	15	9	3	.8	1	0	0	0	*	0
	Sugars:																			
559	Brown, pressed down	1 cup	220	2	820	0	0	0	0	0	212	187	42	7.5	757	0	.02	.07	.4	0
	White:																			
560	Granulated	1 cup	200	1	770	0	0	0	0	0	199	0	0	.2	6	0	0	0	0	0
561		1 tbsp	12	1	45	0	0	0	0	0	12	0	0	*	*	0	0	0	0	0
562		1 packet	6	1	23	0	0	0	0	0	6	0	0	*	*	0	0	0	0	0
563	Powdered, sifted, spooned into cup	1 cup	100	1	385	0	0	0	0	0	100	0	0	.1	3	0	0	0	0	0

Vegetables and vegetable products

No.	Food	Measure																		
	Asparagus, green:																			
	Cooked, drained:																			
	Cuts and tips, 1½- to 2-in. lengths:																			
564	From raw	1 cup	145	94	30	3	*	—	—	—	5	30	73	.9	265	1310	.23	.26	2.0	38
565	From frozen	1 cup	180	93	40	6	*	—	—	—	6	40	115	2.2	396	1530	.25	.23	1.8	41
	Spears, ½-in. diam. at base:																			
566	From raw	4 spears	60	94	10	1	*	—	—	—	2	13	30	.4	110	540	.10	.11	.8	16
567	From frozen	4 spears	60	92	15	2	*	—	—	—	2	13	40	.7	143	470	.10	.08	.7	16
568	Canned, spears, ½-in. diam. at base	4 spears	80	93	15	2	*	—	—	—	3	15	42	1.5	133	640	.05	.08	.6	12
	Beans:																			
	Lima, immature seeds, frozen, cooked, drained:																			
569	Thick-seeded types (Fordhooks)	1 cup	170	74	170	10	*	—	—	—	32	34	153	2.9	724	390	.12	.09	1.7	29

Appendix D
Nutritive Values of the Edible Part of Foods (Continued)

Item No.	Foods, approximate measures, units, and weight (edible part unless footnotes indicate otherwise) — Serving	Weight (g)	Water (%)	Food Energy (Cal.)	Protein (g)	Fat (g)	Saturated (total) (g)	Unsaturated Oleic (g)	Unsaturated Linoleic (g)	Carbohydrate (g)	Calcium (mg)	Phosphorus (mg)	Iron (mg)	Potassium (mg)	Vitamin A value (I.U.)	Thiamin (mg)	Riboflavin (mg)	Niacin (mg)	Ascorbic acid (mg)
570	Thin-seeded types (baby limas), 1 cup	180	69	210	13	*	—	—	—	40	63	227	4.7	709	400	.16	.09	2.2	22
	Snap:																		
	Green:																		
	Cooked, drained:																		
571	From raw (cuts and French style), 1 cup	125	92	30	2	*	—	—	—	7	63	46	.8	189	680	.09	.11	.6	15
	From frozen:																		
572	Cuts, 1 cup	135	92	35	2	*	—	—	—	8	54	43	.9	205	780	.09	.12	.5	7
573	French style, 1 cup	130	92	35	2	*	—	—	—	8	49	39	1.2	177	690	.08	.10	.4	9
574	Canned, drained solids (cuts), 1 cup	135	92	30	2	*	—	—	—	7	61	34	2.0	128	630	.04	.07	.4	5
	Yellow or wax:																		
	Cooked, drained:																		
575	From raw (cuts and French style), 1 cup	125	93	30	2	*	—	—	—	6	63	46	.8	189	290	.09	.11	.6	16
576	From frozen (cuts), 1 cup	135	92	35	2	*	—	—	—	8	47	42	.9	221	140	.09	.11	.5	8
577	Canned, drained solids (cuts), 1 cup	135	92	30	2	*	—	—	—	7	61	34	2.0	128	140	.04	.07	.4	7
	Beans, mature. See Beans, dry (items 509–515) and Blackeye peas, dry (item 516).																		
	Bean sprouts (mung):																		
578	Raw, 1 cup	105	89	35	4	*	—	—	—	7	20	67	1.4	234	20	.14	.14	.8	20
579	Cooked, drained, 1 cup	125	91	35	4	*	—	—	—	7	21	60	1.1	195	30	.11	.13	.9	8
	Beets:																		
	Cooked, drained, peeled:																		
580	Whole beets, 2-in. diam., 2 beets	100	91	30	1	*	—	—	—	7	14	23	.5	208	20	.03	.04	.3	6
581	Diced or sliced, 1 cup	170	91	55	2	*	—	—	—	12	24	39	.9	354	30	.05	.07	.5	10
	Canned, drained solids:																		
582	Whole beets, small, 1 cup	160	89	60	2	*	—	—	—	14	30	29	1.1	267	30	.02	.05	.2	5
583	Diced or sliced, 1 cup	170	89	65	2	*	—	—	—	15	32	31	1.2	284	30	.02	.05	.2	5
584	Beet greens, leaves and stems, cooked, drained, 1 cup	145	94	25	2	*	—	—	—	5	144	36	2.8	481	7400	.10	.22	.4	22
	Blackeye peas, immature seeds, cooked and drained:																		
585	From raw, 1 cup	165	72	180	13	1	—	—	—	30	40	241	3.5	625	580	.50	.18	2.3	28
586	From frozen, 1 cup	170	66	220	15	1	—	—	—	40	43	286	4.8	573	290	.68	.19	2.4	15
	Broccoli, cooked, drained:																		
	From raw:																		
587	Stalk, medium size, 1 stalk	180	91	45	6	1	—	—	—	8	158	112	1.4	481	4500	.16	.36	1.4	162
588	Stalks cut into 1/2-in. pieces, 1 cup	155	91	40	5	*	—	—	—	7	136	96	1.2	414	3880	.14	.31	1.2	140
	From frozen:																		
589	Stalk, 4 1/2 to 5 in. long, 1 stalk	30	91	10	1	*	—	—	—	1	12	17	.2	66	570	.02	.03	.2	22
590	Chopped, 1 cup	185	92	50	5	1	—	—	—	9	100	104	1.3	392	4810	.11	.22	.9	105
	Brussels sprouts, cooked, drained:																		
591	From raw, 7–8 sprouts (1 1/4- to 1 1/2-in. diam.), 1 cup	155	88	55	7	1	—	—	—	10	50	112	1.7	423	810	.12	.22	1.2	135
592	From frozen, 1 cup	155	89	50	5	*	—	—	—	10	33	95	1.2	457	880	.12	.16	.9	126

Nutrients in Indicated Quantity / Fatty Acids

Item No.	Food, approximate measure, and weight		(g)	Water (%)	Food energy	Protein	Fat	Sat.	Oleic	Linoleic	Carbohydrate	Calcium	Phosphorus	Iron	Potassium	Vitamin A	Thiamin	Riboflavin	Niacin	Ascorbic acid
	Cabbage:																			
	Common varieties:																			
	Raw:																			
593	Coarsely shredded or sliced	1 cup	70	92	15	1	*	—	—	—	4	34	20	.3	163	90	.04	.04	.2	33
594	Finely shredded or chopped	1 cup	90	92	20	1	*	—	—	—	5	44	26	.4	210	120	.05	.05	.3	42
595	Cooked, drained	1 cup	145	94	30	2	*	—	—	—	6	64	29	.4	236	190	.06	.06	.4	48
596	Red, raw, coarsely shredded or sliced	1 cup	70	90	20	1	*	—	—	—	5	29	25	.6	188	30	.06	.04	.3	43
597	Savoy, raw, coarsely shredded or sliced	1 cup	70	92	15	2	*	—	—	—	3	47	38	.6	188	140	.04	.06	.2	39
598	Cabbage, celery (also called petsai or wongbok), raw, 1-in. pieces	1 cup	75	95	10	1	*	—	—	—	2	32	30	.5	190	110	.04	.03	.5	19
599	Cabbage, white mustard (also called bokchoy or pakchoy), cooked, drained	1 cup	170	95	25	2	*	—	—	—	4	252	56	1.0	364	5270	.07	.14	1.2	26
	Carrots:																			
	Raw, without crowns and tips, scraped:																			
600	Whole, 7½ by 1⅛ in., or strips, 2½ to 3 in. long	1 carrot or 18 strips	72	88	30	1	*	—	—	—	7	27	26	.5	246	7930	.04	.04	.4	6
601	Grated	1 cup	110	88	45	1	*	—	—	—	11	41	40	.8	375	12,100	.07	.06	.7	9
602	Cooked (crosswise cuts), drained	1 cup	155	91	50	1	*	—	—	—	11	51	48	.9	344	16,280	.08	.08	.8	9
	Canned:																			
603	Sliced, drained solids	1 cup	155	91	45	1	*	—	—	—	10	47	34	1.1	186	23,250	.03	.05	.6	3
604	Strained or junior (baby food)	1 oz (1¾ to 2 tbsp)	28	92	10	*	*	—	—	—	2	7	6	.1	51	3690	.01	.01	.1	1
	Cauliflower:																			
605	Raw, chopped	1 cup	115	91	31	3	*	—	—	—	6	29	64	1.3	339	70	.13	.12	.8	90
	Cooked, drained:																			
606	From raw (flower buds)	1 cup	125	93	30	3	*	—	—	—	5	26	53	.9	258	80	.11	.10	.8	69
607	From frozen (flowerets)	1 cup	180	94	30	3	*	—	—	—	6	31	68	.9	373	50	.07	.09	.7	74
	Celery, Pascal type, raw:																			
608	Stalk, large outer, 8 by 1½ in. at root end	1 stalk	40	94	5	*	*	—	—	—	2	16	11	.1	136	110	.01	.01	.1	4
609	Pieces, diced	1 cup	120	94	20	1	*	—	—	—	5	47	34	.4	409	320	.04	.04	.4	11
	Collards, cooked, drained:																			
610	From raw (leaves without stems)	1 cup	190	90	65	7	1	—	—	—	10	357	99	1.5	498	14,820	.21	.38	2.3	144
611	From frozen (chopped)	1 cup	170	90	50	5	1	—	—	—	10	299	87	1.7	401	11,560	.10	.24	1.0	56
	Corn, sweet:																			
	Cooked, drained:																			
612	From raw, ear 5 by 1¾ in.	1 ear	140[aa]	74	70	2	1	—	—	—	16	2	69	.5	151	310[zz]	.09	.08	1.1	7
	From frozen:																			
613	Ear, 5 in. long	1 ear	229[aa]	73	120	4	1	—	—	—	27	4	121	1.0	291	440[zz]	.18	.10	2.1	9
614	Kernels	1 cup	165	77	130	5	1	—	—	—	31	5	120	1.3	304	580[zz]	.15	.10	2.5	8
	Canned:																			
615	Cream style	1 cup	256	76	210	5	2	—	—	—	51	8	143	1.5	248	840[zz]	.08	.13	2.6	13
	Whole kernel:																			
616	Vacuum pack	1 cup	210	76	175	5	1	—	—	—	43	6	153	1.1	204	740[zz]	.06	.13	2.3	11
617	Wet pack, drained solids	1 cup	165	76	140	4	1	—	—	—	33	8	81	.8	160	580[zz]	.05	.08	1.5	7
	Cowpeas. See Blackeye peas items 585–586.																			
	Cucumber slices, ⅛-in. thick (large, 2⅛-in. diam.; small, 1¾-in. diam.):																			
618	With peel	6 large or 8 small slices	28	95	5	*	*	—	—	—	1	7	8	.3	45	70	.01	.01	.1	3
619	Without peel	6½ large or 9 small pieces	28	96	5	*	*	—	—	—	1	5	5	.1	45	*	.01	.01	.1	3
620	Dandelion greens, cooked, drained	1 cup	105	90	35	2	1	—	—	—	7	147	44	1.9	244	12,290	.14	.17	—	19
621	Endive, curly (including escarole), raw, small pieces	1 cup	50	93	10	1	*	—	—	—	2	41	27	.9	147	1650	.04	.07	.3	5

Appendix D
Nutritive Values of the Edible Part of Foods (Continued)

Item No.	Foods, approximate measures, units, and weight (edible part unless footnotes indicate otherwise)	Serving	Weight (g)	Water (%)	Food Energy (Cal.)	Protein (g)	Fat (g)	Saturated (total) (g)	Oleic (g)	Linoleic (g)	Carbohydrate (g)	Calcium (mg)	Phosphorus (mg)	Iron (mg)	Potassium (mg)	Vitamin A value (I.U.)	Thiamin (mg)	Riboflavin (mg)	Niacin (mg)	Ascorbic acid (mg)
	Kale, cooked, drained:																			
622	From raw (leaves without stems and midribs)	1 cup	110	88	45	5	1	—	—	—	7	206	64	1.8	243	9130	.11	.20	1.8	102
623	From frozen (leaf style)	1 cup	130	91	40	4	1	—	—	—	7	157	62	1.3	251	10,660	.08	.20	.9	49
	Lettuce, raw:																			
	Butterhead, as Boston types:																			
624	Head, 5-in. diam.	1 head	220^hhh	95	25	2	*	—	—	—	4	57	42	3.3	430	1580	.10	.10	.5	13
625	Leaves	1 outer or 2 inner or 3 heart leaves	15	95	*	*	*	—	—	—	*	5	4	.3	40	150	.01	.01	*	1
	Crisphead, as Iceberg:																			
626	Head, 6-in. diam.	1 head	567^iii	96	70	5	1	—	—	—	16	108	118	2.7	943	1780	.32	.32	1.6	32
627	Wedge, 1/4 head	1 wedge	135	96	20	1	*	—	—	—	4	27	30	.7	236	450	.08	.08	.4	8
628	Pieces, chopped or shredded	1 cup	55	96	5	*	*	—	—	—	2	11	12	.3	96	180	.03	.03	.2	3
629	Looseleaf (bunching varieties including romaine or cos), chopped or shredded pieces	1 cup	55	94	10	1	*	—	—	—	2	37	14	.8	145	1050	.03	.04	.2	10
630	Mushrooms, raw, sliced or chopped	1 cup	70	90	20	2	*	—	—	—	3	4	81	.6	290	*	.07	.32	2.9	2
631	Mustard greens, without stems and midribs, cooked, drained	1 cup	140	93	30	3	1	—	—	—	6	193	45	2.5	308	8120	.11	.20	.8	67
632	Okra pods, 3 by 5/8 in., cooked	10 pods	106	91	30	2	*	—	—	—	6	98	43	.5	184	520	.14	.19	1.0	21
	Onions:																			
	Mature:																			
	Raw:																			
633	Chopped	1 cup	170	89	65	3	*	—	—	—	15	46	61	.9	267	*iii	.05	.07	.3	17
634	Sliced	1 cup	115	89	45	2	*	—	—	—	10	31	41	.6	181	*iii	.03	.05	.2	12
635	Cooked (whole or sliced), drained	1 cup	210	92	60	3	*	—	—	—	14	50	61	.8	231	*iii	.06	.06	.4	15
636	Young green, bulb (3/8-in. diam.) and white portion of top	6 onions	30	88	15	*	*	—	—	—	3	12	12	.2	69	*	.02	.01	.1	8
637	Parsley, raw, chopped	1 tbsp	4	85	*	*	*	—	—	—	*	7	2	.2	25	300	*	.01	*	6
638	Parsnips, cooked (diced or 2-in. lengths)	1 cup	155	82	100	2	1	—	—	—	23	70	96	.9	587	50	.11	.12	.2	16
	Peas, green:																			
	Canned:																			
639	Whole, drained solids	1 cup	170	77	150	8	1	—	—	—	29	44	129	3.2	163	1170	.15	.10	1.4	14
640	Strained (baby food)	1 oz (1 3/4 to 2 tbsp)	28	86	15	1	*	—	—	—	3	3	18	.3	28	140	.02	.03	.3	3
641	Frozen, cooked, drained	1 cup	160	82	110	8	*	—	—	—	19	30	138	3.0	216	960	.43	.14	2.7	21
642	Peppers, hot, red, without seeds, dried (ground chili powder, added seasonings)	1 tsp	2	9	5	*	*	—	—	—	1	5	4	.3	20	1300	*	.02	.2	*
	Peppers, sweet (about 5 per lb, whole), stem and seeds removed:																			
643	Raw	1 pod	74	93	15	1	*	—	—	—	4	7	16	.5	157	310	.06	.06	.4	94
644	Cooked, boiled, drained	1 pod	73	95	15	1	*	—	—	—	3	7	12	.4	109	310	.05	.05	.4	70
	Potatoes, cooked:																			

Nutrients in Indicated Quantity

Fatty Acids

Unsaturated

Food composition table (continuation; column headers appear on a preceding page). Item numbers 645–677.

Item No.	Food, approximate measure	Measure	Grams	Water (%)	Food energy (cal)	Protein (g)	Fat (g)	Saturated fat (g)	Oleic (g)	Linoleic (g)	Carbohydrate (g)	Calcium (mg)	Phosphorus (mg)	Iron (mg)	Potassium (mg)	Vitamin A (IU)	Thiamin (mg)	Riboflavin (mg)	Niacin (mg)	Ascorbic acid (mg)
645	Baked, peeled after baking (about 2 per lb, raw)	1 potato	156	75	145	4	*	—	—	—	33	14	101	1.1	782	*	.15	.07	2.7	31
	Boiled (about 3 per lb, raw):																			
646	Peeled after boiling	1 potato	137	80	105	3	*	—	—	—	23	10	72	.8	556	*	.12	.05	2.0	22
647	Peeled before boiling	1 potato	135	83	90	3	*	—	—	—	20	8	57	.7	385	*	.12	.05	1.6	22
	French-fried, strip, 2 to 3½ in. long:																			
648	Prepared from raw	10 strips	50	45	135	2	7	1.7	1.2	3.3	18	8	56	.7	427	*	.07	.04	1.6	11
649	Frozen, oven-heated	10 strips	50	53	110	2	4	1.1	.8	2.1	17	5	43	.9	326	*	.07	.01	1.3	11
650	Hashed brown, prepared from frozen	1 cup	155	56	345	3	18	4.6	3.2	9.0	45	28	78	1.9	439	*	.11	.03	1.6	12
	Mashed, prepared from— Raw:																			
651	Milk added	1 cup	210	83	135	4	2	.7	.4	*	27	50	103	.8	548	40	.17	.11	2.1	21
652	Milk and butter added	1 cup	210	80	195	4	9	5.6	2.3	.2	26	50	101	.8	525	360	.17	.11	2.1	19
653	Dehydrated flakes (without milk), water, milk, butter, and salt added	1 cup	210	79	195	4	7	3.6	2.1	.2	30	65	99	.6	601	270	.08	.08	1.9	11
654	Potato chips, 1¾ by 2½ in. oval cross section	10 chips	20	2	115	1	8	2.1	1.4	4.0	10	8	28	.4	226	*	.04	.01	1.0	3
655	Potato salad, made with cooked salad dressing	1 cup	250	76	250	7	7	2.0	2.7	1.3	41	80	160	1.5	798	350	.20	.18	2.8	28
656	Pumpkin, canned	1 cup	245	90	80	2	2	—	—	—	19	61	64	1.0	588	15,680	.07	.12	1.5	12
657	Radishes, raw (prepackaged) stem ends, rootlets cut off	4 radishes	18	95	5	*	*	—	—	—	1	5	6	.2	58	*	.01	.01	.1	5
658	Sauerkraut, canned, solids and liquid	1 cup	235	93	40	2	*	—	—	—	9	85	42	1.2	329	120	.07	.09	.5	33
	Southern peas. See Blackeye peas (items 585–586).																			
	Spinach:																			
659	Raw, chopped	1 cup	55	91	15	2	*	—	—	—	2	51	28	1.7	259	4460	.06	.11	.3	28
	Cooked, drained:																			
660	From raw	1 cup	180	92	40	5	1	—	—	—	6	167	68	4.0	583	14,580	.13	.25	.9	50
	From frozen:																			
661	Chopped	1 cup	205	92	45	6	1	—	—	—	8	232	90	4.3	683	16,200	.14	.31	.8	39
662	Leaf	1 cup	190	92	45	6	1	—	—	—	7	200	84	4.8	688	15,390	.15	.27	1.0	53
663	Canned, drained solids	1 cup	205	91	50	6	1	—	—	—	7	242	53	5.3	513	16,400	.04	.25	.6	29
	Squash, cooked:																			
664	Summer (all varieties), diced, drained	1 cup	210	96	30	2	*	—	—	—	7	53	53	.8	296	820	.11	.17	1.7	21
665	Winter (all varieties), baked, mashed	1 cup	205	81	130	4	1	—	—	—	32	57	98	1.6	945	8610	.10	.27	1.4	27
	Sweet potatoes: Cooked (raw, 5 by 2 in.; about 2½ per lb):																			
666	Baked in skin, peeled	1 potato	114	64	160	2	1	—	—	—	37	46	66	1.0	342	9230	.10	.08	.8	25
667	Boiled in skin, peeled	1 potato	151	71	170	3	1	—	—	—	40	48	71	1.1	367	11,940	.14	.09	.9	26
668	Candied, 2½ by 2-in. piece	1 piece	105	60	175	1	3	2.0	.8	.1	36	39	45	.9	200	6620	.06	.04	.4	11
	Canned:																			
669	Solid pack (mashed)	1 cup	255	72	275	5	1	—	—	—	63	64	105	2.0	510	19,890	.13	.10	1.5	36
670	Vacuum pack, piece 2¾ by 1 in.	1 piece	40	72	45	1	*	—	—	—	10	10	16	.3	80	3120	.02	.02	.2	6
	Tomatoes:																			
671	Raw, 2³⁄₅-in. diam. (3 per 12 oz pkg.)	1 tomato	135[kkk]	94	25	1	*	—	—	—	6	16	33	.6	300	1110	.07	.05	.9	28[lll]
672	Canned, solids and liquid	1 cup	241	94	50	2	*	—	—	—	10	14[mmm]	46	1.2	523	2170	.12	.07	1.7	41
673	Tomato catsup	1 cup	273	69	290	5	1	—	—	—	69	60	137	2.2	991	3820	.25	.19	4.4	41
674	Tomato catsup	1 tbsp	15	69	15	*	*	—	—	—	4	3	8	.1	54	210	.01	.01	.2	2
	Tomato juice, canned:																			
675	Cup	1 cup	243	94	45	2	*	—	—	—	10	17	44	2.2	552	1940	.12	.07	1.9	39
676	Glass (6 fl oz)	1 glass	182	94	35	2	*	—	—	—	8	13	33	1.6	413	1460	.09	.05	1.5	29
677	Turnips, cooked, diced	1 cup	155	94	35	1	*	—	—	—	8	54	37	.6	291	*	.06	.08	.5	34
	Turnip greens, cooked, drained:																			

Appendix D
Nutritive Values of the Edible Part of Foods (Continued)

Nutrients in Indicated Quantity

Item No.	Foods, approximate measures, units, and weight (edible part unless footnotes indicate otherwise) / Serving	Weight (g)	Water (%)	Food Energy (Cal.)	Protein (g)	Fat (g)	Fatty Acids — Saturated (total) (g)	Unsaturated Oleic (g)	Unsaturated Linoleic (g)	Carbohydrate (g)	Calcium (mg)	Phosphorus (mg)	Iron (mg)	Potassium (mg)	Vitamin A value (I.U.)	Thiamin (mg)	Riboflavin (mg)	Niacin (mg)	Ascorbic acid (mg)
678	From raw (leaves and stems), 1 cup	145	94	30	3	*	—	—	—	5	252	49	1.5	—	8270	.15	.33	.7	68
679	From frozen (chopped), 1 cup	165	93	40	4	*	—	—	—	6	195	64	2.6	246	11,390	.08	.15	.7	31
680	Vegetables, mixed, frozen, cooked, 1 cup	182	83	115	6	1	—	—	—	24	46	115	2.4	348	9010	.22	.13	2.0	15

Miscellaneous items

Baking powders for home use:
Sodium aluminum sulfate:

Item No.	Serving	Weight (g)	Water (%)	Food Energy (Cal.)	Protein (g)	Fat (g)	Saturated (total) (g)	Unsat. Oleic (g)	Unsat. Linoleic (g)	Carbohydrate (g)	Calcium (mg)	Phosphorus (mg)	Iron (mg)	Potassium (mg)	Vitamin A value (I.U.)	Thiamin (mg)	Riboflavin (mg)	Niacin (mg)	Ascorbic acid (mg)
681	With monocalcium phosphate monohydrate. 1 tsp	3.0	2	5	*	*	0	0	0	1	58	87	—	5	0	0	0	0	0
682	With monocalcium phosphate monohydrate, calcium sulfate. 1 tsp	2.9	1	5	*	*	0	0	0	1	183	45	—	—	0	0	0	0	0
683	Straight phosphate, 1 tsp	3.8	2	5	*	*	0	0	0	1	239	359	—	6	0	0	0	0	0
684	Low sodium, 1 tsp	4.3	2	5	*	*	0	0	0	2	207	314	—	471	0	0	0	0	0
685	Barbecue sauce, 1 cup	250	81	230	4	17	2.2	4.3	10.0	20	53	50	2.0	435	900	.03	.03	.8	13

Beverages, alcoholic:

| 686 | Beer, 12 fl oz | 360 | 92 | 150 | 1 | 0 | 0 | 0 | 0 | 14 | 18 | 108 | * | 90 | — | .01 | .11 | 2.2 | — |

Gin, rum, vodka, whisky:

687	80-proof, 1½-fl oz jigger	42	67	95	—	—	0	0	0	*	—	—	—	1	—	—	—	—	—
688	86-proof, 1½-fl oz jigger	42	64	105	—	—	0	0	0	*	—	—	—	1	—	—	—	—	—
689	90-proof, 1½-fl oz jigger	42	62	110	—	—	0	0	0	*	—	—	—	1	—	—	—	—	—

Wines:

| 690 | Dessert, 3½-fl oz glass | 103 | 77 | 140 | * | 0 | 0 | 0 | 0 | 8 | 8 | — | — | 77 | — | .01 | .02 | .2 | — |
| 691 | Table, 3½-fl oz glass | 102 | 86 | 85 | * | 0 | 0 | 0 | 0 | 4 | 9 | 10 | .4 | 94 | — | * | .01 | .1 | — |

Beverages, carbonated, sweetened, nonalcoholic:

692	Carbonated water, 12 fl oz	366	92	115	0	0	0	0	0	29	—	—	—	—	0	0	0	0	0
693	Cola type, 12 fl oz	369	90	145	0	0	0	0	0	37	—	—	—	—	0	0	0	0	0
694	Fruit-flavored sodas and Tom Collins mixer. 12 fl oz	372	88	170	0	0	0	0	0	45	—	—	—	—	0	0	0	0	0
695	Ginger ale, 12 fl oz	366	92	115	0	0	0	0	0	29	—	—	—	0	0	0	0	0	0
696	Root beer, 12 fl oz	370	90	150	0	0	0	0	0	39	—	—	—	0	0	0	0	0	0

Chili powder. See Peppers, hot, red (item 642).
Chocolate:

| 697 | Bitter or baking, 1 oz | 28 | 2 | 145 | 3 | 15 | 8.9 | 4.9 | .4 | 8 | 22 | 109 | 1.9 | 235 | 20 | .01 | .07 | .4 | 0 |

Semisweet, see Candy, chocolate (item 539).

| 698 | Gelatin, dry, 1, 7-g envelope | 7 | 13 | 25 | 6 | * | 0 | 0 | 0 | 0 | — | — | — | — | — | — | — | — | — |
| 699 | Gelatin dessert prepared with gelatin dessert powder and water. 1 cup | 240 | 84 | 140 | 4 | 0 | 0 | 0 | 0 | 34 | — | — | — | — | — | — | — | — | — |

No.	Food, approximate measure	Grams	Water (%)	Food energy (Cal.)	Protein (g)	Fat (g)	Saturated (g)	Oleic (g)	Linoleic (g)	Carbohydrate (g)	Calcium (mg)	Phosphorus (mg)	Iron (mg)	Potassium (mg)	Vitamin A (IU)	Thiamin (mg)	Riboflavin (mg)	Niacin (mg)	Ascorbic acid (mg)
700	Mustard, prepared, yellow — 1 tsp or individual serving pouch or cup	5	80	5	*	*	—	—	—	*	4	4	.1	7	—	—	—	—	—
	Olives, pickled, canned:																		
701	Green — 4 medium or 3 extra large or 2 giant	16	78	15	*	2	.2	1.2	.1	*	8	2	.2	7	40	—	—	—	—
702	Ripe, Mission — 3 small or 2 large	10	73	15	*	2	.2	1.2	.1	*	9	1	.1	2	10	*	*	*	—
	Pickles, cucumber:																		
703	Dill, medium, whole, 3¾ in long, 1¼-in diam. — 1 pickle	65	93	5	1	*	—	—	—	1	17	14	.7	130	70	*	.01	*	4
704	Fresh-pack, slices 1½-in diam., ¼ in thick. — 2 slices	15	79	10	*	*	—	—	—	3	5	4	.3	—	20	*	*	*	1
705	Sweet, gherkin, small, whole, about 2½ in long, ¾-in diam. — 1 pickle	15	61	20	*	*	—	—	—	5	2	2	.2	—	10	*	*	*	1
706	Relish, finely chopped, sweet — 1 tbsp	15	63	20	*	*	—	—	—	5	3	2	.1	—	—	—	—	—	—
707	Popsicle, 3-fl oz size — 1 popsicle	95	80	70	0	0	0	0	0	18	0	—	*	—	0	0	0	0	0
	Soups:																		
	Canned, condensed:																		
	Prepared with equal volume of milk:																		
708	Cream of chicken — 1 cup	245	85	180	7	10	4.2	3.6	1.3	15	172	152	.5	260	610	.05	.27	.7	2
709	Cream of mushroom — 1 cup	245	83	215	7	14	5.4	2.9	4.6	16	191	169	.5	279	250	.05	.34	.7	1
710	Tomato — 1 cup	250	84	175	7	7	3.4	1.7	1.0	23	168	155	.8	418	1,200	.10	.25	1.3	15
	Prepared with equal volume of water:																		
711	Bean with pork — 1 cup	250	84	170	8	6	1.2	1.8	2.4	22	63	128	2.3	395	650	.13	.08	1.0	3
712	Beef broth, bouillon, consomme — 1 cup	240	96	30	5	0	0	0	0	3	*	31	.5	130	*	*	.02	1.2	—
713	Beef noodle — 1 cup	240	93	65	4	3	.6	.7	.8	7	7	48	1.0	77	50	.05	.07	1.0	*
714	Clam chowder, Manhattan type (with tomatoes, without milk) — 1 cup	245	92	80	2	3	.5	.4	1.3	12	34	47	1.0	184	880	.02	.02	1.0	—
715	Cream of chicken — 1 cup	240	92	95	3	6	1.6	2.3	1.1	8	24	34	.5	79	410	.02	.05	.5	*
716	Cream of mushroom — 1 cup	240	90	135	2	10	2.6	1.7	4.5	10	41	50	.5	98	70	.02	.12	.7	*
717	Minestrone — 1 cup	245	90	105	5	3	.7	.9	1.3	14	37	59	1.0	314	2350	.07	.05	1.0	—
718	Split pea — 1 cup	245	85	145	9	3	1.1	1.2	.4	21	29	149	1.5	270	440	.25	.15	1.5	1
719	Tomato — 1 cup	245	91	90	2	2	.5	.5	1.0	16	15	34	.7	230	1000	.05	.05	1.2	12
720	Vegetable beef — 1 cup	245	92	80	3	2	—	—	—	10	12	49	.7	162	2700	.05	.05	1.0	—
721	Vegetarian — 1 cup	245	92	80	2	2	—	—	—	13	20	39	1.0	172	2940	.05	.05	1.0	—
	Dehydrated:																		
722	Bouillon cube, ½ in. — 1 cube	4	4	5	1	*	—	—	—	*	—	—	—	4	—	—	—	—	—
	Mixes:																		
	Unprepared:																		
723	Onion — 1½-oz pkg.	43	3	150	6	5	1.1	2.3	1.0	23	42	49	.6	238	30	.05	.03	.3	6
	Prepared with water:																		
724	Chicken noodle — 1 cup	240	95	55	2	1	—	—	—	8	7	19	.2	19	50	.07	.05	.5	*
725	Onion — 1 cup	240	96	35	1	1	—	—	—	6	10	12	.2	58	*	*	*	*	2
726	Tomato vegetable with noodles — 1 cup	240	93	65	1	1	—	—	—	12	7	19	.2	29	480	.05	.02	.5	5
727	Vinegar, cider — 1 tbsp	15	94	*	*	0	0	0	0	1	1	1	.1	15	—	—	—	—	—
728	White sauce, medium, with enriched flour — 1 cup	250	73	405	10	31	19.3	7.8	.8	22	288	233	.5	348	1150	.12	.43	.7	2
	Yeast:																		
729	Baker's, dry, active — 1 pkg	7	5	20	3	*	—	—	—	3	3	90	1.1	140	*	.16	.38	2.6	*

Note: Dash (—) denotes lack of reliable data for a constituent believed to be present in a measurable amount. * signifies a trace amount of nutritive value.

Source: U.S. Department of Agriculture. Home and Garden Bulletin No. 72, rev. ed. (Washington, D.C.: U.S. Government Printing Office. 1981).

a Vitamin A value is largely from beta-carotene used for coloring. Riboflavin value for items 40–41 apply to products with added riboflavin.
b Applies to product without added vitamin A, value is 500 International Units (I.U.).
c Applies to product without added Vitamin A added.
d Applies to product without added Vitamin A. Without added Vitamin A, value is 20 International Units (I.U.).

Appendix D
Nutritive Values of the Edible Part of Foods (Continued)

[e]Yields 1 qt of fluid milk when reconstituted according to package directions.

[f]Applies to product with added Vitamin A.

[g]Weight applies to product with label claim of $1^1/_3$ cups equal 3.2 oz.

[h]Applies to products made from thick shake mixes and that do not contain added ice cream. Products made from milk shake mixes are higher in fat and usually contain added ice cream.

[i]Content of fat, vitamin A, and carbohydrate varies. Consult the label when precise values are needed for special diets.

[j]Applies to product made with milk containing no added vitamin A.

[k]Based on year-round average.

[l]Based on average Vitamin A content of fortified margarine. Federal specifications for fortified margarine require a minimum of 15,000 International Units (I.U.) of vitamin A per pound.

[m]Fatty acid values apply to product made with regular-type margarine.

[n]Dipped in egg, milk or water, and breadcrumbs; fried in vegetable shortening.

[o]If bones are discarded, value for calcium will be greatly reduced.

[p]Dipped in egg, breadcrumbs, and flour or batter.

[q]Prepared with tuna, celery, salad dressing (mayonnaise type), pickle, onion, and egg.

[r]Outer layer of fat on the cut was removed to within approximately $1/_2$ in. of the lean. Deposits of fat within the cut were not removed.

[s]Crust made with vegetable shortening and enriched flour.

[t]Regular-type margarine used.

[u]Value varies greatly.

[v]About one-fourth of the outer layer of fat on the cut was removed. Deposits of fat within the cut were not removed.

[w]Vegetable shortening used.

[x]Also applies to pasteurized apple cider.

[y]Applies to product without ascorbic acid. For value of product with added ascorbic acid, refer to label.

[z]Based on product claim of 45% of U.S. RDA in 6 fl oz.

[aa]Based on product with label claim of 100% of U.S. RDA in 6 fl oz.

[bb]Weight includes peel and membranes between sections. Without these parts, the weight of the edible portion is 123 g for item 246 and 118 g for item 247.

[cc]For white-fleshed varieties, value is about 20 International Units (I.U.) per cup; for red-fleshed varieties, 1080 I.U.

[dd]Weight includes seeds. Without seeds, weight of the edible portion is 123 g for item 246 and 118 g for item 247.

[ee]Applies to product without added ascorbic acid. With added ascorbic acid, based on claim that 6 fl oz of reconstituted juice contain 45% or 50% of the U.S RDA, value in milligrams is 108 or 120 for a 6 floz can (item 258), 36 or 40 for 1 cup of diluted juice (item 259).

[ff]For products with added thiamin and riboflavin but without added ascorbic acid, values in milligrams would be .60 for thiamin, .80 for riboflavin, and trace for ascorbic acid. For products with ascorbic acid, value varies with the brand. Consult the label.

[gg]Weight includes rind. Without rind, the weight of the edible portion is 272 g for item 271 and 149 g for item 272.

[hh]Represents yellow-fleshed varieties, value is 50 International Units (I.U.) for 1 peach. **90** I.U. for 1 cup of slices.

[ii]Value represents products with added ascorbic acid. For products without added ascorbic acid, value in milligrams is 116 for a 10 oz container, 103 for 1 cup.

[jj]Weight includes pits. After removal of the pits, the weight of the edible portion is 258 g for item 302, 133 g for item 303, 43 g for item 304, and 213 g for item 305.

[kk]Weight includes rind and seeds. Without rind and seeds, weight of the edible portion is 426 g.

[ll]Made with vegetable shortening.

[mm]Applies to product made with white cornmeal. With yellow cornmeal, value is 30 International Units (I.U.).

[nn]Applies to white varieties. For yellow varieties, value is 150 International Units (I.U.).

[oo]Applies to products that do not contain disodium phosphate. If disodium phosphate is an ingredient, value is 162 mg.

[pp]Value may range from less than 1 mg to about 8 mg depending on the brand. Consult the label.

[qq]Applies to product with added nutrient. Without added nutrient, value is trace.

[rr]Value varies with the brand. Consult the label.

[ss]Excepting angelfood cake, cakes were made from mixes containing vegetable shortening, icings, with butter.

[tt]Excepting spongecake, vegetable shortening used for cake portion; butter, for icing. If butter or margarine used for cake portion, vitamin A values would be higher.

[uu]Applies to product made with sodium-aluminum-sulfate-type baking powder. With a low-sodium baking powder containing potassium, value would be about twice the amount shown.

[vv]Equal weights of flour, sugar, eggs and vegetable shortening.

[ww]Products are commercial unless otherwise specified.

[xx]Made with enriched flour and vegetable shortening, except for macaroons, which do not contain vegetable shortening.

[yy]Icing made with butter.

[zz]Applies to yellow varieties, white varieties contain only a trace.

[aaa]Contains vegetable shortening and butter.

[bbb]Made with corn oil.

[ccc]Made with regular margarine.

[ddd]Applies to product made with yellow cornmeal.

[eee]Made with enriched degermed cornmeal and enriched flour.

[fff]Product may or may not be enriched with riboflavin. Consult the label.

[ggg]Weight includes cob. Without cob, weight is 77 g for item 612, 126 g for item 613.

[hhh]Weight includes refuse of outer leaves and core. Without these parts, weight is 163 g.

[iii]Weight includes core. Without core, weight is 539 g. [jjj]Value based on white-fleshed varieties. For yellow-fleshed varieties, value in International Units (I.U.) is 70 for item 633, 50 for item 634, and 80 for item 635.

[kkk]Weight includes cores and stem ends. Without these parts, weight is 123 g.

[lll]Based on year-round average. For tomatoes marketed from November through May, value is about 12 mg; from June through October, 32 mg.

[mmm]Applies to product without calcium salts added. Value for products with calcium salts added may be as much as 63 mg for whole tomatoes, 241 mg for cut forms.

[nnn]Weight includes pits. Without pits, weight is 13 g for item 701, 9 g for item 702.

[ooo]Value may vary from 6 to 60 mg.

Appendix E
Nutrients in Vegetarian Foods[a]

Food[b]	Weight (g)	Water (%)	Energy (kcal)	Protein (g)	Fat (g)	Carbohydrate (g)	Calcium (mg)	Phosphorus[c] (mg)	Iron (mg)	Potassium (mg)	Zinc (mg)	Vitamin A[d] (RE)	Thiamin (mg)	Riboflavin (mg)	Niacin (mg)	Vitamin C (mg)	Folacin (µg)
Bamboo shoots, raw, cut into 1-in.-long pieces (¾ cup)	113	91.0	31	3.0	0.4	5.9	15	67	0.6	605	[0.32]	2	0.17	0.08	0.7	5	[13–72]
Beans and peas, mature seeds, dry, cooked (½ cup except soybeans and peanuts)																	
Black beans (turtle beans)	[100]	77.8	85	5.6	0.4	15.3	30	95	1.7	195	[0.67–0.84]	1	0.09	0.04	0.4	(0)	49
Black-eyed peas (cowpeas)	125	80.0	95	6.4	0.4	17.5	22	119	1.7	287	1.09	2	0.20	0.05	0.5	(0)	74
Broad beans (fava beans)	[100]	72.9	119	7.1	1.6	19.0	35	109	1.5	219	0.90	0	0.09	0.08	0.7	0	104
Garbanzo beans (chickpeas)	85	58.1	145	8.0	2.0	25.0	47	162	2.9	277	1.48	0	0.09	0.04	0.4	0	42
Kidney beans, red	91	67.1	116	7.6	0.5	21.0	(18–33)	112	3.4	363	1.00	1	0.10[e]	0.05	0.7	(0)	66
Lentils, whole	100	72.0	106	7.8	(0)	19.5	25	119	2.1	249	1.00	2	0.07	0.06	0.6	0	32
Lima beans	95	64.1	131	7.8	0.6	24.3	28	147	3.0	582	1.16	[1]	0.13	0.06	0.7	(0)	114
Navy peas (beans)	36	63.1	143	8.9	0.6	26.2	69	156	2.6	298	1.08	0	(0.14–0.27)	0.06	(0.5–0.8)	0	81
Peanuts, roasted, whole, parts (4 tbsp)	100	1.8	210	9.3	18.0	6.8	27	144	0.8	243	1.08	[1]	0.12	0.05	6.2	(0)	52
Pinto beans	100	65.9	131	7.7	0.5	24.5	48	163	3.3	473	1.30	[1]	0.25	0.05	0.4	(0)	[59–106]
Soybeans (⅓ cup)	60	71.0	78	6.6	3.4	6.5	44	107	1.6	324	0.72	2	0.13	0.05	0.4	0	[17–40]
Split peas without seed coat	100	70.0	115	8.0	0.3	20.8	11	89	1.7	296	0.85	4	0.15	0.09	0.9	(0)	7
Bean sprouts, raw (1 cup)																	
Alfalfa	[105]	93.3	27	3.0	0.4	3.3	23	57	0.8	63	0.69	16	0.07	0.13	0.4	8	[12]
Mung	105	88.8	37	4.0	0.2	6.9	(20–59)	[39–67]	(1.4–2.6)	[234–378]	0.95	2	0.14	0.14	0.8	20	[12]
Soy	105	86.3	48	6.5	1.5	5.6	50	70	1.1	[63–378]	0.86	8	0.24	0.21	0.8	14	[12]
Bean sprouts, cooked (1 cup)																	
Mung	125	91.0	35	4.0	0.3	6.5	21	60	1.1	195	0.64	3	0.11	0.13	0.9	8	[12]
Soy	125	89.0	48	6.6	1.8	4.6	54	63	0.9	[234]	0.88	10	0.20	0.19	0.9	5	[12]
Broccoli, boiled, drained, stalks, ½-in. pieces (½ cup)	78	91.3	20	2.4	0.3	3.5	68	48	0.6	207	0.12	194	0.07	0.16	0.6	70	44
Bulgur wheat, dry[f] (2 tbsp)	21	10.0	75	2.4	0.3	16.2	6	72	0.8	49	0.45	(0)	0.06	0.03	1.0	2	2
Carrot juice (½ cup)	[122]	89.0	49	1.0	0.2	11.3	29	50	0.6	350	0.20	2,575	0.11	0.06	0.5	10	5
Cheese (1 oz)																	
Brick	28	41.8	105	6.6	8.4	0.8	191	128	0.1	38	0.74	86	(0)	0.10	(0)	0	6
Camembert	28	52.5	85	5.6	6.9	0.2	110	98	0.1	53	0.68	71	0.01	0.14	0.2	0	18
Edam	28	42.1	101	7.1	7.9	0.4	207	152	0.1	53	1.06	72	0.01	0.11	(0)	0	5
Gorgonzola	28	42.1	111	7.1	9.0	0.3	149	109	[0.0–0.2]	[26–61]	[0.59–1.60]	[103]	0.01	0.09	0.2	0	9
Gouda	28	42.1	101	7.1	7.8	0.6	198	155	0.1	34	1.11	49	0.01	0.10	(0)	0	6
Gruyère	28	33.6	117	8.5	9.2	0.1	287	172	[0.0–0.2]	23	[0.59–1.60]	[105]	0.02	0.08	(0)	0	3
Liederkranz	28	52.9	87	4.8	7.5	0.3	[110]	[98]	[0.0–0.2]	[26–61]	[0.59–1.60]	[91]	[0.01]	[0.18]	0.1	0	34
Limburger	28	48.9	93	5.7	7.7	0.2	141	111	(0)	36	0.60	[110]	0.02	0.14	0.1	0	16
Muenster	28	42.1	104	6.6	8.5	0.3	203	133	0.1	38	0.80	90	(0)	0.09	0.1	0	3
Parmesan, grated	28	17.9	129	11.8	8.5	1.1	390	229	0.3	30	0.90	60	0.01	0.11	0.1	0	2
Roquefort, blue	28	40.0	105	6.1	8.7	0.6	188	111	0.2	26	0.59	90	0.01	0.17	0.2	0	14
Swiss, pasteurized, processed	28	42.9	95	7.0	7.1	0.6	219	216	0.2	61	[1.0–1.3]	65	(0)	0.08	(0)	0	2
Flour																	
Buckwheat, dark (3 tbsp)	18.4	12.0	61	2.2	-0.5	13.3	6	64	0.5	(59)	-0.48	(0)	0.11	0.03	0.5	(0)	(8–30)
Buckwheat, light (3 tbsp)	18.4	12.0	64	1.2	0.2	14.6	2	16	0.2	59	0.48	(0)	0.02	(0.01)	(0.1)	(0)	(8–30)
Rye, medium, sifted, spooned into cup (3 tbsp)	16.5	11.0	58	1.9	0.3	12.4	(5)	43	0.4	34	0.22	(0)	0.05	0.02	0.4	(0)	13
Soybean, full fat, not stirred (¼ cup)	21.0	8.0	90	7.8	4.3	6.5	42	119	1.8	353	[0.29–1.02]	2	0.18	0.07	0.5	0	67
Soybean, full fat, stirred (¼ cup)	17.5	8.0	74	6.4	3.6	5.3	35	98	1.5	291	[0.25–0.85]	2	0.15	0.06	0.4	0	56
Goat's milk (1 cup)	244	87.5	163	7.8	9.8	11.2	315	259	0.2	439	-0.86	(117)	0.10	0.27	0.7	2	2
Grains—see bulgur wheat, flour, millet, oats, rice.																	
Humous (hommous, hummus) (1 tbsp)	84	63.0	185	6.6	11.3	13.2	43	181	2.9	223	1.30	11	0.16	0.07	0.8	8	37
Kale, leaves without stems, cooked, drained (½ cup)	55	87.8	22	(2.5)	(0.4)	3.4	103	32	0.9	(122)	[0.39]	457	0.06	0.10	0.9	51	21
Kefir (1 cup)	233	82.3	160	9.3	4.5	8.8	350	319	0.5	205	0.89	155	0.45	0.44	0.3	6	20

Millet, cooked (½ cup)	95	86.2	54	1.4	0.5	10.8	3	47	1.1	64	0.42	(0)	0.10	0.06	0.4	(0)	10
Miso (3 tbsp)	50	42.9	102	6.2	3.1	13.5	34	71	1.8	79	3.25	0	0.03	0.07	0.7	0	[22]
Nuts																	
Almonds, shelled, whole (¼ cup)	36	4.7	212	6.6	19.3	6.9	83	179	1.7	275	(0.92–1.29)	0	0.09	0.33	1.3	(0)	34
Cashews, roasted in oil, whole kernels (¼ cup)	35	5.2	196	6.0	16.0	10.3	13	131	1.3	163	1.53	4	0.15	0.09	0.6	(0)	24
Pignolia nuts (pine nuts) (6 tbsp)	67	5.6	374	21.1	32.2	7.9	[91]	[311]	[3.6]	[498]	[1.25–3.43]	(0)	0.43	[0.40]	[1.5]	(0)	[16–71]
Pistachios, shelled (¼ cup)	35	5.3	216	7.0	19.5	6.9	48	181	2.7	353	0.83	8	0.24	[0.21]	0.5	0	20
Oats, dry (¼ cup)	20	8.3	78	2.9	1.5	13.7	11	81	0.9	71	0.68	(0)	0.12	0.03	0.2	(0)	11
Onions, green, raw, bulb, entire top (⅛ cup)	13	89.4	5	0.2	(0)	1.0	6	5	0.1	29	[0.01]	(25)	0.01	0.01	0.1	4	[2]
Orange, whole, 2⅝-in. diameter (1 orange)	143	86.4	66	1.0	(0.3)	16.9	60	24	0.3	(290)	0.03	(28)	0.14	0.06	0.6	(63)	66
Peanut butter (1 tbsp)	16	1.7	94	4.0	8.1	3.0	9	61	0.3	100	0.46	(0)	0.02	0.02	2.4	0	13
Peanuts—see beans and peas.																	
Pita bread (Arabic bread, Syrian bread) (½ of a 2½-oz loaf)	35.4	31.2	99	3.7	0.6	19.5	29	36	0.9	42	0.28	(0)	0.27	0.13	1.7	0	[9–21]
Rice																	
Brown, cooked, long grain, hot (⅓ cup)	65	70.3	77	1.6	0.4	16.6	8	47	0.3	46	(0.39–0.73)	(0)	0.06	0.01	0.9	(0)	3
Wild, cooked (½ cup)	[100]	76.0	92	3.6	0.2	19.0	5	85	1.1	55	1.17	(0)	0.11	0.16	1.6	(0)	35
Seeds																	
Pumpkin seeds (squash seeds), dry, hulled	35	4.4	194	10.2	16.4	5.3	18	401	3.9	[334]	[1.3–2.4]	3	0.09	0.07	0.9	(0)	[32]
Sesame seeds, dry, hulled	32	5.5	188	6.0	17.2	5.6	36	188	0.8	[334]	1.90	[2–3]	0.04	0.04	1.6	0	32
Sunflower kernels, dry, hulled	36	4.8	203	8.7	17.2	7.2	44	304	2.6	334	1.64	2	0.71	0.08	2.0	(0)	84
Soymilk (unfortified) (½ cup)	100	90.7	45	2.9	3.1	2.2	10	52	0.4	4	0.18	0	0.28	0.60	0.2	0	28
Squash, yellow (½ cup)	105	95.3	16	1.1	0.2	3.3	27	27	0.4	148	0.19	46	0.06	0.09	0.9	12	11
Tahini (tahini butter) (1 tsp)	7	2.5	45	1.3	4.0	1.0	7	59	0.6	29	0.32	(0)	0.04	0.02	0.3	0	7
Tofu (soybean curd)[g] (1 piece 2½ × 2¾ × 1 in.)	120	84.8	86	9.4	5.0	2.9	154	151	2.3	50	0.88	0	0.07	0.04	0.1	0	[55]
Tomato sauce, canned (½ cup)	125	89.1	39	1.6	0.4	9.1	14	43	1.1	486	(0.25–0.31)	133	0.10	0.06	1.4	22	11
Water chestnuts, raw (4 chestnuts)	58	78.3	46	0.8	0.1	11.1	2	38	0.4	291	0.23	0	0.08	0.12	0.6	2	[13]
Wheat berries, cooked (⅓ cup)	50	86.4	28	(0.8–1.1)	0.2	5.7	3	30	0.3	29	(0.37–0.51)	(0)	0.04	0.01	0.4	(0)	6
Wheat germ, toasted, without sugar (1 tbsp)	6	4.2	23	1.8	0.7	3.0	3	70	0.5	57	0.86	1	0.11	0.05	0.3	1	20
Yeast, brewer's, dry (1 tbsp)	8	5.0	25	3.0	(0)	3.0	17	140	1.4	152	0.59	(0)	1.25	0.34	3.0	(0)	313[h]

[a]Zero in parentheses indicates that the amount of a nutrient, if present, is probably too small to measure. Numbers and ranges in parentheses denote values obtained from food sources that provided information on a food apparently identical to the food listed here. A range is given when two or more values were found that differed by more than 20%. Numbers and ranges in brackets denote values ascribed to the food from values for a similar food or food group. Whenever water percentages are given, estimates of nutrient amounts were adjusted for water content. When no water percentages are given, nutrients were calculated on the basis of weight only.

[b]Edible portions unless otherwise indicated.

[c]Most of the phosphorus in nuts, legumes, and outer layers of cereal grains is present as phytic acid.

[d]When vitamin A (I.U.) was reported for animal products, the value given was divided by 3.33 to derive RE (Retinol equivalents); when for plant products, by 10.0.

[e]Dark red kidney beans may have more thiamin per ½-cup serving.

[f]Bulgur values are for 2 tbsp dry, hard, red winter wheat as indicated. For 2 tbsp canned unseasoned wheat (56% water), all values are about 40% of those shown here except those for thiamin and riboflavin, which are about 15% of those shown here.

[g]Tofu has varying protein and water contents. Differences depend on method of preparation, type of coagulant, and grade and protein content of beans. Calcium and magnesium contents of tofu also vary considerably, according to the coagulant used. Sea salt coagulant is high in magnesium.

[h]The availability of folacin in yeast is significantly lower than in other foods, perhaps because of the conjugase inhibitors in yeast.

Source: Deloris D. Trusdale, Eleanor N. Whitney, and Phyllis B. Acosta, "Nutrients in Vegetarian Foods," Copyright The American Dietitic Association. Reprinted by permission from Journal of the American Dietetic Association, *84 (1984):28–35.*

Appendix F
Energy Expenditure in Household, Recreational, and Sports Activities (in kcal/min)

Activity	kcal/min	\[Kilograms\] 40 / \[Pounds\] 89	46 / 101	50 / 110	53 / 117	56 / 123	59 / 130	62 / 137	65 / 143	68 / 150	71 / 157	74 / 163	77 / 170	80 / 176	83 / 183	86 / 190	89 / 196	92 / 203	95 / 209	98 / 216
Archery	0.065	2.6	3.0	3.3	3.4	3.6	3.8	4.0	4.2	4.4	4.6	4.8	5.0	5.2	5.4	5.6	5.8	6.0	6.2	6.4
Badminton	0.097	3.9	4.7	4.9	5.1	5.4	5.7	6.0	6.3	6.6	6.9	7.2	7.5	7.8	8.1	8.3	8.6	8.9	9.2	9.5
Basketball	0.138	5.5	6.3	6.9	7.3	7.7	8.1	8.6	9.0	9.4	9.8	10.2	10.6	11.0	11.5	11.9	12.3	12.7	13.1	13.5
Billiards	0.042	1.7	1.9	2.1	2.2	2.4	2.5	2.6	2.7	2.9	3.0	3.1	3.2	3.4	3.5	3.6	3.7	3.9	4.0	4.1
Boxing																				
in ring	0.222	8.9	10.2	6.9	7.3	7.7	8.1	8.6	9.0	9.4	9.8	10.2	10.6	11.0	11.5	11.9	12.3	12.7	13.1	13.5
sparring	0.138	5.6	6.3	11.1	11.8	12.4	13.1	13.8	14.4	15.1	15.8	16.4	17.1	17.8	18.4	19.1	19.8	20.4	21.1	21.8
Canoeing																				
leisure	0.044	1.8	2.0	2.2	2.3	2.5	2.6	2.7	2.9	3.0	3.1	3.3	3.4	3.5	3.7	3.8	3.9	4.0	4.2	4.3
racing	0.103	4.1	4.7	5.2	5.5	5.8	6.1	6.4	6.7	7.0	7.3	7.6	7.9	8.2	8.5	8.9	9.2	9.5	9.8	10.1
Card playing	0.025	1	1.1	1.3	1.3	1.4	1.5	1.6	1.6	1.7	1.8	1.9	1.9	2.0	2.1	2.2	2.2	2.3	2.4	2.5
Carpentry, general	0.052	2.1	2.4	2.6	2.8	2.9	3.1	3.2	3.4	3.5	3.7	3.8	4.0	4.2	4.3	4.5	4.6	4.8	4.9	5.1
Carpet sweeping (F)	0.045	1.8	2.1	2.3	2.4	2.5	2.7	2.8	2.9	3.1	3.2	3.3	3.5	3.6	3.7	3.9	4.0	4.1	4.3	4.4
Carpet sweeping (M)	0.048	1.9	2.2	2.4	2.5	2.7	2.8	3.0	3.1	3.3	3.4	3.6	3.7	3.8	4.0	4.1	4.3	4.4	4.6	4.7
Cleaning (F)	0.062	2.5	2.9	3.1	3.3	3.5	3.7	3.8	4.0	4.2	4.4	4.6	4.8	5.0	5.1	5.3	5.5	5.7	5.9	6.1
Cleaning (M)	0.058	2.3	2.7	2.9	3.1	3.2	3.4	3.6	3.8	3.9	4.1	4.3	4.5	4.6	4.8	5.0	5.2	5.3	5.5	5.7
Climbing hills																				
with no load	0.121	4.8	5.6	6.1	6.4	6.8	7.1	7.5	7.9	8.2	8.6	9.0	9.3	9.7	10.0	10.4	10.8	11.1	11.5	11.9
with 5-kg load	0.129	5.2	5.9	6.5	6.8	7.2	7.6	8.0	8.4	8.8	9.2	9.5	9.9	10.3	10.7	11.1	11.5	11.9	12.3	12.6
with 10-kg load	0.140	5.6	6.4	7.0	7.4	7.8	8.3	8.7	9.1	9.5	9.9	10.4	10.8	11.2	11.6	12.0	12.5	12.9	13.3	13.7
with 20-kg load	0.147	5.9	6.8	7.4	7.8	8.2	8.7	9.1	9.6	10.0	10.4	10.9	11.3	11.8	12.2	12.6	13.1	13.5	14.0	14.4
Coal mining																				
drilling coal, rock	0.094	3.8	4.3	4.7	5.0	5.3	5.5	5.8	6.1	6.4	6.7	7.0	7.2	7.5	7.8	8.1	8.4	8.6	8.9	9.2
erecting supports	0.088	3.5	4.0	4.4	4.7	4.9	5.2	5.5	5.7	6.0	6.2	6.5	6.8	7.0	7.3	7.6	7.8	8.1	8.4	8.6
shoveling coal	0.108	4.3	5.0	5.4	5.7	6.0	6.4	6.7	7.0	7.3	7.7	8.0	8.3	8.6	9.0	9.3	9.6	9.9	10.3	10.6
Cooking (F)	0.045	1.8	2.1	2.3	2.4	2.5	2.7	2.8	2.9	3.1	3.2	3.3	3.5	3.6	3.7	3.9	4.0	4.1	4.3	4.4
Cooking (M)	0.048	1.9	2.2	2.4	2.5	2.7	2.8	3.0	3.1	3.3	3.4	3.6	3.7	3.8	4.0	4.1	4.3	4.4	4.6	4.7
Croquet	0.059	2.4	2.7	3.0	3.1	3.3	3.5	3.7	3.9	4.0	4.2	4.4	4.5	4.7	4.9	5.1	5.3	5.4	5.6	5.8
Dancing																				
ballroom	0.051	2.0	2.3	2.6	2.7	2.9	3.0	3.2	3.3	3.5	3.6	3.8	3.9	4.1	4.2	4.4	4.5	4.7	4.8	5.0
choreographed				8.4	8.9	9.4	9.9	10.4	10.9	11.4	11.9	12.4	12.9	13.4	13.9	14.4	15.0	15.5	16.0	16.5
"twist," "wiggle"	0.168	6.7	7.7	5.2	5.5	5.8	6.1	6.4	6.7	7.0	7.3	7.6	7.9	8.2	8.5	8.9	9.2	9.5	9.8	10.1
Digging trenches	0.145	5.8	6.7	7.3	7.7	8.1	8.6	9.0	9.4	9.9	10.3	10.7	11.2	11.6	12.0	12.5	12.9	13.3	13.8	14.2
Drawing (standing)	0.036	1.4	1.7	1.8	1.9	2.0	2.1	2.2	2.3	2.4	2.6	2.7	2.8	2.9	3.0	3.1	3.2	3.3	3.4	3.5
Eating (sitting)	0.023	1.0	1.1	1.2	1.2	1.3	1.4	1.4	1.5	1.6	1.6	1.7	1.8	1.8	1.9	2.0	2.0	2.1	2.2	2.3
Electrical work	0.058	2.3	2.7	2.9	3.1	3.2	3.4	3.6	3.8	3.9	4.1	4.3	4.5	4.6	4.8	5.0	5.2	5.3	5.5	5.7
Farming																				
barn cleaning	0.135	5.4	6.2	6.8	7.2	7.6	8.0	8.4	8.8	9.2	9.6	10.0	10.4	10.8	11.2	11.6	12.0	12.4	12.8	13.2
driving harvester	0.040	1.6	1.8	2.0	2.1	2.2	2.4	2.5	2.6	2.7	2.8	3.0	3.1	3.2	3.3	3.4	3.6	3.7	3.8	3.9
driving tractor	0.037	1.5	1.7	1.9	2.0	2.1	2.2	2.3	2.4	2.5	2.6	2.7	2.8	3.0	3.1	3.2	3.3	3.4	3.5	3.6
feeding cattle	0.085	3.4	3.9	4.3	4.5	4.8	5.0	5.3	5.5	5.8	6.0	6.3	6.5	6.8	7.1	7.3	7.6	7.8	8.1	8.3
feeding animals	0.065	2.6	3.0	3.3	3.4	3.6	3.8	4.0	4.2	4.4	4.6	4.8	5.0	5.2	5.4	5.6	5.8	6.0	6.2	6.4
forking straw bales	0.138	5.5	6.3	6.9	7.3	7.7	8.1	8.6	9.0	9.4	9.8	10.2	10.6	11.0	11.5	11.9	12.3	12.7	13.1	13.5
milking by hand	0.054	2.2	2.5	2.7	2.9	3.0	3.2	3.3	3.5	3.7	3.8	4.0	4.2	4.3	4.5	4.6	4.8	5.0	5.1	5.3
milking by machine	0.023	1.0	1.1	1.2	1.2	1.3	1.4	1.4	1.5	1.6	1.6	1.7	1.8	1.8	1.9	2.0	2.0	2.1	2.2	2.3
shoveling grain	0.085	3.4	3.9	4.3	4.5	4.8	5.0	5.3	5.5	5.8	6.0	6.3	6.5	6.8	7.1	7.3	7.6	7.8	8.1	8.3
Field hockey	0.134	5.4	6.2	6.7	7.1	7.5	7.9	8.3	8.7	9.1	9.5	9.9	10.3	10.7	11.1	11.5	11.9	12.3	12.7	13.1
Fishing	0.062	2.5	2.9	3.1	3.3	3.5	3.7	3.8	4.0	4.2	4.4	4.6	4.8	5.0	5.1	5.3	5.5	5.7	5.9	6.1
Food shopping (F)	0.062	2.5	2.9	3.1	3.3	3.5	3.7	3.8	4.0	4.2	4.4	4.6	4.8	5.0	5.1	5.3	5.5	5.7	5.9	6.1
Food shopping (M)	0.058	2.3	2.7	2.9	3.1	3.2	3.4	3.6	3.8	3.9	4.1	4.3	4.5	4.6	4.8	5.0	5.2	5.3	5.5	5.7
Football	0.132	5.3	6.1	6.6	7.0	7.4	7.8	8.2	8.6	9.0	9.4	9.8	10.2	10.6	11.0	11.4	11.7	12.1	12.5	12.9
Forestry																				
ax chopping, fast	0.297	11.9	13.7	14.9	15.7	16.6	17.5	18.4	19.3	20.2	21.1	22.0	22.9	23.8	24.7	25.5	26.4	27.3	28.2	29.1
ax chopping, slow	0.085	3.4	3.9	4.3	4.5	4.8	5.0	5.3	5.5	5.8	6.0	6.3	6.5	6.8	7.1	7.3	7.6	7.8	8.1	8.3
barking trees	0.123	4.9	5.7	6.2	6.5	6.9	7.3	7.6	8.0	8.4	8.7	9.1	9.5	9.8	10.2	10.6	10.9	11.3	11.7	12.1

Appendix F (*Continued*)

		Kilograms																		
		40	46	50	53	56	59	62	65	68	71	74	77	80	83	86	89	92	95	98
											Pounds									
Activity	kcal/min	89	101	110	117	123	130	137	143	150	157	163	170	176	183	190	196	203	209	216
carrying logs	0.186	7.4	8.6	9.3	9.9	10.4	11.0	11.5	12.1	12.6	13.2	13.8	14.3	14.9	15.4	16.0	16.6	17.1	17.7	18.2
felling trees	0.132	5.3	6.1	6.6	7.0	7.4	7.8	8.2	8.6	9.0	9.4	9.8	10.2	10.6	11.0	11.4	11.7	12.1	12.5	12.9
hoeing	0.091	3.6	4.2	4.6	4.8	5.1	5.4	5.6	5.9	6.2	6.5	6.7	7.0	7.3	7.6	7.8	8.1	8.4	8.6	8.9
planting by hand	0.109	4.4	5.0	5.5	5.8	6.1	6.4	6.8	7.1	7.4	7.7	8.1	8.4	8.7	9.0	9.4	9.7	10.0	10.4	10.7
sawing by hand	0.122	4.9	5.6	6.1	6.5	6.8	7.2	7.6	7.9	8.3	8.7	9.0	9.4	9.8	10.1	10.5	10.9	11.2	11.6	12.0
sawing, power	0.075	3.0	3.5	3.8	4.0	4.2	4.4	4.7	4.9	5.1	5.3	5.6	5.8	6.0	6.2	6.5	6.7	6.9	7.1	7.4
stacking firewood	0.088	3.5	4.0	4.4	4.7	4.9	5.2	5.5	5.7	6.0	6.2	6.5	6.8	7.0	7.3	7.6	7.8	8.1	8.4	8.6
trimming trees	0.129	5.2	5.9	6.5	6.8	7.2	7.6	8.0	8.4	8.8	9.2	9.5	9.9	10.3	10.7	11.1	11.5	11.9	12.3	12.6
weeding	0.072	2.9	3.3	3.6	3.8	4.0	4.2	4.5	4.7	4.9	5.1	5.3	5.5	5.8	6.0	6.2	6.4	6.6	6.8	7.1
Furriery	0.083	3.3	3.8	4.2	4.4	4.6	4.9	5.1	5.4	5.6	5.9	6.1	6.4	6.6	6.9	7.1	7.4	7.6	7.9	8.1
Gardening																				
digging	0.126	5.0	5.8	6.3	6.7	7.1	7.4	7.8	8.2	8.6	8.9	9.3	9.7	10.1	10.5	10.8	11.2	11.6	12.0	12.3
hedging	0.077	3.1	3.5	3.9	4.1	4.3	4.5	4.8	5.0	5.2	5.5	5.7	5.9	6.2	6.4	6.6	6.9	7.1	7.3	7.5
mowing	0.112	4.5	5.2	5.6	5.9	6.3	6.6	6.9	7.3	7.6	8.0	8.3	8.6	9.0	9.3	9.6	10.0	10.3	10.6	11.0
raking	0.054	2.2	2.5	2.7	2.9	3.0	3.2	3.3	3.5	3.7	3.8	4.0	4.2	4.3	4.5	4.6	4.8	5.0	5.1	5.3
Golf	0.085	3.4	3.9	4.3	4.5	4.8	5.0	5.3	5.5	5.8	6.0	6.3	6.5	6.8	7.1	7.3	7.6	7.8	8.1	8.3
Gymnastics	0.066	2.6	3.0	3.3	3.5	3.7	3.9	4.1	4.3	4.5	4.7	4.9	5.1	5.3	5.5	5.7	5.9	6.1	6.3	6.5
Horse-grooming	0.128	5.1	5.9	6.4	6.8	7.2	7.6	7.9	8.3	8.7	9.1	9.5	9.9	10.2	10.6	11.0	11.4	11.8	12.2	12.5
Horse-racing																				
galloping	0.137	5.5	6.3	6.9	7.3	7.7	8.1	8.5	8.9	9.3	9.7	10.1	10.6	11.0	11.4	11.8	12.2	12.6	13.0	13.4
trotting	0.110	4.4	5.1	5.5	5.8	6.2	6.5	6.8	7.2	7.5	7.8	8.1	8.5	8.8	9.1	9.5	9.8	10.1	10.5	10.8
walking	0.041	1.6	1.9	2.1	2.2	2.3	2.4	2.5	2.7	2.8	2.9	3.0	3.2	3.3	3.4	3.5	3.6	3.8	3.9	4.0
Ironing (F)	0.033	1.3	1.5	1.7	1.7	1.8	1.9	2.0	2.1	2.2	2.3	2.4	2.5	2.6	2.7	2.8	2.9	3.0	3.1	3.2
Ironing (M)	0.064	2.6	2.9	3.2	3.4	3.6	3.8	4.0	4.2	4.4	4.5	4.7	4.9	5.1	5.3	5.5	5.7	5.9	6.1	6.3
Judo	0.195	7.8	9.0	9.8	10.3	10.9	11.5	12.1	12.7	13.3	13.8	14.4	15.0	15.6	16.2	16.8	17.4	17.9	18.5	19.1
Knitting, sewing (F)	0.022	1.0	1.0	1.1	1.2	1.2	1.3	1.4	1.4	1.5	1.6	1.6	1.7	1.8	1.8	1.9	2.0	2.0	2.1	2.2
Knitting, sewing (M)	0.023	1.0	1.1	1.2	1.2	1.3	1.4	1.4	1.5	1.6	1.6	1.7	1.8	1.8	1.9	2.0	2.0	2.1	2.2	2.3
Locksmith	0.057	2.3	2.6	2.9	3.0	3.2	3.4	3.5	3.7	3.9	4.0	4.2	4.4	4.6	4.7	4.9	5.1	5.2	5.4	5.6
Lying at ease	0.022	1.0	1.0	1.1	1.2	1.2	1.3	1.4	1.4	1.5	1.6	1.6	1.7	1.8	1.8	1.9	2.0	2.0	2.1	2.2
Machine-tooling																				
machining	0.048	1.9	2.2	2.4	2.5	2.7	2.8	3.0	3.1	3.3	3.4	3.6	3.7	3.8	4.0	4.1	4.3	4.4	4.6	4.7
operating lathe	0.052	2.1	2.4	2.6	2.8	2.9	3.1	3.2	3.4	3.5	3.7	3.8	4.0	4.2	4.3	4.5	4.6	4.8	4.9	5.1
operating punch press	0.088	3.5	4.0	4.4	4.7	4.9	5.2	5.5	5.7	6.0	6.2	6.5	6.8	7.0	7.3	7.6	7.8	8.1	8.4	8.6
tapping and drilling	0.065	2.6	3.0	3.3	3.4	3.6	3.8	4.0	4.2	4.4	4.6	4.8	5.0	5.2	5.4	5.6	5.8	6.0	6.2	6.4
welding	0.052	2.1	2.4	2.6	2.8	2.9	3.1	3.2	3.4	3.5	3.7	3.8	4.0	4.2	4.3	4.5	4.6	4.8	4.9	5.1
working sheet metal	0.048	1.9	2.2	2.4	2.5	2.7	2.8	3.0	3.1	3.3	3.4	3.6	3.7	3.8	4.0	4.1	4.3	4.4	4.6	4.7
Marching, rapid	0.142	5.7	6.5	7.1	7.5	8.0	8.4	8.8	9.2	9.7	10.1	10.5	10.9	11.4	11.8	12.2	12.6	13.1	13.5	13.9
Mopping floor (F)	0.062	2.5	2.9	3.1	3.3	3.5	3.7	3.8	4.0	4.2	4.4	4.6	4.8	5.0	5.1	5.3	5.5	5.7	5.9	6.1
Mopping floor (M)	0.058	2.3	2.7	2.9	3.1	3.2	3.4	3.6	3.8	3.9	4.1	4.3	4.5	4.6	4.8	5.0	5.2	5.	5.5	5.7
Painting, inside	0.034	1.4	1.6	1.7	1.8	1.9	2.0	2.1	2.2	2.3	2.4	2.5	2.6	2.7	2.8	2.9	3.0	3.1	3.2	3.3
Painting, outside	0.077	3.1	3.5	3.9	4.1	4.3	4.5	4.8	5.0	5.2	5.5	5.7	5.9	6.2	6.4	6.6	6.9	7.1	7.3	7.5
Planting seedlings	0.070	2.8	3.2	3.5	3.7	3.9	4.1	4.3	4.6	4.8	5.0	5.2	5.4	5.6	5.8	6.0	6.2	6.4	6.7	6.9
Plastering	0.078	3.1	3.6	3.9	4.1	4.4	4.6	4.8	5.1	5.3	5.5	5.8	6.0	6.2	6.5	6.7	6.9	7.2	7.4	7.6
Printing	0.035	1.4	1.6	1.8	1.9	2.0	2.1	2.2	2.3	2.4	2.5	2.6	2.7	2.8	2.9	3.0	3.1	3.2	3.3	3.4
Running, cross-country	0.163	6.5	7.5	8.2	8.6	9.1	9.6	10.1	10.6	11.1	11.6	12.1	12.6	13.0	13.5	14.0	14.5	15.0	15.5	16.0
Running, horizontal																				
11 min, 30 s per mile	0.135	5.4	6.2	6.8	7.2	7.6	8.0	8.4	8.8	9.2	9.6	10.0	10.5	10.9	11.3	11.7	12.1	12.5	12.9	13.3
9 min per mile	0.193	7.7	8.9	9.7	10.2	10.8	11.4	12.0	12.5	13.1	13.7	14.3	14.9	15.4	16.0	16.6	17.2	17.8	18.3	18.9
8 min per mile	0.208	8.3	9.6	10.8	11.3	11.9	12.5	13.1	13.6	14.2	14.8	15.4	16.0	16.5	17.1	17.7	18.3	18.9	19.4	20.0
7 min per mile	0.228	9.1	10.5	12.2	12.7	13.3	13.9	14.5	15.0	15.6	16.2	16.8	17.4	17.9	18.5	19.1	19.7	20.3	20.8	21.4
6 min per mile	0.252	10.1	11.6	13.9	14.4	15.0	15.6	16.2	16.7	17.3	17.9	18.5	19.1	19.6	20.2	20.8	21.4	22.0	22.5	23.1
5 min, 30 s per mile	0.289	11.6	13.3	14.5	15.3	16.2	17.1	17.9	18.8	19.7	20.5	21.4	22.3	23.1	24.0	24.9	25.7	26.6	27.5	28.3
Scraping paint	0.063	2.5	2.9	3.2	3.3	3.5	3.7	3.9	4.1	4.3	4.5	4.7	4.9	5.0	5.2	5.4	5.6	5.8	6.0	6.2
Sitting quietly	0.021	1.0	1.0	1.1	1.1	1.2	1.2	1.3	1.4	1.4	1.5	1.6	1.6	1.7	1.7	1.8	1.9	1.9	2.0	2.1
Skiing, hard snow																				
level, moderate speed	0.119	4.8	5.5	6.0	6.3	6.7	7.0	7.4	7.7	8.1	8.4	8.8	9.2	9.5	9.9	10.2	10.6	10.9	11.3	11.7
level, walking	0.143	5.7	6.6	7.2	7.6	8.0	8.4	8.9	9.3	9.7	10.2	10.6	11.0	11.4	11.9	12.3	12.7	13.2	13.6	14.0
uphill, maximum speed	0.274	11.0	12.6	13.7	14.5	15.3	16.2	17.0	17.8	18.6	19.5	20.3	21.1	21.9	22.7	23.6	24.4	25.2	26.0	26.9

Appendix F (*Continued*)

Activity	kcal/min	40 / 89	46 / 101	50 / 110	53 / 117	56 / 123	59 / 130	62 / 137	65 / 143	68 / 150	71 / 157	74 / 163	77 / 170	80 / 176	83 / 183	86 / 190	89 / 196	92 / 203	95 / 209	98 / 216
Skiing, soft snow																				
leisure (F)	0.111	4.4	5.1	4.9	5.2	5.5	5.8	6.1	6.4	6.7	7.0	7.3	7.5	7.8	8.1	8.4	8.7	9.0	9.3	9.6
leisure (M)	0.098	3.9	4.5	5.6	5.9	6.2	6.5	6.9	7.2	7.5	7.9	8.2	8.5	8.9	9.2	9.5	9.9	10.2	10.5	10.9
Skindiving, as frogman																				
considerable motion	0.276	11.0	12.7	13.8	14.6	15.5	16.3	17.1	17.9	18.8	19.6	20.4	21.3	22.1	22.9	23.7	24.6	25.4	26.2	27.0
moderate motion	0.206	8.2	9.5	10.3	10.9	11.5	12.2	12.8	13.4	14.0	14.6	15.2	15.9	16.5	17.1	17.7	18.3	19.0	19.6	20.2
Snowshoeing, soft snow	0.166	6.6	7.6	8.3	8.8	9.3	9.8	10.3	10.8	11.3	11.8	12.3	12.8	13.3	13.8	14.3	14.8	15.3	15.8	16.3
Squash	0.212	8.5	9.8	10.6	11.2	11.9	12.5	13.1	13.8	14.4	15.1	15.7	16.3	17.0	17.6	18.2	18.9	19.5	20.1	20.8
Standing quietly (F)	0.025	1.0	1.2	1.3	1.3	1.4	1.5	1.6	1.6	1.7	1.8	1.9	1.9	2.0	2.1	2.2	2.2	2.3	2.4	2.5
Standing quietly (M)	0.027	1.1	1.2	1.4	1.4	1.5	1.6	1.7	1.8	1.8	1.9	2.0	2.1	2.2	2.2	2.3	2.4	2.5	2.6	2.6
Steel mill, working in																				
fettling	0.089	3.6	4.1	4.5	4.7	5.0	5.3	5.5	5.8	6.1	6.3	6.6	6.9	7.1	7.4	7.7	7.9	8.2	8.5	8.7
forging	0.100	4.0	4.6	5.0	5.3	5.6	5.9	6.2	6.5	6.8	7.1	7.4	7.7	8.0	8.3	8.6	8.9	9.2	9.5	9.8
hand rolling	0.137	5.5	6.3	6.9	7.3	7.7	8.1	8.5	8.9	9.3	9.7	10.1	10.6	11.0	11.4	11.8	12.2	12.6	13.0	13.4
merchant mill rolling	0.145	5.8	6.7	7.3	7.7	8.1	8.6	9.0	9.4	9.9	10.3	10.7	11.2	11.6	12.0	12.5	12.9	13.3	13.8	14.2
removing slag	0.178	7.1	8.2	8.9	9.4	10.0	10.5	11.0	11.6	12.1	12.6	13.2	13.7	14.2	14.8	15.3	15.8	16.4	16.9	17.4
tending furnace	0.126	5.0	5.8	6.3	6.7	7.1	7.4	7.8	8.2	8.6	8.9	9.3	9.7	10.1	10.5	10.8	11.2	11.6	12.0	12.3
tipping molds	0.092	3.7	4.2	4.6	4.9	5.2	5.4	5.7	6.0	6.3	6.5	6.8	7.1	7.4	7.6	7.9	8.2	8.5	8.7	9.0
Stock clerking	0.054	2.2	2.5	2.7	2.9	3.0	3.2	3.3	3.5	3.7	3.8	4.0	4.2	4.3	4.5	4.6	4.8	5.0	5.1	5.3
Swimming																				
backstroke	0.169	6.8	7.8	8.5	9.0	9.5	10.0	10.5	11.0	11.5	12.0	12.5	13.0	13.5	14.0	14.5	15.0	15.5	16.1	16.6
breast stroke	0.162	6.5	7.5	8.1	8.6	9.1	9.6	10.0	10.5	11.0	11.5	12.0	12.5	13.0	13.4	13.9	14.4	14.9	15.4	15.9
crawl, fast	0.156	6.2	7.8	7.8	8.3	8.7	9.2	9.7	10.1	10.6	11.1	11.5	12.0	12.5	12.9	13.4	13.9	14.4	14.8	15.3
crawl, slow	0.128	5.1	5.9	6.4	6.8	7.2	7.6	7.9	8.3	8.7	9.1	9.5	9.9	10.2	10.6	11.0	11.4	11.8	12.2	12.5
side stroke	0.122	4.9	5.6	6.1	6.5	6.8	7.2	7.6	7.9	8.3	8.7	9.0	9.4	9.8	10.1	10.5	10.9	11.2	11.6	12.0
treading, fast	0.170	6.8	7.8	8.5	9.0	9.5	10.0	10.5	11.1	11.6	12.1	12.6	13.1	13.6	14.1	14.6	15.1	15.6	16.2	16.7
treading, normal	0.062	2.5	2.9	3.1	3.3	3.5	3.7	3.8	4.0	4.2	4.4	4.6	4.8	5.0	5.1	5.3	5.5	5.7	5.9	6.1
Tailoring																				
cutting	0.041	1.6	1.9	2.1	2.2	2.3	2.4	2.5	2.7	2.8	2.9	3.0	3.2	3.3	3.4	3.5	3.6	3.8	3.9	4.0
hand-sewing	0.032	1.3	1.5	1.6	1.7	1.8	1.9	2.0	2.1	2.2	2.3	2.4	2.5	2.6	2.7	2.8	2.8	2.9	3.0	3.1
machine-sewing	0.045	1.8	2.1	2.3	2.4	2.5	2.7	2.8	2.9	3.1	3.2	3.3	3.5	3.6	3.7	3.9	4.0	4.1	4.3	4.4
pressing	0.062	2.5	2.9	3.1	3.3	3.5	3.7	3.8	4.0	4.2	4.4	4.6	4.8	5.0	5.1	5.3	5.5	5.7	5.9	6.1
Typing																				
electric	0.027	1.1	1.2	1.4	1.4	1.5	1.6	1.7	1.8	1.8	1.9	2.0	2.1	2.2	2.2	2.3	2.4	2.5	2.6	2.6
manual	0.031	1.2	1.4	1.6	1.6	1.7	1.8	1.9	2.0	2.1	2.2	2.3	2.4	2.5	2.6	2.7	2.8	2.9	2.9	3.0
Walking, normal pace																				
asphalt road	0.080	3.2	3.7	4.0	4.2	4.5	4.7	5.0	5.2	5.4	5.7	5.9	6.2	6.4	6.6	6.9	7.1	7.4	7.6	7.8
fields and hillsides	0.082	3.3	3.8	4.1	4.3	4.6	4.8	5.1	5.3	5.6	5.8	6.1	6.3	6.6	6.8	7.1	7.3	7.5	7.8	8.0
grass track	0.081	3.2	3.7	4.1	4.3	4.5	4.8	5.0	5.3	5.5	5.8	6.0	6.2	6.5	6.7	7.0	7.2	7.5	7.7	7.9
plowed field	0.077	3.1	3.5	3.9	4.1	4.3	4.5	4.8	5.0	5.2	5.5	5.7	5.9	6.2	6.4	6.6	6.9	7.1	7.3	7.5
Wallpapering	0.048	1.9	2.2	2.4	2.5	2.7	2.8	3.0	3.1	3.3	3.4	3.6	3.7	3.8	4.0	4.1	4.3	4.4	4.6	4.7
Window cleaning (F)	0.059	2.4	2.7	3.0	3.1	3.3	3.5	3.7	3.8	4.0	4.2	4.4	4.5	4.7	4.9	5.1	5.3	5.4	5.6	5.8
Window cleaning (M)	0.058	2.3	2.7	2.9	3.1	3.2	3.4	3.6	3.8	3.9	4.1	4.3	4.5	4.6	4.8	5.0	5.2	5.3	5.5	5.7
Writing (sitting)	0.029	1.2	1.3	1.5	1.5	1.6	1.7	1.8	1.9	2.0	2.1	2.1	2.2	2.3	2.4	2.5	2.6	2.7	2.8	2.8

Note: Symbols (M) and (F) denote experiments for males and females, respectively.

Source: William D. McArdle, Frank I. Katch, and Victor L. Katch, Exercise Physiology: Energy, Nutrition, and Human Performance, 2d ed. (Philadelphia: Lea & Febiger, 1986), pp. 642–649. Used by permission of the publisher. Original data from E. W. Bannister and S. R. Brown, "The Relative Energy Requirements of Physical Activity," in H. B. Falls, ed., Exercise Physiology, Academic Press, New York, 1968; E. T. Howley and M. E. Glover, "The Calorie Costs of Running and Walking One Mile for Men and Women," Medicine and Science in Sports, 6: *235, 1974; R. Passmore and J. V. G. A. Durin, "Human Energy Expenditure,"* Physiological Reviews, 35: *801, 1955.*

Appendix G
Construction of a *t* Scale

Computation of *t* Scores from Raw Scores

1. Compute the mean and standard deviation for the data.

$$M = \frac{\Sigma x}{N}$$

where

Σx = sum of raw scores
N = total number of scores

$$SD = \sqrt{\frac{N \Sigma x^2 - (\Sigma x)^2}{N(N - 1)}}$$

where

$N \Sigma x^2$ = total number of scores times the sum of x^2
$(\Sigma x)^2$ = sum of $(x)^2$

2. Divide the standard deviation by 10.
3. Construct a table of numbers from 20 to 80. Begin by placing 50 in the center of the page and numbering upward to 80 and downward to 20. Place the mean of the raw scores opposite 50 at the center of the table.
4. Add the value obtained in step 2 to the mean and to each subsequent number to represent *t* scores 51 to 80. Conversely, subtract the constant found in step 2 from the mean and from each number to represent *t* scores 49 to 20.
5. Round off the scores in order to correspond to the actual raw scores.

Note: Rarely will raw scores for any test exceed 80 or fall below 20 on a *t* scale. In cases where the raw scores need higher or lower *t* scale values, the *t* score numbers can be extended from 1 to 100.

Appendix H
Miscellaneous Exercises

These exercises are designed primarily to strengthen or stretch muscles that if underexercised or underdeveloped will contribute to postural abnormalities and back problems.

1. Head Resister (Figure H.1)

Objective: To strengthen the neck muscles.
Instructions: Clasp fingers behind head, with elbows pointing forward. Force the head backward while pulling hands forward to resist the backward movement of the head. Hold position for 5 to 10 seconds.

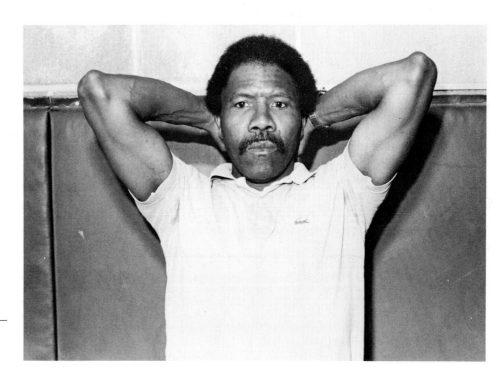

Figure H.1
Head resister.

2. Shoulder Stretch (Figure H.2)

Objective: To develop flexibility in the shoulder joint.

Instructions: From a standing position, reach over the right shoulder with the right hand and touch the fingers of the left hand, which is placed behind the back with palms facing away from the body. Repeat with left hand.

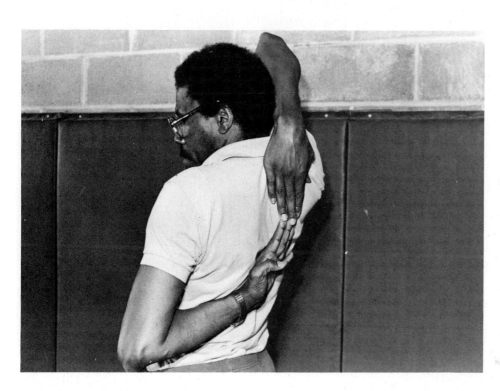

Figure H.2
Shoulder stretch.

3. Abdominal Tightener (Figure H.3)

Objective: To strengthen the abdominal muscles.

Instructions: Contract the abdominal muscles as you inhale. Hold position for 10 to 15 seconds while breathing normally.

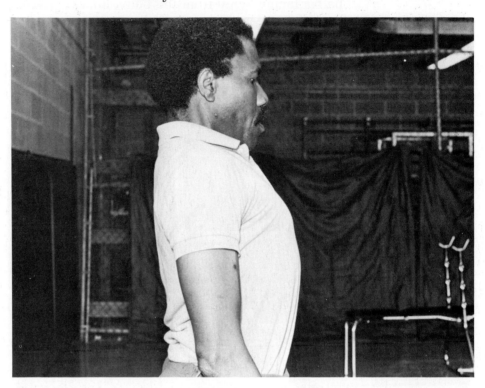

Figure H.3
Abdominal tightener.

4. Curl and Tuck (Figure H.4)

Objective: To strengthen the abdominals and hip flexor muscles.

Instructions: Lying on the back with knees slightly bent and arms outstretched overhead, curl up with the upper body and drag the heels along the floor to arrive in a seated tuck position with the hands clasped behind the knees. Hold for 10 to 30 seconds before returning to the starting position. Inhale in the lying position; exhale as you tuck.

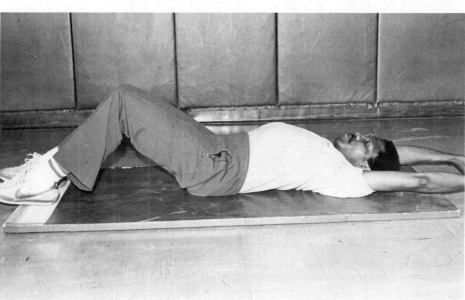

(a)

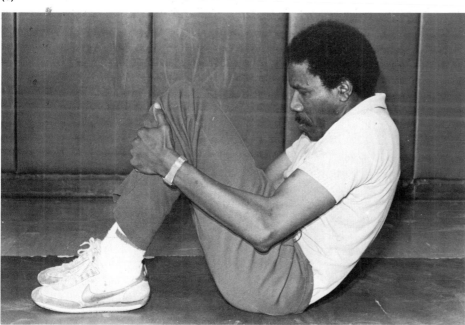

(b)

Figure H.4
Curl and tuck: (a) start, (b) finish.

5. Pelvic Tilt (Figure H.5)

Objective: To strengthen the abdominals and stretch the back muscles (erector spinae).

Instructions: From a lying position on the back with the knees bent and feet flat on floor, contract the abdominals and buttocks and press the lower back against the floor. Hold contracted position for 10 to 30 seconds, then relax. Repeat 3 times. Exhale as you contract. Do not hold your breath.

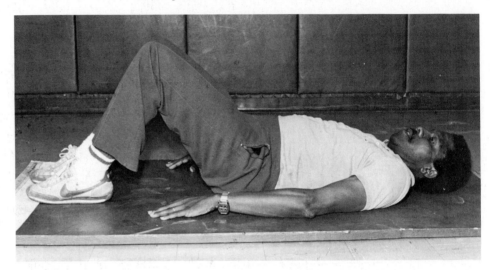

Figure H.5
Pelvic tilt

6. Supine Single-Leg Extension (Figure H.6)

Objective: To increase the flexibility of the muscles in the lumbar spine area (lower back).

Instructions: From a supine (face-up) position with knees bent, bring one knee to your chest, then extend the knee and foot toward the ceiling. Hold this position for 3 to 5 seconds. Return to the starting position by bringing the knee back to the chest and then to the floor. Repeat with the other leg. Keep the lower back flat against the floor throughout the exercise.

Alternate: A more strenuous exercise is the Supine Double-Leg Extension. It is performed by drawing both knees to the chest, then extending both legs toward the ceiling while keeping the lower back flat against the floor.

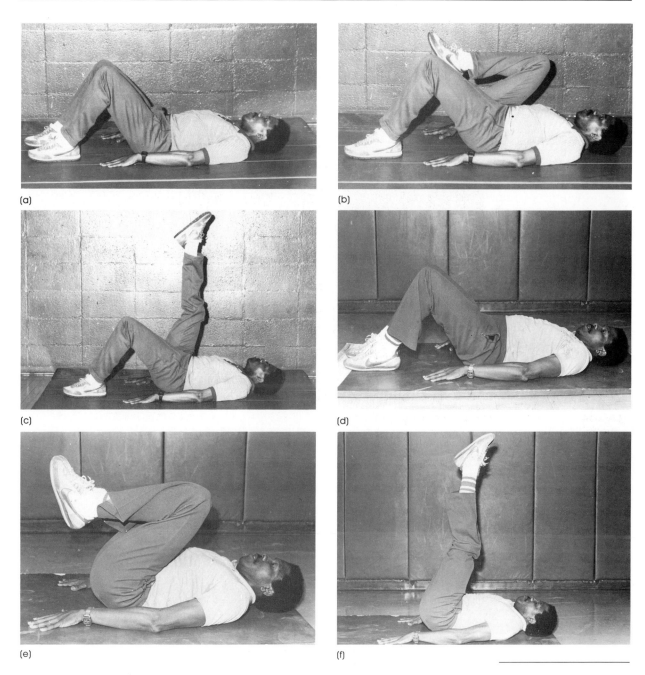

(a)

(b)

(c)

(d)

(e)

(f)

Figure H.6
Supine single-leg
extension: (a) start, (b)
intermediate, (c) finish.
Alternate: (d) start, (e)
intermediate, (f) finish.

7. Buttocks Lift (Figure H.7)

Objective: To strengthen the gluteal muscles.

Instructions: From a lying position flat on the back with the feet close to the buttocks, contract the gluteal muscles and lift the buttocks as high off the floor as possible. Do not raise the back from the floor. Hold position for 5 seconds and relax. Repeat 3 to 5 times.

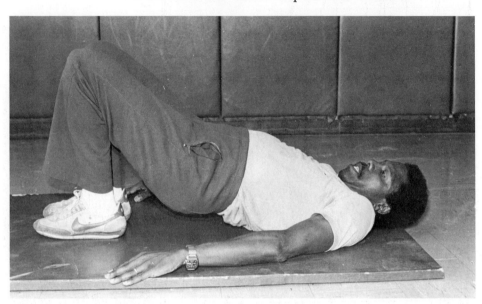

Figure H.7
Buttocks lift.

8. Wall Squat (Figure H.8)

Objective: To strengthen the quadriceps muscle.

Instructions: From a standing position about 6 inches from a wall, gradually lower the body until a sitting position is reached (knees bent to a 90-degree angle). Keep the back straight and do not place all the body weight on the wall (use the wall only to keep the body straight).

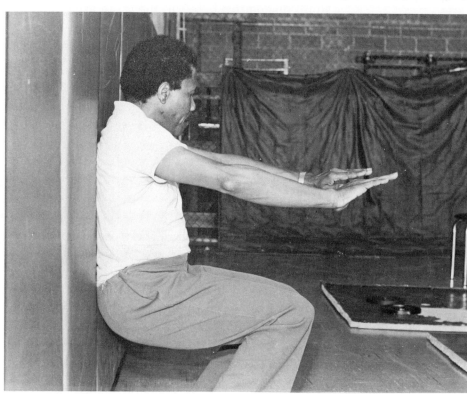

Figure H.8
Wall squat.

9.   Groin Stretcher (Figure H.9)

Objective: To increase the flexibility of the abductor muscles of the inner thighs.

Instructions: From a sitting position with the knees bent and feet turned so that the soles are touching, move the feet as close to the crotch as possible. Stretch the groin muscles by slowly pushing down on the knees until a slight discomfort is felt in the groin area. Hold for 10 to 30 seconds.

Note: This exercise may also be performed by bending forward at the waist (with a rounded back) and clasping the hands around the toes.

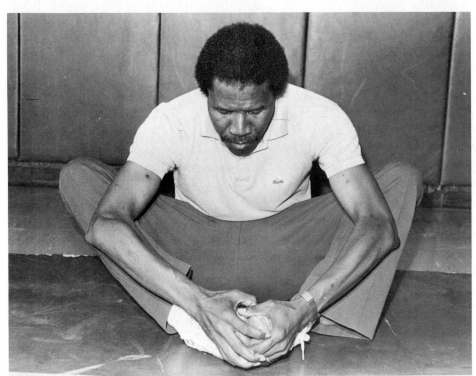

Figure H.9
Groin stretcher.

10. Lunge (Figure H.10)

Objective: To increase the flexibility of the hip flexor muscles.
Instructions: From a position with the right leg bent in front of the
                    body and the left leg nearly straight and the heel of
                    the left foot off the floor, shift the weight forward on
                    the right leg. Hold the position for 3 to 5 seconds, then
                    relax and repeat with the other leg. (Place the hands
                    on the floor outside the bent front leg for balance.)

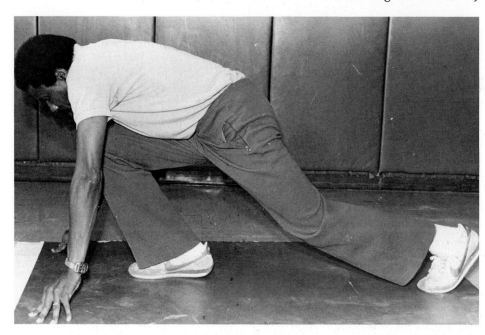

Figure H.10
Lunge.

11. Shin Pull (Figure H.11)

Objective: To stretch the muscles at the front of the lower leg (tibialis anterior).

Instructions: From a seated position with the legs straight in front, flex the ankles and point the toes toward the knees. Hold position 5 to 10 seconds, then relax and repeat.

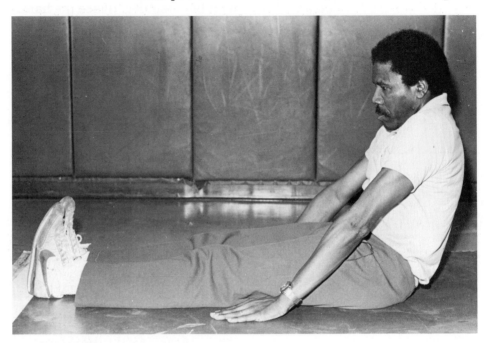

Figure H.11
Shin pull.

12.   Heel Raise (Figure H.12)

Objective: To strengthen the muscles at the back of the lower leg (gastrocnemius and soleus).

Instructions: Standing with the feet shoulder-width apart, bounce gently on the toes, bending the knees slightly and keeping the heels from touching the floor.

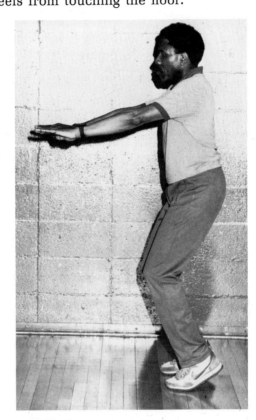

Figure H.12
Heel raise.

13.   Achilles Stretcher (Figure H.13)

Objective: To increase the flexibility of the heel cord area (primarily the Achilles tendon).

Instructions: Standing with the balls of the feet on a book, thick board, bleacher seat, or some other solid object, slowly lower the heel as far as possible below the top surface of the object used to stand on. Do not let the heels touch the floor. Hold position for 10 to 30 seconds.

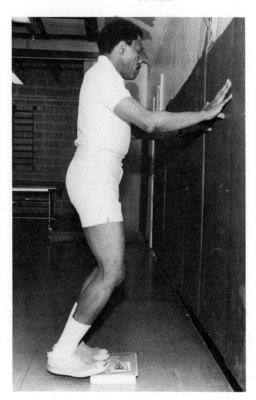

Figure H.13
Achilles stretcher.

Appendix I
Fitness Forms

Aerobic Exercise Record Form

NAME_____ GOAL:_____ DATE FOR GOAL_____

DATE	ACTIVITY	DURATION	THR*	RHR+

*Target Heart Rate

+Resting Heart Rate

Physical Fitness Test Battery Record Form

Name_____ Age_____Sex_____ Date_____

Body Weight_____Height_____Percent Body Fat_____

Anthropometric Measurements

Bust/Chest_____ in.
Hips   _____ in.
Waist   _____ in.
Thighs (R)_____ in. (L)_____ in.
Upper Arm (R)_____ in. (L)_____ in.

Strength	Raw Score	T-Score
Dominant-hand Grip Strength		
Nondominant-hand Grip Strength	_____ kg.	_____
Bench Press	_____ lbs.	_____

Muscular Endurance

	Raw Score	T-Score
Sit-ups (Bent Knee)	_____ no.	_____
Pull-ups	_____ no.	_____
Flexed-arm Hang	_____ sec.	_____
Push-ups	_____ no.	_____
Modified Push-ups	_____ no.	_____
Squat Thrusts	_____ no.	_____

Flexibility

	Raw Score	T-Score
Sit-and-Reach	_____ ins.	_____
Back Arch	_____ ins.	_____

Cardiorespiratory Endurance (Use one of the two tests.)

Resting Heart Rate   _____ Beats per Minute
12-minute Run-Walk   _____ Distance covered in
                                    miles _____
Step Test   _____ Recovery
                                    Index _____

Physical Fitness Profile Record Form

Date _____

Name _____ Age _____ Sex _____

Body weight _____ Height _____ Percent body fat _____

Composite evaluation of all fitness components:

	Raw Score	t Score*	Classification†
Strength			
Dominant-hand grip strength	_____kg	_____	_____
Nondominant-hand grip strength	_____kg	_____	_____
Bench press	_____lb	_____	_____
Muscular Endurance			
Sit-ups (bent-knee)	_____no.	_____	_____
Pull-ups *or*	_____no.	_____	_____
Flexed-arm hang	_____no.	_____	_____
Squat thrusts	_____no.	_____	_____
Flexibility			
Sit and reach	_____in.	_____	_____
Back arch	_____in.	_____	_____
Cardiorespiratory Endurance			
12-minute run-walk	_____ (distance covered)		
		_____	_____

Sum of *t* scores = _____

Average of *t* scores = _____   _____

(Divide sum of *t* scores by number of tests to get average *t* score.)   Overall Classification

_____

*Tables 5.16 and 5.17 contain *t* scores for some of the test items included here.

†Rate each test according to the classification scale in Table 5.18.

Eating Behavior Record Form

Name_____ Day & Date_____

	ANTECEDENT EVENTS (when, where, time and mood before & during eating)	Food Consumption			CONSEQUENT EVENTS (activities & mood following eating)
		Food	Amount	Calories	
BREAKFAST					
INBETWEEN					
LUNCH					
INBETWEEN					
DINNER					
AFTER DINNER					

Total Calories = _____

Source: Adapted from Craighead/Kazdin/Mahoney: Behavior Modification: Principles, Issues, and Applications, Copyright © 1976 by Houghton Mifflin Company. Adapted with permission.

Two-Week Weight Information Form

Name_____

Body frame_____(S)_____(M)_____(L)_____

Beginning weight _____   Date_____

Desired weight   _____   Date_____

Day	Date	Beginning weight	Current weight	Difference
1 M	____	_____	_____	_____
2 Tu	____	_____	_____	_____
3 W	____	_____	_____	_____
4 Th	____	_____	_____	_____
5 F	____	_____	_____	_____
6 S	____	_____	_____	_____
7 Su	____	_____	_____	_____
8 M	____	_____	_____	_____
9 Tu	____	_____	_____	_____
10 W	____	_____	_____	_____
11 Th	____	_____	_____	_____
12 F	____	_____	_____	_____
13 S	____	_____	_____	_____
14 Su	____	_____	_____	_____

Daily Weight Graph Form

Name_____

Body frame___(S)_____(M)_____(L)_____

Beginning weight_____ Date_____

Desired weight_____ Date_____

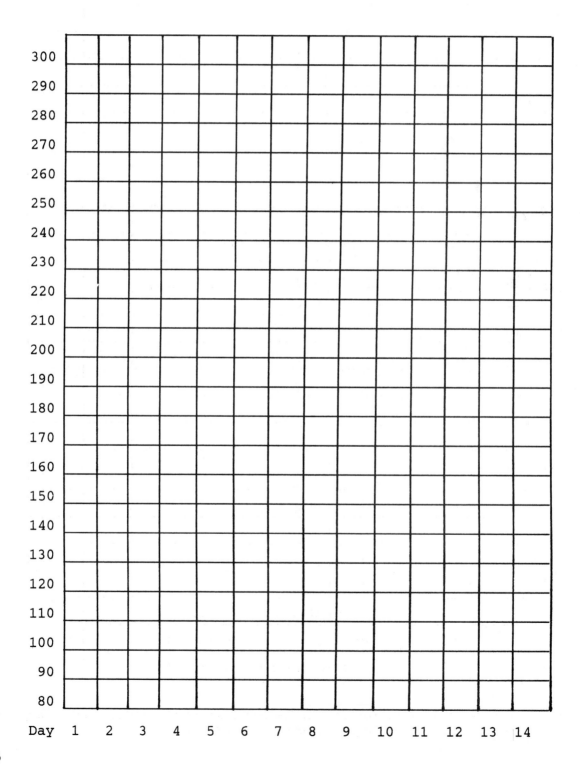

Day   1   2   3   4   5   6   7   8   9   10 11 12 13 14

Activity Record Form

Name		1/2 MET	Wt. 1/2 hr MET	1/2 MET	Total METS per hr
A.M. 6:00			6:30		
7:00			7:30		
8:00			8:30		
9:00			9:30		
10:00			10:30		
11:00			11:30		
12:00			12:30		
P.M. 1:00			1:30		
2:00			2:30		
3:00			3:30		
4:00			4:30		
5:00			5:30		
6:00			6:30		
7:00			7:30		
8:00			8:30		
9:00			9:30		
10:00			10:30		
11:00			11:30		
12:00			12:30		
A.M. 1:00			1:30		
2:00			2:30		
3:00			3:30		
4:00			4:30		
5:00			5:30		
Total METS per day (add down)					
Multiply by your 1/2-hr MET value					
Total Calories burned this day					

Source: From Thin and Fit: Your Personal Lifestyle *by Dorothy E. Dusek.* © *1982 by Wadsworth, Inc. Reprinted by permission of Wadsworth Publishing Company, Belmont, California 94002.*

Weight Training Record Form

Name_____ Body Weight_____

Exercise		Dates										
	lb											
	RM											
	lb											
	RM											
	lb											
	RM											
	lb											
	RM											
	lb											
	RM											
	lb											
	RM											
	lb											
	RM											
	lb											
	RM											
	lb											
	RM											
	lb											
	RM											
	lb											
	RM											

Calisthenic Exercise Program Record Form

Name _____ Body Weight _____

Class _____ Section _____ Date _____

Exercise	Target Muscle Group	Repetitions & Sets	
1.			
2.			
3.			
4.			
5.			
6.			
7.			
8.			
9.			
10.			
11.			
12.			
13.			
14.			

Appendix J
Instructions for Large Group Fitness Testing*

Grip Strength (See Figure 5.4)

Instructions

1. Provide at least one dynamometer for each 10 to 15 persons to be tested.
2. Assign one tester for each group to score and record the test results.
3. Make sure that the dynamometer is on the zero setting before the first person uses it.
4. Use some type of chalk on the hands to prevent them from slipping when squeezing the dynamometer.
5. Adjust the grip of the dynamometer so that it fits the hands of the person being tested.
6. Hold the dynamometer in one hand (use the dominant hand first). With the dial set at zero and the bar adjusted for a comfortable grip, apply as much gripping force on the dynamometer as possible with one maximal contraction of the muscles involved. The hand with the dynamometer may be moved during the performance of the test.
7. The hand with the dynamometer is not allowed to be placed against the body, and the free hand cannot be used to assist the hand with the dynamometer in any way.
8. Reset the dial to zero on the dynamometer after each trial.

Scoring instructions

1. Read the dial and record the results in kilograms as indicated by the dial pointer. Record scores only for trials in which the correct procedure is used.
2. Allow two trials, and record the best score (use the Grip Strength Record Chart below). Test the entire group on one hand before testing the other hand. See Table 5.6 for grip strength norms.

Grip Strength Record Chart

Name _____   Date _____

Dominant hand: Trial 1 _____ kg

                                                        Best score _____ kg

                       Trial 2 _____ kg

Nondominant
hand: Trial 1 _____ kg

                                                        Best score _____ kg

                       Trial 2 _____ kg

*The purpose and description of the tests and test norms appear in Chapter 5.

Instructions

1. Assign a tester to observe and record the scores for the subjects.
2. Adjust the weight at the highest number of pounds each person feels he or she can lift once. (A few trial runs might be scheduled before the testing day in order for the participants to get some idea of the weight they can handle.)
3. Instruct the individuals to perform the bench press as indicated in the description of the exercise.
4. If a person fails to lift the selected weight or lifts the weight and feels that additional weight can be lifted, permit two additional adjustments in weight selection.

Scoring instructions

1. Record the greatest amount of weight the person is able to lift.
2. Recognize only scores in which the individuals perform the test using the correct procedure, and record the scores in the Physical Fitness Test Battery Profile Chart in Table 5.1.

Bench Press (See Figure 5.5)

Instructions

1. Divide the group in half. One group assists the other to perform the test.
2. Instruct the participants to assume the starting position on their backs. The assistants should assume their positions as indicated in the description.
3. On the signal to start, the participants should perform as many sit-ups as possible in two minutes.
4. The assistants should count (silently to themselves) the number of sit-ups performed by the persons being tested and record the score on the Physical Fitness Test Battery Profile Chart in Table 5.1.
5. Instruct the groups to exchange places, with the persons being tested becoming the assistants and vice versa. Have the remaining individuals perform the test and the assistants count and record the scores.

Bent-Knee Sit-ups (See Figure 5.6)

Scoring instructions

1. Count each correctly performed sit-up as one.
2. *Do not count* an attempt during which the participant fails to reach a full sit-up position (with the knees touching the elbows and the back in a vertical position).

Pull-ups (See Figure 5.7)*

Instructions

1. Set the bar at a height so the majority of the group will be able to grasp the bar and assume a "dead hang" position. Adjust the height of the bar for extremely tall individuals, and use a chair for those who can't jump and grasp the bar. (Exceptionally tall individuals whose feet will touch the ground should be instructed to bend their legs back at the knees before performing the pull-up.)
2. Assign a spotter to assist the person in grasping the bar and in assuming the "dead hang" position and to keep count of the number of pull-ups being performed.
3. On the command "Begin," instruct the person to assume the correct starting position and execute as many pull-ups as possible. The pull-ups must be performed continuously; resting between pull-ups is not permitted.

Scoring instructions

1. Count the total number of pull-ups performed by the individual, assigning one for each correctly executed pull-up.
2. *Do not count* it as a pull-up if the person (a) fails to raise the chin above the bar, (b) swings or kicks the legs to help raise the body, or (c) fails to come to a "dead hang" after each pull-up.
3. Record the score for the correctly performed pull-ups in the Physical Fitness Profile Chart in Table 5.1.

Flexed-Arm Hang (See Figure 5.8)

Instructions

1. Assign two spotters to assist the persons in assuming the proper flexed-arm hanging position. A chair or some other object may be used for the subjects to attain the proper starting position.
2. Set the bar at a height so that the hanging position can be assumed with the elbows flexed, the body close to the bar, and the chin above the bar.
3. Assign an assistant with a stopwatch to keep track of the time that each person maintains the flexed-arm hang.
4. Instruct the spotters to assist the person in attaining the flexed-arm hanging position. Once the participant is in position and free of the grasp of the spotters, the timer is instructed to start the stopwatch.

Scoring instructions

1. Keep the time (in seconds or minutes and seconds) that the person maintains a proper flexed-arm hang.
2. *Do not count* the time if the person (a) fails to get the chin above the bar, (b) uses kicking and jerking movements to help keep the chin above the bar, (c) rests the chin on the bar, or (d) tilts the body back so that the chin is away from its correct position over the bar.

*Anyone who cannot perform one pull-up should use the flexed-arm hang (Figure 5.8) instead.

Instructions

Push-ups (See Figure 5.9) **and** Modified Push-ups (See Figure 5.10)

1. Divide the group in half. One group assists the other group to perform the test.
2. Instruct the persons being tested to assume the starting position (front-leaning support position) with the assistants kneeling to the side and slightly in front of the persons being tested. Each assistant should place one hand near the chest of the person being tested.
3. On the signal "Ready," the participants are to assume the front-leaning position, and on the signal "Start," they are to perform as many push-ups or modified push-ups as possible in the alloted time.
4. The instructor or assistant should keep the time with a stopwatch.
5. Instruct the groups to exchange places, with the persons being tested becoming the assistants and vice versa. Have the remaining individuals perform the test and the assistants count and record the scores.

Scoring instructions

1. Instruct the assistants to count the number of push-ups or modified push-ups performed by the persons being tested (counting one for each time the person correctly executes the push-up or modified push-up).
2. *Do not count* it as a push-up or modified push-up if the person (a) fails to extend the arms fully, (b) fails to touch the assistant's hand, or (c) fails to keep the body straight throughout the push-up or modified push-up.

Instructions

Squat Thrusts (See Figure 5.11)

1. Divide the group in half. One group assists the other group to perform the test.
2. Instruct the persons being tested to assume the starting position, with the assistants standing in front of them to count and record the number of correctly performed squat thrusts.
3. On the signal "Start," the subjects are to perform as many squat thrusts as possible in 30 seconds.
4. The instructor or an assistant should keep the time with a stopwatch.
5. Instruct the groups to exchange places after the first group completes the test. Have the remaining individuals perform the test and have the assistants count and record the scores.

Scoring instructions

1. Instruct the assistants to count the number of squat thrusts performed by the persons being tested (counting one for each time the person comes to a standing position).
2. *Do not count* it as a squat thrust if the person (a) fails to extend the legs fully in the front support position, (b) goes straight from the standing position to the front support position, (c) fails to return to the squat position before standing, or (d) fails to come to a complete standing position at the end of each repetition.

Sit and Reach (See Figure 5.12)

Instructions

1. Assign one assistant to test 10 to 15 individuals. Instruct the assistant in the proper procedure for testing.
2. Provide a few minutes for the persons being tested to warm up before the test by stretching and bending the muscles that will be used during the test.
3. With an assistant holding the person's knees down and on the signal "Start," perform the sit-and-reach motion as described for the test.
4. Hold the position for three seconds.

Scoring instructions

1. Have the assistant measure the distance reached with the fingertips on the ruler to the nearest quarter inch.
2. Allow two trials, and record the results of the longest distance reached.
3. *Do not count* it if the person (a) fails to keep the knees straight, (b) bounces while reaching, or (c) fails to hold the flexed position for three seconds.

Back Arch (See Figure 5.13)

Instructions

1. Assign one assistant to test 10 to 15 individuals. Instruct the assistant in the proper procedure for testing.
2. Allow the persons being tested to warm up for a few minutes before they are tested.
3. With an assistant holding down the legs and buttocks of the person being tested, and on the signal to start, perform the back arch as described.
4. Hold the position for three seconds.

Scoring instructions

1. Have the assistants measure the distance from the floor to the chin (to the nearest quarter inch).
2. Allow two trials, and record the results of the longest distance measured.
3. *Do not count* it if the person (a) raises the hips off the floor or (b) fails to hold the arched position for three seconds.

Instructions

1. Assume a relaxed, sitting position and remain in that position for 3 to 5 minutes.
2. At the end of the resting period, have each person locate his or her pulse (instruct each person to locate the pulse at the same site—carotid or radial artery).
3. With the instructor or an assistant holding a stopwatch to keep the time, give the signal to begin, and have the individuals count their pulse rate for 30 seconds. This number is doubled to get the heart rate for one minute.

Scoring instructions

1. Allow three trials to get accurate pulse counts.
2. Disregard the highest and lowest pulse counts and record the middle count.
3. Invalidate the results if the heart rate varies more than two beats for any one of the three counts.
4. Permit individuals to take the heart rate until an accurate count is made.
5. Record the results in Table 5.1 and evaluate your score according to the Norms for Resting Heart Rate in Chapter 5.

Note: Individuals might be instructed to take their resting heart rate when they awaken and are still in a reclining position. This should provide the most accurate count of the resting heart rate.

Determining the Resting Heart Rate (See Figure 5.14)

Instructions

1. Mark off a running surface for the 12-minute run-walk. A quarter-mile track is ideal. However, any appropriately measured surface will suffice.
2. Give each person a slip of paper and instruct each of them to write his or her last name and first initial on the paper.
3. Divide the group in half. One group assists the other group to perform the test.
4. Instruct the group that is to run first to line up at the starting line. Each assistant is to count the number of laps his or her partner runs in the 12 minutes.
5. Assign a person with a stopwatch to time the 12-minute run-walk.
6. On the signal to start, the persons being tested are to cover as many laps as possible in the 12 minutes. They may use a combination of running and walking.
7. Inform the persons being tested to attempt to maintain a constant pace for the entire 12 minutes.
8. After the first group completes the run and their scores are recorded by the assistants, have the other group run. The group that was tested will now act as assistants to count laps and record the scores.

Twelve-Minute Run-Walk (See Figure 5.15)

Scoring instructions

1. Instruct each of the assistants to keep a continuous count of the distance being covered by marking a tally on the slip of paper each time his or her partner reaches the starting line. Record the number of laps or the distance covered to the nearest ⅛ mile (refer to Figure 5.15 and the information in the box on this page for a clarification of the scoring and recording procedures).

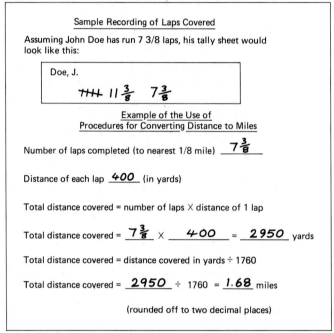

Sample Recording of Laps Covered

Assuming John Doe has run 7 3/8 laps, his tally sheet would look like this:

Doe, J.

TTTT II 11 $\frac{3}{8}$ 7$\frac{3}{8}$

Example of the Use of
Procedures for Converting Distance to Miles

Number of laps completed (to nearest 1/8 mile) __7$\frac{3}{8}$__

Distance of each lap __400__ (in yards)

Total distance covered = number of laps × distance of 1 lap

Total distance covered = __7$\frac{3}{8}$__ × __400__ = __2950__ yards

Total distance covered = distance covered in yards ÷ 1760

Total distance covered = __2950__ ÷ 1760 = __1.68__ miles

(rounded off to two decimal places)

2. Record the number of miles covered in Table 5.1, and evaluate the results according to the norms in Table 5.14.

Step Test (See Figure 5.16)

Instructions

1. Divide the group in half. One group assists the other group to perform the test.
2. Instruct the persons being tested to face the bench and assume the starting position.
3. Assign an assistant to monitor and record the postexercise heart rate of each person being tested.
4. The instructor or an assistant with a stopwatch is responsible for calling out the stepping cadence.
5. On the signal "Begin," the watch is started and the persons being tested are to step up and down on the 18-inch bench for three minutes or as long as they can. If the right foot is used to step up first, it must be followed by the left foot. The lead foot may be changed one time. Straighten out the knees completely when stepping up on the bench. (The call by the instructor or assistant is "up, up; down, down.") The persons being tested must maintain a 30-steps-per-minute cadence. Those who are not able to maintain this cadence should be instructed to discontinue the test.

6. On the signal "Stop," given at the end of three minutes, all persons taking the test are to sit on the bench facing the assistants.

7. Instruct each assistant to locate the pulse of his or her partner and indicate that the first of three postexercise heart rate counts will be taken one minute after the completion of the step test. The time periods for the recovery heart rate are as follows:

1–1½ minutes in recovery
2–2½ minutes in recovery
3–3½ minutes in recovery

8. When preparing to take the recovery heart rates, instruct the assistants to locate the pulse about ten seconds before the signal to begin. Refer to "Determining the Resting Heart Rate" for instructions on taking the pulse rate. Caution the persons taking the test and the assistants to remain quiet during the time the heart rate recovery times are being taken.

9. Reverse the groups, and have the assistants take the test and the other group act as assistants.

Scoring instructions

1. Instruct the assistants to record the following recovery heart rate information in a physical fitness notebook (or on small index cards).

Step test _____ (minutes performed)   Date _____
Heart rates in recovery: (number of beats)   Time _____
     1–1½ min _____   Bench height _____(in.)
     2–2½ min _____
     3–3½ min _____
     Total _____ (Recovery index)

Evaluating cardiorespiratory endurance is accomplished by comparing the recovery index with the norms in Table 5.15. Transfer the heart rate recovery index from the notebook or file cards to the Physical Fitness Profile Chart in Table 5.1.

2. Calculate the recovery index only for persons who perform the step test for the entire three minutes. Record the time for such persons in the blank space following "Step test" on the heart rate information sheet, and record the recovery heart rate in the spaces provided.

3. *Do not* calculate the recovery index for persons who fail to complete the entire three minutes on the step test. Record the time for such persons in the blank space following "Step test" as you did for persons who completed the test.

4. Inform the person to stop and sit down if (a) he or she fails to maintain a stepping rate of 30 steps per minute (according to the person calling out the stepping cadence), (b) he or she does not step up completely on the bench (come to a momentary standing position with the knees straight), or (c) he or she changes the lead foot more than once during the test.

5. Invalidate the scores for persons whose pulse rate was counted improperly (that is, contrary to the instructions for taking the pulse rate). A pulse count would not be accepted, for instance, if it were not taken during the specific time periods indicated in the instructions.

Appendix K
Aerobic Dance Workout

Warm-up activities consist of the following bending, twisting, and stretching movements (others could be included to meet individual needs):

Warm-up (5–10 minutes)

1. Stand in a straddle position, feet about shoulder-width apart, toes straight ahead, and arms at the sides. Keep elbows straight and lift both arms up over the head (8 counts). Then push the right arm up, stretching the right side. Then the left side. Repeat right and left for 8 counts. Lower both arms back down to the side (8 counts). Keeping the knees locked, bend forward slowly as far as you can go, reaching for the floor, letting the arms and head hang loose (8 counts). Hold that position for 8 counts. Lift the upper body, starting with the abdomen (midsection) and continuing until you are in a standing position (8 counts). Keep the shoulders relaxed and down. Repeat the entire movement, starting from the top again.
2. Assume a wide straddle position with the toes turned out. Bring the right arm over the head, bending the upper body to the left side (stretching the right side), and move the left arm across the body (to the right) and gently bounce. Repeat the movement to the left side and gently bounce (8 counts). Extend both arms out to the side and bend the upper torso forward so that it is parallel to the floor. Keep the back flat and the knees locked and gently bounce (8 counts). Come back up to a standing position, place hands on the hips, and arch backward. Move the head back and bounce gently (8 counts). Start the entire movement again from the top and perform 4 counts, then repeat everything again for 2 counts, and again for 1 count (complete 4 sets).
3. Move head down, up (8 counts—hereafter, count is given in parentheses).
    Move head side to side (8).
    Turn head right and left (8).
    Circle head to the right (4).
    Circle head to the left (4).
    Repeat head circles right and left.
    Move right shoulder up, down (8).
    Move left should up, down (8).
    Move both shoulders up, down (8).
    Move right shoulder forward and back (8).
    Move left shoulder forward and back (8).
    Move both shoulders forward and back (8).
    Perform forward arm circles with both arms extended to the side (8).
    Perform backward arm circles (8).
    Perform waist twist right and left with both arms extended to the side (8).
    Bend forward and touch right toe with left hand and left toe with right hand (swing arms and turn at the waist) (8).

4. Jog forward (8).
    Jog backward (8).
    Repeat jogs twice.
    Jump with feet together (8).
    Jump with feet apart (8).
    Repeat jumps with feet together (8).
    Perform Jumping Jacks (8) twice.

Conditioning Bout (15–20 minutes)

The conditioning bout is the aerobic part of the workout, which should be performed continuously for the entire time period. It can be performed at a low, moderate, or high intensity level. The step patterns include jogging, running, hopping, skipping, jumping, and kicking steps.

1. Assume a standing position with feet together. Moving to the right, side-step right, tap left toe on floor (8 counts). (See Figure K.1.) Perform 4 times.

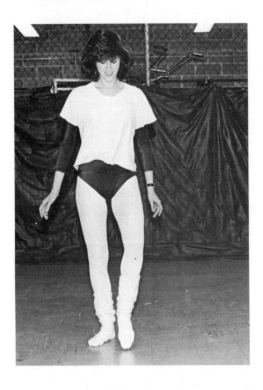

Figure K.1
Step right; tap left toe on floor.

2. Side-step left, tap right toe on floor (8, 4×).
3. Side-step right, feet together, side-step, tap left foot on floor (4 counts: 1-2-3-4) (8, 4×).
4. Side-step left, feet together, side-step, tap right foot on floor (4 counts: 1-2-3-4) (8, 4×).
5. Side-step right, feet together, side-step, jump (8, 4×).
6. Repeat left, same as 5 (8, 4×).

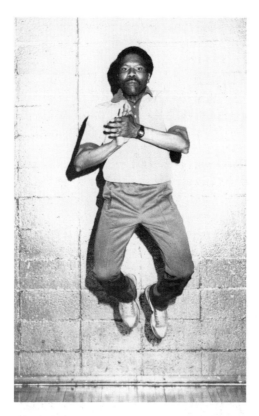

Figure K.2
Jump; clap hands on
jump.

7. Side-step to the right, jump (clap hands on the jump) (8, 4×). (See Figure K.2.)
8. Side-step to the left, jump and clap hands (8, 4×).
9. Jog in place (8, 4×). (See Figure K.3.)

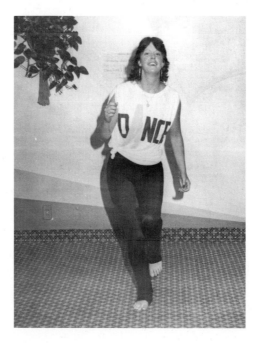

Figure K.3
Jog in place.

10. Run forward three steps and hop, starting with right foot; run backward three steps and hop, starting with left foot (8).

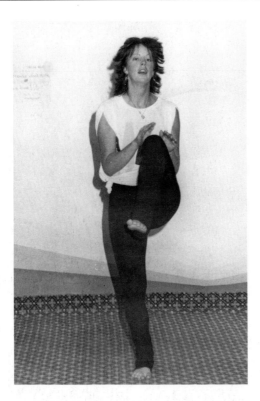

Figure K.4
Skip, touching the
knee with both hands.

11. Skip (step hop, alternating feet, bringing the knee up high and hitting the knee with both hands) (8, 2×). (See Figure K.4.)

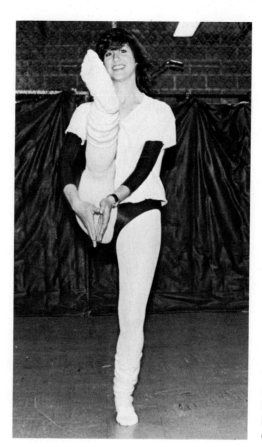

Figure K.5
Kick leg and clap
hands under leg (right
and left).

12. Hop on right foot, kick left leg high, and clap hands under leg (8, 2×). (See Figure K.5.)
13. Repeat on left foot. Alternate kicks (8, 2×).
14. Jog in place (8, 4×). Swing both arms behind you when on the right foot; swing arms in front and clap hands when on left foot.
15. Perform pendulum side-kicks: Hop in place on right foot, kick left leg to left side, swing body to right side. Move arms in the opposite direction of upper body movement (8, 2×).
16. Repeat on the left foot, and continue motion from one foot to the other (8, 2×).

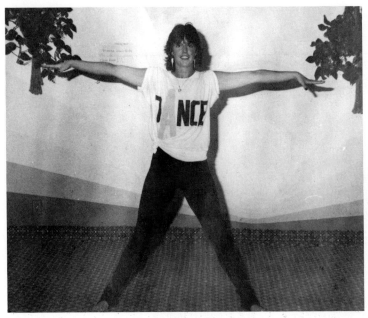

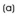

(a)

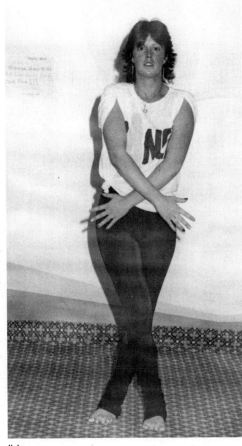

(b)

Figure K.6
Crisscross jump: (a) arms out, (b) arms crossed.

17. Perform crisscross jumps: Swing both arms up and out to the side as you straddle jump, and cross arms in front of body as your feet cross in front and in back (8, 2×). (See Figure K.6.)

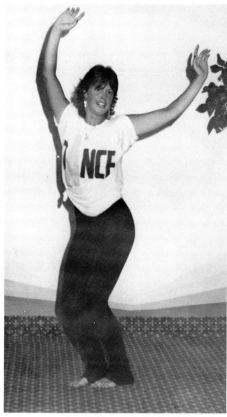

(a)

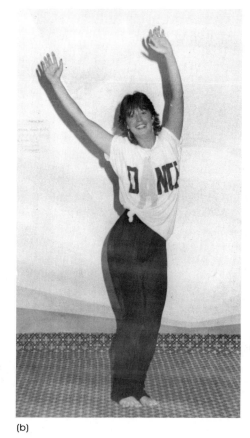

(b)

Figure K.7
Jump twist: (a) right,
(b) left.

18. Perform jump-twists: With arms over the head, jump in place, turning the feet from side to side. Turn arms in the opposite direction (8, 2×). (See Figure K.7.)

19. Perform the Charleston heel hit: Jump on both feet, then kick the right foot up in back and touch with the right hand (8, 2×). (See Figure K.8.)

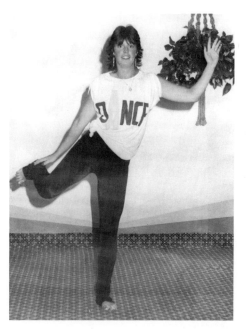

Figure K.8
Charleston heel hit.

20. Repeat to the left. Alternate right and left (8, 2×).
21. Jog in place, kick feet as high up as possible in the back, and shoot the arms straight out in front of the body as if punching. Extend right arm and then left (8, 2×). (See Figure K.9.)

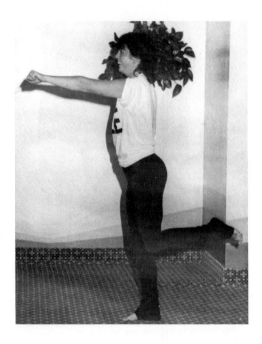

Figure K.9
Jog in place, kick feet high in the back, punch with the arms right and left.

Note: These steps may be repeated as many times as desired.
IMPORTANT! Check the pulse rate immediately after the conditioning bout.

Cool-down (5–10 minutes)

1. Walk slowly for one or two minutes (have students count the pulse rate immediately after the conditioning bout).
2. Place the feet in a straddle position and keep them flat on the floor. Bend the knees and lower the body down on 4 counts and up on 4 counts. Move the hands from the side of the body up over the head as you bend your knees and down again to the side as you straighten your legs. (Repeat four times.)
3. Sit on the floor with the legs in a straddle position. Put both hands on the head with elbows out. Bend to the right side as far as you can, then repeat to the left side (4×).
4. Put the soles of the feet together. Hold the ankles and bend forward. Try to take your head to your feet slowly on 4 counts. Hold this position, breathing in and out for 4 counts. Straighten the back on 4 counts (4×).

5. Lie on the back. Bend both knees up to the chest, extend the legs out, and lower them to the floor on 4 counts (4×).
6. Remain on the back with both arms over the head. Lift the back and bring the arms up over the head, forward and reaching for your toes and holding (4 counts, 4×).
7. Lie on back; breathe deeply and relax for a few minutes (imagine yourself in your favorite vacation spot).

Acclimatization A process whereby the body makes the necessary physiological adjustments to cope with a stressful environment such as extreme heat or high altitude.

Aerobic Dance An aerobic activity that uses dance movements performed to the rhythmic beat of popular music for the purpose of developing cardiorespiratory endurance.

Aerobic Metabolism A process of energy production in the body in which adequate oxygen is available.

Afferent Neurons Motor nerve cells that relay information from the central nervous system to the muscles and glands.

Agonist A muscle that is primarily responsible for a body movement. See also *antagonist.*

Amenorrhea Delayed menstruation or an absence of normal menstrual blood flow.

Anaerobic Metabolism A process of energy production in the body that takes place without adequate oxygen; muscular contraction cannot take place for more than a few minutes during anaerobic metabolism because of the buildup of lactic acid that causes muscle fatigue.

Angina Pectoris A form of heart attack characterized by a pain in the chest and left arm caused by a temporary lack of adequate oxygen to the heart muscle.

Anorexia Nervosa An extreme eating disorder associated with an abnormal fear of becoming obese, and resulting in unconventional eating habits and sometimes an avoidance of food. This disorder is most prevalent among teenage girls. See also *bulimia.*

Antagonist A muscle that relaxes during the contraction of an agonist, or prime mover; the triceps muscle is the antagonist during flexion of the forearm. See also *agonist.*

Anthropometric Measurement The measurement of body parts such as hips and thighs to help assess general body physique.

Arteriosclerosis Hardening of the arteries. See also *atherosclerosis.*

Assessment Evaluation or measurement, such as the evaluation of body composition.

Asthma A respiratory disease in which the lungs become clogged due to mucosal swelling and thick mucus; the condition usually results in labored breathing.

Atherosclerosis A form of arteriosclerosis characterized by a buildup of fatty tissue in one or more coronary arteries that causes a thickening and narrowing of such vessels. See also *arteriosclerosis.*

ATP (Adenosine Triphosphate) A high energy phosphate found in the cells that provides energy for muscular activity.

Atrophy A wasting away or decrease in the size of a body part due to lack of use. For example, the size of the leg muscle will become smaller after being immobilized in a cast for several months.

Ballistic Stretching A form of stretching using quick, forceful movements.

Basal Metabolic Rate (BMR) The minimal energy requirement necessary for the body to perform essential processes during the resting state.

Behavior Modification A form of behavior management in which reinforcement strategies are used to foster positive behaviors.

Bicycle Ergometer A stationary bicycle that can be used to measure work performance. See also *treadmill.*

Body Building A competitive sport in which weight training or progressive resistance exercises are used to develop muscle definition and an aesthetically appealing physique.

Body Composition The relative structural components of the body, namely, lean body mass or muscle, fatty tissue, and bone.

Bulimia An eating disorder characterized by eating binges followed by a purging or cleansing of the body through regurgitation, use of laxatives and/or diuretics, or some other method. This disorder is most prominent among college-age women. See also *anorexia nervosa.*

Bursitis An inflammation of the bursa (sac containing synovial fluid) within a joint; commonly, the knee, shoulder, and elbow joints are affected.

Calisthenics Generalized exercises such as push-ups, jumping jacks, and squat thrusts that are used to develop selected fitness components, including muscular endurance and flexibility.

Calorie A unit of measure for the rate of heat or energy production in the body. A small calorie is the amount of heat needed to raise one gram of water one degree Celsius. A large Calorie (more commonly termed a kilocalorie and abbreviated as kcal) is equal to 1,000 small calories; it is the amount of heat needed to raise one kilogram of water one degree Celsius.

Carbohydrate Loading Carbohydrate (or glycogen) loading is a procedure designed to saturate the muscles and liver with glycogen stores to enhance participation in endurance activities.

Carbohydrates The food group that is the primary energy source for vigorous, aerobic-type activities. Sugars comprise the simple carbohydrates and starches are the complex carbohydrates; these substances are found in the body in the form of glucose and glycogen.

Cardiac Output (CO) The amount of blood pumped out of the left ventrical in one minute; normally about 5 liters/min under resting conditions. It is a product of stroke volume times heart rate. See also *stroke volume.*

Cardiac Rehabilitation Any of the various methods used to restore the physical, social, psychological and emotional well-being of a post-cardiac patient.

Cardiorespiratory Endurance A primary component of physical fitness, cardiorespiratory endurance is the ability of the heart, blood vessels, and lungs to function at their optimal capacity, to enable one to perform aerobic activities such as running, lap swimming, and cross country skiing. This term and cardiorespiratory fitness are used interchangeably.

Cardiovascular Disease Disease of the heart and blood vessels.

Cholesterol A white, crystalline alcohol molecule that is a necessary component of the body, especially needed for cell structure and for the development of steroid hormones. It is produced in the body (principally by the liver) and also ingested through certain foods in the diet such as fatty meats and dairy products.

Circuit Training A training technique that involves performing a series of exercises or activities arranged in a logical sequence at different stations. The objective is to complete the circuit as quickly as possible or to perform as many repetitions of the exercise as possible in a set time period.

Concentric Contraction An isotonic contraction in which the muscle shortens.

Continuous Training A method of training whereby the activity is sustained at a constant tempo for a period of time (15 minutes is recommended as the minimum time for the development of cardiorespiratory endurance).

Coronary Arteries The arteries that supply blood to the heart muscle.

Coronary Heart Disease (CHD) A degenerative disease of the heart caused by a buildup of fatty substances and cholesterol in the inner walls of the coronary arteries. See also *arteriosclerosis* and *atherosclerosis.*

Creeping Obesity The gradual accumulation of fat tissue over a period of time (in some cases over several years) that leads to obesity.

Cystic Fibrosis An inherited generalized body disease, characterized by chronic lung impairment, a deficiency of pancreatic enzymes, and an abnormally high concentration of salt in the sweat.

Diabetes Mellitus A disorder of carbohydrate metabolism due to a malfunction of the insulin mechanism, resulting in an abnormally high concentration of blood sugar.

Diastolic Blood Pressure The blood pressure in the arteries during the relaxation phase of the heartbeat.

Dysmenorrhea Painful menstruation manifested mainly by cramps.

Eccentric Contraction An isotonic contraction in which the muscle lengthens.

ECG (or EKG) An electrocardiogram used to measure the electrical activity of the heart. See also *exercise stress test.*

Efferent Neurons Sensory nerve cells that carry messages from sense receptors in the muscles and glands to the central nervous system.

Endorphins Naturally occuring peptides in the brain with morphinelike properties that help to reduce pain.

Energy Balance Also called calorie balance, it is a concept in weight control that indicates that the energy produced or calories consumed is equal to the energy expended through physical activity.

Epilepsy A symptom of a disfunction of the nervous system within the brain, characterized by short, periodic episodes of motor, sensory, or psychological malfunction.

Exercise Prescription A recommended exercise workout including the intensity, duration, frequency, and type or mode of activity.

Exercise Stress Test A work test, using either a bicycle ergometer or treadmill in conjunction with an ECG, to determine the degree to which the body can adjust to increased metabolic demands, and whether any pathological conditions of the heart exist.

External Respiration The exchange of gases (oxygen and carbon dioxide) between the alveoli of the lungs and the pulmonary blood capillaries.

Fat A food compound formed from glycerol and fatty acids; it is the body's most concentrated source of energy.

Fat Weight The amount of body weight that is fat, as distinguished from muscle and bones.

Flexibility The range of motion in a joint.

Food Exchange Lists A grouping of foods into lists or categories with food servings of similar nutrient content and caloric value.

Frostbite Injury to body tissue due to exposure to cold.

Glucose The product of carbohydrate breakdown, it is transported in the blood and is metabolized in the cells.

Glycogen The form in which glucose molecules are stored in the liver and muscle cells.

Health A dynamic state of complete physical, mental, and social well-being; not merely the absence of disease or infirmity.

Heart Rate The number of times the heart beats per minute.

Heat Exhaustion A condition characterized by cool, sweaty skin, profuse perspiration, and loss of salt that results in muscle cramps, nausea, and dizziness. This condition results from overexertion in an extremely hot environment.

Heat Stroke A condition characterized by a profound increase in body temperature (up to 106°F), dry, hot skin, disorientation, shock, and coma. It results from a breakdown of the heat regulatory mechanisms while the body is in an extremely hot environment. Heat stroke is a serious medical emergency that can lead to death.

Hemoglobin An iron-containing protein in red blood cells that is involved with the transport of oxygen and carbon dioxide throughout the circulatory system.

High Density Lipoprotein A protein-lipid complex in the blood that facilitates the transportation of cholesterol from body cells to the liver for elimination from the body.

High Density Lipoprotein-Cholesterol (HDL-Cholesterol) One of the major classes of plasmalipoprotein and a transporter of cholesterol in the blood. High HDL-Cholesterol is thought to be protective against coronary heart disease.

HR max The maximal heart rate that an individual can attain during the most strenuous exercise or work task.

Hyperlipidemia Elevated levels of serum triglyceride and/or serum cholesterol.

Hyperlipoproteinemia (HLP) Elevated levels of lipoproteins.

Hypertension An elevated blood pressure that is higher than normal; that is, a systolic pressure of 140mm Hg and above and a diastolic pressure of 90 and above. It is commonly referred to as high blood pressure.

Hyperthermia An abnormally elevated body temperature.

Hypertrophy An enlargement of cell tissue (for example, the increase in size of the biceps muscle resulting from progressive resistance workouts).

Hypokinetic Disease A condition characterized by aches and pains, headaches, and stiff neck that results, in part, from insufficient exercise or movement.

Hypothermia An abnormally low body temperature.

Hypoxia A lack of adequate oxygen.

Insulin A hormone secreted by the pancreas that controls the blood glucose level.

Insulin-dependent Diabetes Diabetes mellitus in which insulin is needed to help control the condition. It commonly occurs in Type I or juvenile-onset diabetes.

Internal Respiration The exchange of oxygen and carbon dioxide at the muscle tissue level.

Interval Training A training technique whereby exercise bouts of near maximal intensity are alternated with periods of rest or light activity such as walking or stretching.

Isokinetic Training A training technique in which a muscle contracts at a set speed and against a resistance that is equal to the force of contraction throughout the movement.

Isometric Training A training technique whereby the joints do not move through a full range of motion and there is no significant change in length in the contracting muscle. An example is a person in a front-leaning position prior to performing a push-up.

Isotonic Training A training technique in which the contracting muscle changes in length and movement occurs in the affected body parts. Performing a push-up is an example.

Jogging Moving continuously at a pace slightly slower than a run (11 to 12 minutes per mile). See also *running*.

Juvenile Onset Diabetes A type of diabetes mellitus that requires externally administered insulin. This type of diabetes, also referred to as Type I diabetes and insulin-dependent diabetes, usually occurs before adulthood, although it may first appear in older adults.

Kilocalorie A large Calorie. See also *calorie*.

Kilogram A unit of mass in the metric system; one kilogram is equivalent to 2.2 pounds.

Lactation The secretion of milk by the mammary glands.

Lactic Acid The end product of anaerobic metabolism that results from the incomplete oxidation of glucose during muscular work. A buildup of lactic acid will cause a cessation of muscle contractions if the concentration is high enough.

Lacto-ovo-vegetarian A class of vegetarians who use dairy products and eggs in addition to plant foods in their diets.

Lacto-vegetarian A category of vegetarians who use only dairy products in addition to plant foods.

Lean Body Mass The body weight that is composed of muscle tissue rather than fat tissue; also referred to as lean body weight.

Lipid An organic compound that is usually insoluble in water, but soluble in alcohol, ether, chloroform and other fat solvents; examples are fats, fatty acids and phospholipids.

Lipoprotein A protein-lipid complex that carries cholesterol and triglycerides in the bloodstream.

Low-density Lipoprotein A protein carrier that seems to pick up cholesterol and deposit it in body cells; thus it is implicated in the increase incidence of CHD.

Low-density Lipoprotein-cholesterol (LDL-Cholesterol) A protein carrier of cholesterol in the bloodstream. High ratios of LDL to cholesterol are associated with increased incidences of coronary heart disease.

Lumbar Lordosis An exaggerated forward curvature of the vertebral column (spine) in the lower (lumbar) region of the back.

Maturity Onset Diabetes A form of diabetes mellitus that usually occurs in people who are over 40 and overweight. It is also referred to as Type II diabetes and noninsulin-dependent diabetes.

Maximal Heart Rate See HR max.

Maximal Oxygen Uptake (VO$_2$ max) The greatest amount of oxygen that the body can take in and use as an energy source during heavy muscular work. Also referred to as the maximal oxygen consumption, maximal oxygen intake, or max VO$_2$, the maximal oxygen uptake is one of the best physiological indexes of aerobic capacity or cardiorespiratory endurance.

Mean A term used in statistics, referred to as the arithmetic average (computed by adding all scores and dividing by the total number of scores).

MET A unit of measure for energy expenditure; one met is the amount of energy expenditure at rest. Two or more mets are multiples of the resting metabolic rate.

Metabolism The sum of all the biochemical reactions that occur within an organism; also, the process by which food is transformed into energy to be used by the organism.

Mitochondria Structural components within the cells where ATP is produced during aerobic metabolism.

Motivation The desire or drive to achieve a goal in order to satisfy a need. One might be motivated, for example, to exercise in order to improve one's level of physical fitness to satisfy the need for increased health.

Muscular Endurance The ability of a muscle or muscle group to exert repetitive contractions against a resistance or to hold a static contraction for a period of time.

Myocardial Infarction Death of a part of the heart muscle due to an absence of blood flow to that area for an extended period of time. Also referred to as a heart attack.

Myocardium The heart muscle.

Negative Addiction A concept that obsessive devotion to exercise can be a negative lifestyle factor when it is engaged in to the detriment of family, friends, and even one's own health.

Neuron A nerve cell.

Norm A value that is considered to be representative of a specified group. Norms are usually based on the scores of a large group of individuals.

Nutrients The chemicals obtained from food to permit proper functioning of the body.

Nutrition The food that is eaten and the manner in which the body uses it.

Obesity An excessive amount of body fat; the percentage of body fat indicative of obesity for males and females is 25 and 30, respectively.

Optimal Fitness The highest level of fitness any individual can attain; it can vary from individual to individual.

Osteoporosis Increased porosity or thinning of bone.

Overload Principle A major principle of training whereby a stress or intensity greater than normal is placed on a body system in order to create a training effect. One example is to increase the amount of weight during weight training to increase muscle strength.

Overweight Body weight that is more than normal according to height-weight tables.

Physical Fitness The ability of the heart, lungs, blood vessels, muscles, and bones to function at their optimal level. This is the health-related fitness approach.

Principle of Progression A principle of training based on the concept that an activity should be started at a level of intensity and/or duration appropriate for an individual, and that the increase in these variables should be systematic and progressive enough to establish a training effect.

Principle of Specificity A principle that dictates that the training effect will be realized only when the activity and methods of training are specific to the outcome desired.

Progressive Resistance Exercise The concept of increasing the resistance and/or repetitions when working with weights to improve strength and muscular endurance; also referred to as weight training.

Protein Primary food source that provides the basic structural properties of cells; proteins are made up of amino acids linked by peptide bonds.

Protein Complementing The practice, usually among vegetarians, of using foods which contain complementing proteins in order to get all of the essential nutrients (for example, combining one food that is high in an essential amino acid with another food low in that amino acid but high in another essential amino acid).

Rating of Perceived Exertion (RPE) A rating, based on an intuitive feeling of the strenuousness of an exercise task, that numerically expresses heart rate response to the task.

Reinforcement A principle of learning that stresses strengthing the connection between a stimulus and response by reinforcing a satisfying stimulus to increase the likelihood of the desired response being repeated. Immediate reinforcement of a positive nature is desired as opposed to delayed reinforcement which is negative or aversive.

Repetition A single complete execution of an exercise task.

Repetitions Maximum (RM) A concept used in weight training to denote the maximum weight that can be lifted for a designated number of repetitions.

Resting Heart Rate The number of times the heart beats per minute during the basal, or resting, state.

Running The act of moving continuously at an 8 to 10 minute mile pace. See also *jogging*.

Set In weight training, the number of consecutive repetitions of an exercise performed or executed. (For example, performing six arm curls three times would represent three sets of six repetitions each.)

Sprain A stretch or tear of a ligament (tough connective tissue that connects bones to each other).

Standard Deviation A measure of variability that indicates the dispersion or spread of approximately two-thirds of a distribution of scores about the mean. See also mean.

State Anxiety A temporary state of extreme worry or fear caused by a stressor at that time.

Static Stretching Slow, rhythmical sustained stretching movements. This type of stretching is recommended, rather than quick, jerky stretching movements (ballistic stretching).

Steady State A physiological state during an exercise task when the oxygen consumption is sufficient to meet the oxygen requirement of the task. It is necessary to reach a steady state when performing aerobic exercise tasks such as running two miles or lap swimming for 30 minutes.

Strain A stretch or tear of a muscle or tendon (fibrous tissue that connects muscles to bones).

Strength The ability of a muscle or muscle group to exert a maximal force against a resistance (a single contraction).

Stress Any condition or situation that upsets the internal equilibrium (homeostasis) of the body.

Stressor Any psychological or physiological condition that disrupts the homeostatic balance of the body; anything that produces stress.

Stretch Reflex The automatic reflex action of a muscle that causes it to contract when it is suddenly stretched beyond its normal length in a forceful, jerky motion. The stretch reflex comes into action during ballistic stretching.

Stroke Volume The amount of blood pumped out of the left ventrical in each beat or stroke. See also *cardiac output*.

Systolic Blood Pressure The blood pressure caused by the force exerted by the arterial blood flow against the walls of the blood vessels during the contraction phase of the heart beat.

Target Heart Rate The intensity level at which an exercise is performed; it is usually at a level high enough to produce a training effect. See also *training effect.*

Target Heart Rate Range A range of the percentage of maximal heart rate indicating the lower and upper levels of intensity at which one exercises to produce the desired training effect. The lower level (or threshold stimulus) necessary for a training effect is 70 percent of the maximum heart rate. The upper level of the target heart rate range is 90 percent of the maximum heart rate.

Threshold Stimulus The lowest level of intensity in terms of heart rate at which a training effect will be realized.

Training Effect The improved physiological changes that acrue due to participation in various physical activities. In aerobic activities such as bicycle riding or cross country skiing, for example, the heart rate must be raised to 70 percent or more of the maximum heart rate to produce a training effect on the cardiovascular and respiratory systems. See also *target heart rate.*

Trait Anxiety A prolonged state of extreme fear or worry that is characteristic of a certain personality type.

Treadmill A motor-driven conveyor belt designed so that the speed of the belt and the incline are adjustable to provide varying workloads. Like the bicycle ergometer, it can be used to measure work capacity.

Triclycerides A chemical name for fats; they constitute the major storage form of fat. They also provide the primary means for transporting fat in the blood. Research studies link high levels of triglycerides with atherosclerosis.

T-Score A standard statistical score that permits the comparison and interpretation of raw scores from dissimilar data. For example, sit-up scores measured in numbers can be standardized and compared to scores made on a twelve minute run-walk, which is measured in time (minutes and seconds).

Type A Personality A term used to describe individuals who exhibit personality traits of impatience, extreme competitiveness, time consciousness, and anxiety proneness. These individuals do not handle stress effectively.

Unsaturated Fats A liquid type of fat that may be either polyunsaturated (found in vegetable oils such as soybean and sunflower) or monosaturated (such as peanut and olive oils).

Valsalva Maneuver A maneuver, usually associated with weight lifting, in which a forceful exhalation is made against a closed glottis (the narrowest part of the larynx for passage of air through the trachea) to produce the maximum application of force for a short duration. This procedure is not recommended since it diminishes blood supply to the brain and causes dizziness, disorientation, and sometimes fainting when heavy weights are used.

Vegan A true vegetarian who eats only plant foods.

Vegetarian A person whose diet, for various reasons, is limited to foods from vegetable or plant sources. See also *lacto-ovo-vegetarian, lacto-vegetarian* and *vegan.*

Wellness A term that denotes dynamic, optimal fitness; the highest level of health.

Wind-chill Factor Consideration of the wind velocity along with the absolute temperature to arrive at a true temperature determination.

Work Capacity The readiness of the body to make physiological adjustments to metabolic demands that exceed the resting requirement. When one works to exhaustion at an exercise task, one is said to be working at the maximum physical working capacity. The level of working capacity is associated with the level of physical fitness; the higher the level of physical fitness, the higher the working capacity.

Note: t after a page number indicates the entry is discussed in a table.